The **10**
Secrets of
**Healthy
Ageing**

DRAWN
FROM
COLLECTION

D0210538

OTHER BOOKS BY PATRICK HOLFORD

patrick HOLFORD
and Jerome Burne

The 10
Secrets of
Healthy
Ageing

HOW TO LIVE LONGER, LOOK YOUNGER AND FEEL GREAT

piatkus

PIATKUS

First published in Great Britain in 2012 by Piatkus

Copyright © Patrick Holford and Jerome Burne 2012

The moral right of the authors has been asserted.

All rights reserved.
No part of this publication may be reproduced, stored in a retrieval system, or transmitted
in any form or by any means, without the prior permission in writing of the publisher,
nor be otherwise circulated in any form of binding or cover other than that in which it is
published and without a similar condition including this condition being imposed on the
subsequent purchaser.

A CIP catalogue record for this book
is available from the British Library.

ISBN 978-0-7499-5654-7

Typeset in 11.5/15pt Minion by Phoenix Photosetting, Chatham, Kent
Printed and bound in Great Britain by CPI (UK) Ltd, Croydon, CR0 4YY

Papers used by Piatkus are from well-managed forests
and other responsible sources.

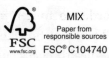

MIX
Paper from
responsible sources
FSC® C104740
www.fsc.org

Piatkus
An imprint of
Little, Brown Book Group
100 Victoria Embankment
London EC4Y 0DY

An Hachette UK Company
www.hachette.co.uk

www.piatkus.co.uk

With this book you are entitled to
A FREE ONLINE bioage AND HEALTH CHECK.

Go to www.patrickholford.com to get your free bioage and Health Check today.
Plus £5 OFF YOUR 100% HEALTH PROGRAMME (Special price £19.95). To
obtain your discount use the following special code: 10SECUK512. See opposite
for further information on what this offer entitles you to and how to access your
100% Health Programme.

YOUR FREE ONLINE bioage AND HEALTH CHECK

HOW ARE YOU AGEING?

Are you getting older in good shape or accumulating symptoms, weight and health issues with every passing year? Find out whether your biological age is greater or lesser than your chronological age, and how to reverse the trend.

You really can wake up full of energy with a clear mind and a balanced mood, you can maintain a healthy weight and stay disease-free well into your nineties. Having worked with over 100,000 people, we know what changes are going to most rapidly transform how you feel. The **100% Health Programme** is the most comprehensive and genuinely effective way of taking a major step towards 100% Health. It includes your free **bio**age **Health Check**.

Go to www.patrickholford.com to get your free online bioage Health Check. This will tell you just how healthy you are. Once you have completed your online health check, use your special discount code (provided opposite) to save £5 on your personalised 100% Health Programme (normally £24.95). This is the ultimate online personal health profile, showing you what your perfect diet and daily supplement programme should be and which lifestyle changes will make the most difference.

The **100% Health Programme** provides: a full set of results on how well your body systems and processes are working • an in-depth report on your health • your perfect recipes • your own library of special health reports • your action plan and personal supplement programme • full lifestyle analysis, including exercise, stress, sleep and pollution levels.

For an extra £9.95 a month you can also receive: weekly support and guidance from Patrick • a free reassessment to chart your progress, month by month • telephone access to a nutritional therapist • your questions answered by Patrick plus all the benefits of membership (see back pages).

ABOUT THE AUTHORS

Patrick Holford BSc, DipION, FBANT, NTCRP is a leading spokesman on nutrition in the media, specialising in the field of mental health. He is the author of over 30 books, translated into over 20 languages and selling over a million copies worldwide, including *The Optimum Nutrition Bible, The Low GL-Diet Bible, Optimum Nutrition for the Mind* and *The 10 Secrets of 100% Healthy People*.

Patrick started his academic career in the field of psychology. He then became a student of two of the leading pioneers in nutrition medicine and psychiatry – the late Dr Carl Pfeiffer and Dr Abram Hoffer. In 1984 he founded the Institute for Optimum Nutrition (ION), an independent educational charity, with his mentor, twice Nobel Prize winner Dr Linus Pauling, as patron. ION has been researching and helping to define what it means to be optimally nourished for the past 25 years and is one of the most respected educational establishments for training nutritional therapists. At ION, Patrick was involved in groundbreaking research showing that multivitamins can increase children's IQ scores – the subject of a *Horizon* documentary in the 1980s. He was one of the first promoters of the importance of zinc, antioxidants, high-dose vitamin C, essential fats, low-GL diets and homocysteine-lowering B vitamins and their importance in mental health and Alzheimer's disease prevention.

Patrick is Chief Executive Officer of the Food for the Brain Foundation and director of the Brain Bio Centre, the Foundation's treatment centre that specialises in helping those with mental issues ranging from depression to schizophrenia. He is an honorary fellow of the British Association of Nutritional Therapy, as well as a member of the Nutrition Therapy Council and the Complementary and Natural Healthcare Council. He is also Patron of the Irish and South African Associations of Nutritional Therapy.

Jerome Burne is an award-winning medical and health journalist who, over the last 20 years, has been writing for most of the UK nationals about the latest developments in health and cutting-edge research. He is co-author of *Food is Better Medicine than Drugs*, with Patrick. He was an early champion of probiotics and higher doses of vitamin D and was one of the first in the UK to write about epigenetics – the ability of the environment to directly affect genes.

Jerome has queried the benefits of the widespread prescription of cholesterol-lowering statins to people without heart disease and was one of the first UK journalists to cover the links between the SSRI drugs and suicide in children. He wrote one of the first features investigating the excessive and ineffective prescribing of anti-psychotic medication to elderly patients with dementia and was consultant on the 2010 *Panorama* programme on the slow official response to the finding that the diabetes drug Avandia raised the risk of heart disease.

CONTENTS

Part Three:
YOUR ANTI-AGEING ACTION PLAN   275

ACKNOWLEDGEMENTS

This book is a team effort – not only of Jerome and Patrick but also the people who support us, leading an anti-social lifestyle of early mornings and late nights. Immense thanks to Patrick's wife, Gaby, for her support and encouragement! Also, to Jo Muncaster, Patrick's super-efficient assistant, and to his daughter, Jade, for help with the references and tracking down useful resources. Special thanks also to Gill Pyrah, Jerome's wife, for her thoughtful comments on the big picture, sharp eye for the details and for making him laugh a lot. Thanks also to Jerome's teenage daughters, Georgia and Kitty, for actually listening to discussions about ageing.

We'd also like to thank the very talented Brian Russell for his illustrations, Lynn Alford-Burow for her help researching solutions for eye problems, David Alpert from the International Institute for Anti-Ageing, for sharing his research and ideas about anti-ageing, Jillian Stewart and Jan Cutler for their help with editing, and Gill Bailey and Tim Whiting at Piatkus for their support and encouragement to publish this book and get it to as many people as possible.

We would both like to acknowledge the help we get from the experts, not only for their years of invaluable research, but also their willingness to answer our questions. This includes Professor David Smith, Dr Marion Gluck, Dr Malcolm Carruthers, Professor Bruce Ames, Dr Fedon Lindberg, Dr Des Fernandes, Dr Rollin McCraty, Dr Michael Dixon and Dr David Beales.

DISCLAIMER

Although all the nutrients and dietary changes referred to in this book have been proven safe, those seeking help for specific medical conditions are advised to consult a qualified nutrition therapist, clinical nutritionist, doctor or equivalent health professional. The recommendations given in this book are solely intended as education and information, and should not be taken as medical advice. Neither the authors nor the publisher accept liability for readers who choose to self-prescribe.

All supplements should be kept out of the reach of infants and children.

GUIDE TO ABBREVIATIONS, MEASURES AND REFERENCES

Vitamins

1 gram (g) = 1,000 milligrams (mg) = 1,000,000 micrograms (mcg, also written as μg)

Most vitamins are measured in milligrams or micrograms. Vitamins A, D and E used to be measured in International Units (iu), a measurement designed to standardise the various forms of these vitamins, which have different potencies.

6mcg of beta-carotene, the vegetable precursor of vitamin A is, on average, converted into 1mcg of retinol, the animal form of vitamin A. So, 6mcg of beta-carotene is called 1mcgRE (RE stands for retinol equivalent). Throughout this book beta-carotene is referred to in mcgRE.

1mcg of retinol (1mcgRE) = 3.3iu of vitamin A
1mcgRE of beta-carotene = 6mcg of beta-carotene
100iu of vitamin D = 2.5mcg or 1mcg of vitamin D = 40iu
100iu of vitamin E = 67mg
1 pound (lb) = 16 ounces (oz)
2.2lb = 1 kilogram (kg)
1 pint = 0.6 litres
1.76 pints = 1 litre
In this book 'calories' means kilocalories (kcals)

References and further reading

In each part of the book, you'll find numbered references. These refer to research papers listed in the References section beginning on page 357, and are there for readers who want to study this subject in depth. More details on most of these studies can be found on the internet, at PubMed, a service of the US National Library of Medicine (see http://www.ncbi.nlm.nih.gov/pubmed/).

On pages 382–83 you will find a list of the best books to read to enable you to dig deeper into the topics covered. You will also find that many of the topics touched on in this book are covered in detail in feature articles available at www.patrickholford.com. If you want to stay up to date with all that is new and exciting in this field, I recommend you subscribe to my 100% Health newsletter, details of which are on the website www.patrickholford.com.

INTRODUCTION: HOW TO SURF THE SILVER TSUNAMI

Dr Abram Hoffer was one of my (Patrick's) heroes and teachers. He was a Canadian biochemist and psychiatrist, and a pioneer of nutritional medicine – especially in the treatment of schizophrenia using the B vitamin niacin. His disease-free old age proved an inspiration when I finally had to admit, at 55 years old, that I was ageing. Now, I hope that this book will pass on to you my optimism about the possibility of ageing well.

Dr Hoffer died in 2009 at the age of 91. He had practised psychiatry until the age of 88 but continued to advise people about their health until about two weeks before his death. He was very careful about what he ate, avoiding sugar and refined foods, and he took a cocktail of vitamins, minerals and essential fats every day. Four days before his death he started to feel unwell. Two days later he checked in to the local hospital. He didn't have cancer, heart disease, diabetes, Alzheimer's, osteoporosis or any other disease as such. His organs just started to shut down and he died peacefully and painlessly.

For the last 30 years I've been a practising nutritional therapist and am the author of over 30 books on how to live healthily, but what I have found more recently is that these ideas really come into their own the older you get. You may have already started to notice a few changes in yourself: perhaps you're not recovering from a hard afternoon's exercise as quickly as you used to, or maybe you're noticing too many new wrinkles, or perhaps, despite the exercise, you're finding the pounds are going on a bit faster than you'd like.

Good nutrition and other lifestyle changes aren't just about protecting your heart or dealing with diabetes, they are about keeping your whole system working well, and that is precisely what you need as you age. We are facing an elderly population time bomb, and helping people to stay healthy for longer is an essential way of defusing it.

I believe it's no accident that two of my other teachers were also healthy and working right up to the end of their lives. Dr Roger Williams discovered two vitamins (B₅ and folic acid) and was the first to talk about how food can change gene expression – a cutting-edge topic we cover later in some detail. He died at 96 and was still writing and teaching at the age of 95. Dr Linus Pauling, twice a Nobel Prize winner, who put high-dose vitamin C for fighting cancer and infections on the map, also died in his nineties. I filmed him only six months before his death, when he was actively researching a new risk factor for heart disease – a type of fat called lipoprotein(a) that predicts heart disease, and which is only just moving into the mainstream; we talk about this in Secret 7. I'll be drawing on their experience and my own to tell you how to make the changes that will help you stay energetic, mentally sharp and physically fit for as long as possible.

HOW YOU AGE ISN'T DOWN TO LUCK OR GENES – IT'S UP TO YOU

Perhaps you feel, if you think about it at all, that ageing is one of those things that just happens and that it's probably the result of your genes. You get what you get. You are either lucky or you're not. But it's not as straightforward as that. The research Jerome and I have uncovered while writing this book shows that while luck obviously plays a part, there's a lot you can do to reduce your chances of drawing the short straw. The science of ageing is advancing fast. Scientists on both sides of the Atlantic are exploring ways that markers for how well you are ageing – found in every cell in your body – can be altered by the kind of exercise you do, the food you eat and the way you handle stress. In fact, as we'll explain later, and as Dr Williams predicted back in the 1960s, your lifestyle can directly change the activities of some genes for better or worse. It's increasingly clear that we can all make changes to the genetic hand we were dealt.

Unfortunately, it is also clear that just relying on the medical profession to keep you healthy until very near the end is not the best strategy. Imagine a house built 50 or more years ago. It would certainly be in need of some repairs. You could leave it like that and deal with the inevitable emergencies by calling highly trained builders or a plumber, but it's much cheaper and more pleasant to employ someone reliable who can maintain it regularly for you. Alternatively, you could read a manual and develop some DIY skills. This book is that manual. Unlike houses, though, our bodies have remarkable powers of recuperation and renewal, and big improvements can be made by supplying the appropriate 'building materials' when supplies start to run short.

Whatever your age, and whether you run marathons or watch a lot of TV, there are going to be times when this manual will come in handy. The kind of broad-brush advice about lifestyle changes you are likely to get from official bodies is along the lines of 'keep an eye on your weight' or 'don't eat too much fat' – it's sensible but not specific. This manual has a lot of very specific instructions, and it will be suitable for you as you start to move into your fifties or beyond, or even if you don't personally need it right now, it could be very handy if you are looking after an older relative. Carers and other health professionals will also find valuable new information here.

SURFING THE SILVER TSUNAMI

We are now facing what has been termed the Silver Tsunami, when the baby boomers – those born between 1946 and 1964 – begin reaching 65. As a result, the number of elderly people is set to soar. Twenty-five years ago there were about 660,000 people over 85 in the UK, and this is the group that is a heavy and costly user of health and other social services. That number has now doubled to 1.4 million and is set to reach 3.6 million by 2035.[1] The cost of this elderly inflation will be crippling and is giving economists and administrators sleepless nights. But it also presents us with a hugely exciting opportunity.

We have the chance to make much better choices about the way we age than our parents, who stumbled into longer lives almost by accident. When they were born, no one expected the average life span would be around 80. As a result, the treatment older people get today is a continuation of a largely pharmaceutical approach to prevention offered to younger people. But, as we'll see, it is often not appropriate.

So, there is an urgent need for the baby boomers to reshape and re-invent what it means to grow old. Just as we've put our stamp on everything else – pop music, sex, jobs, shopping, housing – now we need to create a new vision of ageing.

A popular wish-list for ageing well might include good general health, smooth, firm skin, strong muscles, an efficient immune system, good memory and a healthy brain. And the longer you stay healthy the longer you'll hang on to those benefits as well as cutting your risk of developing one or more of those chronic diseases that afflict us in the West: cancer, diabetes, heart disease and arthritis. The secrets of how to slash your chances of falling prey to the top ten afflictions is what Part Two is all about.

Nobody can promise that everyone will get off scot-free, but if you follow the programmes set out in the book you can be sure of keeping yourself in a healthy well-functioning state longer than you will if you follow the path of long-term elderly decline, which is likely to involve several of the following: heartburn, sleeplessness, muscle pain, depression, nausea, constipation and a fading memory. And that's before you've got to the point where you need a stay in hospital or a nursing home, where a whole new set of hazards lurk, such as neglect, malnutrition (suffered by 30 per cent of old people), superbug infections and avoidable bedsores.

STAYING OFF THE DRUG COCKTAILS

The conventional way to treat your growing list of ailments is with more and more drugs for the symptoms. Although public health advice for looking after yourself is to get 'five a day', the medical version of this is not calculated in portions of fruit and vegetables but in prescriptions: 50 per cent of people over 65 are now getting five drugs a day.[2] That can't be the best solution. The five at 65 is very likely to become ten by 75. Children born today can expect to live to around 90, but on the present course they can also expect to spend a third of their lives on a cocktail of drugs. Meanwhile, deaths attributed to prescribed medication or medical intervention in the USA has become the third leading cause of death,[3] and a UK study in 2004 estimated the number of deaths from prescription drugs given at the correct dosage to be at least 10,000.[4]

Apart from all the problems that come with that scale of prescribing, the National Health Service in the UK is just not going to be able to afford it. By 2030 there will be five million more people over 65 in the UK than there are today. If you are reasonably healthy, the odds that you'll benefit from taking prescription drugs for years to avoid falling ill are very long: 200-plus to 1. And that is without factoring in the risks that they carry.

YOU CAN'T CHEAT DEATH, BUT YOU *CAN* CHEAT ILL HEALTH

We all get older, of course, and, because evolution has designed us to reproduce quickly, our powerful natural repair-and-renewal systems do start to become more haphazard as we age. But research is uncovering more details about how our cells run down and what can be done to bring them up to speed again. There is the drop in performance of the tiny power plants that provide energy for every cell. Clearing the garbage of dead and dying cells becomes less efficient and protein assembly is less accurate, so mistakes start creeping into the processes of living. This is the decline we experience as wrinkles, weaker sight, fatigue, and aches and pains.

Supplementing with vitamins, minerals, essential fats and other essential nutrients is a valuable part of helping all these systems to function effectively. Nevertheless, doctors and dieticians often claim that it's nearly always unnecessary to take supplements and that you can get all the micronutrients you need from 'a healthy balanced diet', but we hope that by the time you've finished reading this book you'll be persuaded that that's not true, particularly when it comes to ageing well. All sorts of surveys show that the older you are the more likely you will be deficient in various vitamins and minerals, so it makes a lot of sense to replace what's missing. It has very recently been officially acknowledged, for example, that older people would get massive benefit from taking vitamin D in amounts that you can't get from your diet, and there is growing evidence that high doses of B vitamins can slow down the rate of brain shrinkage, the prelude to Alzheimer's disease, and osteoporosis.

That's just a start, not least because, as described later, many of the drugs older people are likely to be prescribed can make the minerals and vitamins in your body less available. This is information that could be valuable not only for you as you get older but for any one helping out with their elderly parents. For more detail on this see Chapter 4 where we have a list of some of the drugs that are particularly risky, especially for elderly people, and another showing the key micronutrients that older people, in particular, are likely to be short of.

The remainder of Part One tells you about the latest ideas in anti-ageing research and how they fit in with new findings about genetics. In Part Two we explain how you can apply them to reduce the damage that ageing will be doing to vulnerable parts of your body, such as your joints, bones, skin and eyes, as well as increasing your protection against the likes of heart disease, diabetes and a declining memory. But if you don't want to bother with any of the theory, turn straight to Part Three, which contains your Action Plan for healthy ageing.

GETTING TO GRIPS WITH THE BIOCHEMISTRY

While Patrick's mission has been discovering what works to keep people healthier I (Jerome) have always been more interested in the whys and the hows. For the last 20 years I've been a health and medical journalist writing for most of the UK nationals, usually about what's new or scandalous. I was an early champion of probiotics and higher doses of vitamin D; I've queried the benefits of giving cholesterol-lowering statins to everyone and the widespread prescribing of SSRI antidepressants. I've investigated the hazards of mobile phones and the slow official response to the finding that the diabetes drug Avandia raised the risk of heart disease.

In all that time, however, I never looked at ageing – except to write one of the first pieces about the excessive and totally inappropriate use of anti-psychotic drugs on elderly patients with dementia. Like most people, I thought ageing in general was a pretty dull topic about a depressing decline and loss. That's why researching this book has been such a revelation. Like every health journalist, I'd written about the benefits of various nutrients – the ACE vitamins, omega-3 fats, B vitamins, and so on, but it had always been in connection with a particular condition: were they good for heart disease or brain function or diabetes, for example.

DRUGS AREN'T GOING TO DO IT

As I wrote about how individual body parts begin to decline with age – the blood vessels, the guts, the joints – the same nutritional connections kept cropping up. I wrote about studies that showed that antioxidants and omega-3 fats help with the heart but also with the eyes and with the skin. The very familiar link between excessive blood sugar and diabetes also turned up as a risk factor for cancer; it was connected with bone loss, as well as harming the skin and the eyes. The conclusion is clear. If you want to stay healthy as you age, you need those nutrients, because not only do they cut the risk of particular diseases but they also support your underlying state of health. And ageing is a shorthand way of saying 'a gradual decline in your underlying state of health'. But at the same time it became clear that if you want to keep people healthy for longer as they age, relying on new drugs to fix this or that problem isn't going to do it.

Drugs, unlike nutrients, are loners. They don't get on so well with other drugs and can cause a lot of collateral damage. Nutrients usually need to work in teams to have the best effect, and damaging interactions are rare. Don't get me wrong, drugs can be hugely valuable and they are life-savers in an emergency; you are likely to need some as you get older. But as tools for keeping you healthy, their track record is not so hot, as we cover later.

For some people, 'anti-ageing medicine' means aiming to expand human life span to 100 and beyond. Two gerontologists have a famous on-going bet about whether the oldest person in 2150 will be 130 or 150, and a few radicals talk about living for centuries. This book isn't about how to reach 120 but how to arrive at the end of a normal life span in as healthy a state as possible.

THE ULTRA-MARATHON APPROACH TO AGEING

Healthy ageing is a new field, and there's still a lot to discover. Ideally, much more would be spent both on research, building on what we know about the benefits of diet, exercise and lifestyle changes, and applying what we already know far more effectively. But there's no money in it. Meanwhile, drug companies are pouring billions of dollars into developing new products to slow down some age-related disease. And the more drugs you take the more money they make. It's an approach that leaves you passively waiting for medical and pharmaceutical experts to gather the evidence and then provide the drugs that will stop you from suffering with Alzheimer's or cancer, for example. Patrick and I don't believe that this is the only way to go.

American Dr Richard Lippman, who invented, among other things, the nicotine patch and was nominated for the Nobel Prize in Medicine in 1996 for developing a non-invasive method of measuring free-radical activity in human cells, is an example of what might be called hard-core anti-ageing. Now aged 66, Dr Lippman is enjoying a very active retirement living in Honolulu and occasionally giving lectures on healthy ageing around the world. His philosophy includes taking industrial quantities of minerals, vitamins and other supplements daily, including antioxidants and hormones – probably more than most of us would feel we wanted to take.[5] Like many dedicated anti-agers, what is more, he also swallows some heavyweight drugs to tackle some of the damage done by ageing, including two to treat rheumatoid arthritis, a cancer drug and a drug used in the treatment of diabetes.

Now, that is the kind of drug cocktail that is standard medical treatment, and drug companies are very interested in using drugs with anti-ageing benefits, even though some of those Dr Lippman is using can't be licensed for anti-ageing uses as such yet. He's just using them off-label – taking a drug without a licence to treat that particular condition – which is also medically perfectly acceptable. But does taking this quantity of supplements and drugs really make sense?

AGEING WELL: A LIFE SKILL

The drug-cocktail approach seems the wrong place to start, even though officially it's what's on offer. There's good evidence, as we'll show, that many of the lifestyle changes everyone is familiar with mesh very well with the latest findings about ageing and are effective at slowing it down: what we eat, the micronutrients we take in, the type of exercise we do. Patrick and I believe that learning how to put them together is a new life skill. As part of normal living we acquire all kinds of skills: running a business, bringing up children, creating a garden, cooking. Making sure you age well, with the help of this book, is exactly the same sort of challenge and no more difficult. Taking this approach to prevention could go a long way towards cutting the spiralling costs of the Silver Tsunami in countries such as the UK. If this was already being done, we wouldn't be spending £600 million a year on diabetes drugs. Making that happen, however, involves political changes that are beyond the scope of this book.

TAKE A TEST TO FIND OUT HOW YOU ARE DOING

You can start future-proofing yourself right now. We have created a comprehensive online health check that you can complete to find out how well you are ageing. Turn to Chapter 2 to discover your biological age – which may not be the same as the number of your birthdays. You'll find out which bits of you seem OK and which need some work to prevent something worse happening down the line. Once you've found your weaknesses, we will suggest what you can do to improve them. Then, after a while, you can test again to see if your personal health programme is having an effect.

We'll also stay with you, if you want. You can take an annual online health check-up and become part of a community of people learning the healthy ageing life skill. We hope you'll share experiences and teach each other what really works for adding years to your life and life to your years.

Wishing you the best of health,
Patrick Holford and Jerome Burne

Part One

THE TRUTH ABOUT HEALTHY AGEING

We are not going to tell you how to live forever, or even promise you'll live several decades longer. What we do offer are ways to stay in better shape as you begin, inevitably, to run down. Modern medicine can perform wonders, but it is an expensive and not very effective way of keeping you well or preventing you from falling ill. The hunt is certainly on for new drugs to keep you looking and feeling younger, but they will be a long time coming.

So, what are you going to do right now? We all know the lifestyle advice about diet and exercise for staying healthy and avoiding chronic diseases. The good news is that they work just as well to help you age well. Researchers studying the diets of long-lived rats, monkeys and worms, or watching how their genes change as they get older, are all coming up with the same message.

Whatever sign of ageing you are worried about – wrinkles, weaker muscles, less energy, poor healing and repair – you have a chance to improve them by getting the right food, sufficient nutrients and taking the best exercise. You can't beat ageing, but you can put it off, and the science is on the side of lifestyle. You aren't totally at the mercy of your genes. You have choices. This part tells you why. Later, we'll tell you how.

Chapter 1

THE NEW SCIENCE OF AGEING

Just suppose for a moment that the doctors have told you that your newborn baby has an unusual genetic disorder which means she is going to gradually become weaker and less able to function, until by the age of ten or so she will be in a wheelchair, only able to lead a pretty limited life. You have, however, been told some good news that you can do something about her predicament. There are no drugs that will make a difference but researchers have developed a package for parents which appears to have a fairly good chance of keeping your daughter out of that wheelchair. She has to eat a particular diet, but the ingredients are all widely available; she will need to do some specially designed exercises several times a week and there are a few other compounds that she should be taking. Wouldn't you bust a gut to make sure every part of that package was faithfully carried out?

Even though it wasn't certain she'd be OK, you'd know you owed it to her to make sure she had the best possible chance to stay mobile and healthy.

Now, suppose we are not talking about your vulnerable new baby, but we are talking about you. Right now you may be fine. You may be in reasonable shape but perhaps you're noticing a few changes: occasional twinges, having to suck in your stomach a bit further when checking in the mirror, and so on. But you realise that unless you take control, things are not going to get any better. You've got 20, maybe 50 more years. You want to have the maximum time being engaged and feeling good, and the absolute minimum time on medication or, at worse, drugged to the eyeballs in a care home. No one can afford to retire, anyway, so there is greater pressure than ever to stay healthy!

WHAT HAS THE FUTURE GOT IN STORE FOR YOU?

Most of us tend to leave our health to our doctors. Let's assume you are responsible and health-conscious: you have increasingly regular checks of health markers such as blood pressure and cholesterol. If you aren't yet on a cholesterol-lowering statin plus an aspirin to cut the risk of a dangerous blood clot and a couple of blood-pressure pills, it's likely that they are not so far down the line. Even so, your outlook, if you just keep following the current medical model, is pretty grim. You are looking at a steady decline of all your abilities, an increasing number of diseases and, perhaps worst, years of barely functioning at all.

These are the kind of changes you can expect to be coming your way:

- By 40 you are already starting to lose muscle mass at the rate of about 1 per cent a year, and your tendons and ligaments are becoming less elastic. Only 20 per cent of us in the UK aged between 65 and 74 exercise enough to reverse that.
- By 50 your levels of the hormones needed for the likes of libido, muscle mass and skin repair will have dropped sharply.
- Half of those who reach 65 have signs of osteoarthritis, and every year after the age of 65 one in two will have a bad fall that can cause a fracture, a hospital visit and possibly admission to a nursing home.
- Over 65 is the watershed. This is when 50 per cent of all heart attacks occur, most strokes, three-quarters of cancers and 95 per cent of the deaths from pneumonia.
- The risk of dementia is still relatively low by 65; just 5 per cent will have developed it. But 20 per cent of 80-year-olds will be affected.
- By 80 years, 50 per cent of both men and women will have a hearing problem.

SENTENCED TO BE HOUSEBOUND FOR TEN YEARS

Left unchecked, this catalogue of physical decay means that you will become increasingly reliant on others. Options about where to go and what to do will relentlessly diminish. Since 1998 the average number of disease-free years you can expect has declined, according to the December 2010 issue of the *Journal of Gerontology*. A male aged 20 today can look forward to spending 5.8 years of his life effectively housebound. That means not being able to climb ten steps, walk a quarter of a mile, or bend or kneel without using special equipment. The future for females is even bleaker: 9.8 years virtually immobilised. Even ten years ago, the figures were 3.8 years and 7.3 respectively. And, as more of us live longer, those averages are going to get worse.

What is more, you can't help having noticed that what's in store as the years roll by is pretty unappealing in other ways too. Hospitals have become more dangerous places, where superbug infections are an ever-present risk, along with neglect that is so bad in some cases that it results in bedsores or even fatal dehydration.

I (Jerome) have researched and written about the poor hygiene in hospitals and the complete failure over decades to improve something as basic as the food. I've also interviewed a remarkable campaigner for better conditions in care homes and read her reports of conditions that reveal the shocking complacency of the official inspections which gloss over a scandalous lack of care, isolation and boredom. And even if the home is genuinely caring and supportive, you will be treated by a medical system that tends to respond to older people's gradual decline by prescribing an increasing number of drugs with little evidence that they are appropriate or effective when you reach old age.

DRUGS CAN MAKE THINGS WORSE

If the poor care, poor food and worry about hygiene weren't enough, the drugs you will be getting for relief of your symptoms come trailing a wide variety of unpleasant side effects known as ADRs (adverse drug reactions). What's more, the latest reports indicate that the damage caused by ADRs is rising.

The latest figures from the Royal Society of Medicine shows that the number of hospital admissions associated with ADRs has increased by over 75 per cent since 1991, according to the *New Scientist*.[1] Meanwhile, according to the *Lancet* in 2010: 'Adverse drug reactions have reached epidemic proportions and are increasing at twice the rate of prescriptions … [while] the cost of new medicines is rising unsustainably.'[2]

The situation is even worse than that, however. The ADRs that are known about are the tip of an alarmingly large iceberg. As the *New Scientist* article reports: 'It is estimated that over 90 per cent of ADRs are not reported by doctors and health professionals.' And if you are old, you are more at risk, not only because you are likely to be popping more pills, but because you are going to be frailer and your body will be getting less efficient at detoxification.

AND THERE IS NOTHING TO BE DONE ABOUT IT …

So, not only is what's on offer at the moment pretty unappealing but, as a society, we can't afford it. One estimate is that in the UK by 2050 the cost of caring for the elderly will be three times what it is now. Until 2011 the over-65s made up around 16 per cent of the population, but 43 per cent of the NHS total budget was spent on them and they took up 65 per cent of acute hospital beds.

And what's the very worst thing about this catalogue of highly expensive misery and discomfort? That anyone who knows about ageing medicine realises there is nothing new or surprising about it at all. It is certainly not considered shocking. People get sicker as they get older and all drugs come with risks and benefits. It is just the way things are. This view was set out recently in a book by famed developmental biologist Professor Lewis Wolpert,[3] called: *You're Looking Very Well: The Surprising Nature of Getting Old.*

The figures quoted above, about the various failings at the different ages, come from that book. It is hugely well informed about the ways and history of ageing and does a clear and engaging job of describing the problem, but the conclusion is resolutely stoical: this is what ageing is like, and it must be endured; you can take comfort in small mercies, like the fact that libido doesn't drop off as much as you might expect, but essentially there is nothing to be done. 'There is no such thing as an anti-ageing intervention,' is his clear-eyed conclusion.

... ACTUALLY, THERE IS

We don't agree with him. First though, it is worth clearing up a possible confusion about the meaning of the word 'anti-ageing'. This is often used to mean a drug or treatment that could keep you forever young, in a sort of spooky Dorian Gray way. This is the fantasy territory of fountains of youth and the blood of virgins. And in that sense Wolpert is right. There's been a long list of hopeful candidates, with some of the biggest claims made for hormones, but none has lived up to expectations. There are a number of drug hopefuls in the pipeline, but none is expected very soon.

So, why is the prognosis so bleak? Doctors are only human, and ageing has historically been something of a medical backwater, essentially because it isn't sexy. Gerontology and geriatrics have none of the dramatic glamour of heart surgery or cancer specialists, and funding for really effective prevention is hard to find because it doesn't produce a patentable product. Besides which, prevention also lacks the glamour of a dash to A&E and daily battles to save a life.

But none of this means there is nothing to be done. There isn't nearly as much hard data on what works well for older people – including drug treatments – as there should be. The resources available to test the effectiveness of changing diets or exercise regimes are a fraction of that devoted to drugs. So, most doctors' grip on nutrition is fairly limited, and they are unlikely to recommend more than a few staples of prevention – such as don't smoke, lose weight, and so on.

That's where this book comes in. You are not doomed to become another of the statistics on the path to steady decline. Time and again we see that taking steps to stay in good health can make a massive difference to the way you age. The solution is to start taking control of your own ageing. What's really good about it is that the benefits start appearing very quickly and you'll soon set up a virtuous circle.

THE AGEING REVOLUTION

The Silver Tsunami, when the baby boomers – those born between 1946 and 1964 – turn 65, is adding 150,000 people to the older population almost every year.[4] Already it's heralding an ageing revolution. This is the generation that spearheaded sexual, political and lifestyle revolutions, and now it's ageing that is due for a shake-up, not least because these are the people with the money. This age group spends nearly £100 billion a year and their assets are estimated to be £3.5 trillion, almost half of the UK's total wealth.[5]

The current generation of the elderly had the misfortune to be pioneers. No one expected so many to live as long as they have or had any clear idea about how to help them age in the best possible way. Scientists now know much more about what happens in our bodies as we age, and many are exploring ways to slow it down and keep us healthier for longer.

There are two major changes that need to happen as a result of the ageing revolution:

STEP ONE: GET SERIOUS

Preventative medicine needs to be taken far more seriously – it's still the Cinderella of the NHS, despite giving lip service to 'five-a-day'. That means the responsibility for staying healthy starts with you, which is where this book comes in. It is about the exciting findings from new ageing research that could transform what it means to be old, if you start applying them to your own life.

Of course, we are more likely to get sick as we get older, and medical care is always going to be concentrated at the end of life. But just how fast does our decline have to be, and how much can we cut down on the time spent in that wheelchair? Isn't exploring that worth at least as much time and effort as you would have given that newborn baby we mentioned at the beginning of this chapter?

Already we know that following just some of the regular healthy lifestyle advice can bring very worthwhile benefits. Even ten years ago many researchers believed that having good genes was probably your best bet for ageing well. That's no longer true. One study out of many, for example, found that when over 20,000 men and women aged between 45 and 79 were followed for an average of 11 years those who did just four healthy things lived 14 years longer than those who did none of them.[6] The healthy ones didn't do anything more than follow the most basic and familiar advice: they didn't smoke, they drank moderately, they kept physically active and ate five servings a day of fruit and veg.

There probably isn't a doctor in the country who hasn't given out precisely that healthy-living advice a thousand times. But with only seven to ten minutes for each consultation the hard business of getting people to change their habits often fails. The result is that a condition like diabetes, which is largely caused by diet and responds very well to dietary change, ends up being controlled with drugs.

Secret 3 describes some remarkable results in reducing all the signs of diabetes by following a diet, known as low GL (low glycemic load). It is rather different from the low-fat diet that is normally recommended for people with diabetes and for preventing heart disease and losing weight, and there is growing evidence that it is more effective as well as having specific benefits in slowing down ageing.

Your doctor may not know very much about a low-GL diet, however, because it is rather different from the one usually favoured by the diabetes charities. And it is worth knowing that although doctors will usually recommend diet and exercise as a starting point for handling diabetes, their practices receive bonus payments for putting patients on drugs licensed to treat conditions such as diabetes and heart disease as part of the government's attempts at beating these conditions; they do not receive any payments for keeping patients on a healthy diet and lifestyle regime. Whether this is the best way to ensure that we all age healthily is the topic for another book. Right now you know what is coming your way if you don't start taking action, so it's surely worth the application of considerable energy and resources to avoid it. If you want some specific steps to take right now, turn to Part Three.

STEP 2: THERE'S PLENTY THAT CAN BE DONE

There is certainly no anti-ageing magic bullet, precisely because what happens as you get old is that many abilities decline together. But by dealing with specific problems in turn, it's possible to increase the time you spend out of hospital or marooned in your house unable to go upstairs or venture out.

As you get older, the level of various minerals and vitamins in your body starts to decline. For some micronutrients the level of deficiency can be as high as 90 per cent. So, as you set off on the road to healthy ageing we recommend finding out if you do have any deficiencies and to start replacing them.

Here are short examples of two replacements that can make a big difference to your body as you age. Both are described in much more detail in later chapters. Then we'll go into a little more detail about two changes that are unlikely to be part of any regular healthy-lifestyle advice: vitamin D and the importance of maintaining your muscle mass.

HORMONES: A POWERFUL ALLY THAT YOU MAY BE MISSING

As we get older, the kinds of symptoms people often complain about include feeling tired and not being interested in sex. Very often these can be helped with a supplement of hormones. Even in your forties and fifties the amount of hormones, such as oestrogen and progesterone, in your blood will be considerably less than it was when you were younger.

Hormones are powerful and need to be handled with care, so you will need to find a good practitioner. The type we recommend is known as bio-identical – meaning their chemical structure is exactly the same as your body has been making. (The chemicals in regular HRT are not bio-identical.) (We explain all this in Secret 10.)

HEALTHY BONES NEED MORE THAN CALCIUM

Another classic sign of ageing is that along with thinning hair comes thinning bones. Vitamin D has been known for years to be important for keeping your bones strong and, as we explain below, this is now the new supplement star linked with a wide range of benefits. But to ensure your bones stay strong you need other minerals too, such as magnesium, zinc and boron, which you don't normally hear much about. You'll also discover that milk isn't the best source of calcium and that new research has found that insulin – usually talked about in terms of getting excess glucose out of the bloodstream – is also very much involved in making new bone.

WHY VITAMIN D IS SO IMPORTANT

As we mentioned above, vitamin D is now being more generally recognised as a wonder vitamin, and how much you need to take is currently a highly controversial topic. Everyone agrees you need between 5 and 10 micrograms (mcg) a day to protect your bones, but the big debate is whether taking much higher amounts will also cut your risk of heart disease, diabetes, various cancers including breast and colon, and improve your immune response. In research, elderly patients with very low levels in their blood (below 32nmol/l) were twice as likely to die from heart disease as those with higher amounts (70nmol/l).[7] (For more detail on the different units used to measure vitamin D and how they relate to one another see Part 2, Secret 6.)

Many studies now show that to get a wide range of benefits you need a level of vitamin D in your blood that is much higher than that – between 100 and 150nmol/l. You won't reach that just by getting the officially recommended 10mcg a day and it would be very hard to get it just from food. Raw Atlantic herring, the richest source, contains around 40mcg per 100 grams and you'd need to eat at least two servings of that a day! American figures suggest that only about 10 per cent of the population reach the higher level – most are people who work outdoors, because the body makes its own vitamin D when your skin is exposed to sunshine. For the rest of us that leaves supplements to make up the shortfall.

Leading vitamin D researcher, Dr Cedric Garland of the University of California San Diego School of Medicine, has been using a website (Grassroots Health) to monitor over 3,500 people aged 50 and older who are taking a supplement and has also been checking the levels in their blood. His latest report shows that those who have between 100 and 150nmol/l in the blood are getting between 100 and 200mcg a day.[8]

This is the kind of community-based research that is likely to become increasingly common as interest in healthy ageing grows. Large controlled trials are needed to nail down exactly who benefits and by how much. Vitamin D is certainly not the only way to lower cancer risk[9] but it is likely to be part of any package of protection. Experts are divided about whether much higher doses can be dangerous, but there is good evidence to suggest that amounts below 250mcg are safe.[10]

A few UK cancer experts, such as Professor Angus Dalgleish at St George's, University of London, are currently testing the vitamin D levels in all their patients and prescribing high-dose supplements when levels are low.[11] All of this research is changing the old blanket advice to slap on sun cream the moment you step out of doors. You still need to be careful, but the sun is certainly not the enemy. In the UK in the summer you should be able to make a healthy level with 20 minutes sunbathing, with as much of your body exposed as you can.

MAINTAIN YOUR MUSCLE BY EATING ADEQUATE PROTEIN

The second example of something that is already being tried to allow people to age in a much more healthy and positive way involves building up the muscle you are going to lose if nothing is done. Classic signs of ageing – wrinkles, trembling hands, poor coordination and becoming bent over – are usually thought to be inevitable. That's just what happens when you get old, they say. But actually they are linked, among other things, to a loss of muscle mass, caused by a decline in your hormones and a lack of protein. This means that it can be reversed.

We normally get protein, the building blocks of muscle, from two sources. Some we make and the rest comes from our diet. As we get older we make less and even though we actually need more, older people frequently don't eat enough of it. The classic elderly stoop develops because the muscles that support the spine and shoulders have withered.

This elderly muscle loss is known as sarcopenia and it's worse in people who don't take any exercise. That's why it also showed up in the first astronauts. The cure is exercise. But not, and this is important, the kind that doctors normally recommend – a little light walking or jogging.

To build muscle you need resistance training – and that means weights, springs or 'resistance' exercises that really stress your muscles. That might sound rather extreme for much older people but recently a study from the University of Michigan recommended starting resistance training – using weights – from about the age of 50, if not before. The review found that if you do resistance training for 18–20 weeks you can put on nearly 2½ pounds of lean muscle and increase your strength by 25–30 per cent. If you don't do any exercise after the age of 50 you can expect to lose muscle at the rate of half a pound a year, and the older you get, the faster you'll lose it.[12] In Part Three we describe muscle-building exercises you can do as part of a regular routine.

PUMPING IRON TO PREVENT CANCER

Weight training has also been found to help cancer patients and older people who have nothing obviously wrong but who are suffering from the muscle-wasting disorder called cachexia.[13] Dieticians may recommend a calorie-rich diet, which puts on fat but no muscle.

As we have already explained, the body also needs a good protein supply to build muscle. An easily absorbed source, long used by body builders, is branched chain amino acids (BCAAs). There is obviously a case for giving them as a supplement, but they can also be obtained from meat, whey protein, egg protein, bean protein and high protein dairy products. BCAA, plus exercise, may also come with other benefits, including more efficient muscle function and improvement in diabetes symptoms. There's no proof yet that BCAAs are going to make humans live any longer, but they have been found to improve insulin sensitivity and blood glucose control in elderly people with diabetes.[14]

What you can be certain about is that taking these supplements and muscle strengthening will cause very few adverse side effects.

No one should stop taking drugs without discussing it with their doctor but, given the risks, the case for trying options like vitamins and resistance training first makes a lot of sense.

A NEW SORT OF MEDICINE

Just sticking with the drugs just might, but very probably won't, cut your risk of developing one or more of the chronic diseases of ageing. In Chapter 4, we'll reveal just how many people have to take a preventative drug for just one to benefit – you'll be amazed.

The last decade has seen an explosion of information about what exactly goes on in our bodies as we age. Scientists can now boost the healthy life span of lab animals such as worms, mice, fruit flies, and even monkeys, simply by changing their diet and by giving them compounds found in fruit and vegetables. We think this is a much more promising place to start to build a healthy-ageing programme for yourself.

THE FOOD THAT TURNS GENES ON AND OFF

One of the most groundbreaking discoveries is that all kinds of foods and supplements can actually change the activity of genes linked with illness and ageing; for example, a high carbohydrate diet that pushes up the amount of sugar in the blood can change how fast lab animals age.

This in turn is related to the discovery that cutting your calories can turn on a gene that is linked to all kinds of health benefits, such as the repair of DNA and better resistance to stress. Having high levels of insulin is turning out to be really bad if you want to age well. This is why in Secret 3 we advocate eating a low-GL diet, which keeps blood sugar levels and insulin down – something that brings many health benefits very quickly.

This approach is also different because you will be aiming to make changes to parts of your body that you may never have heard of before – such as mitochondria, which make energy; telomeres, which may predict how well you are ageing; and a nasty combo of proteins and sugar called advanced glycation end-products, or AGEs for short, which can gum up your body's works. We will be showing you how to get rid of them in Chapter 5.

USING THE HEALTHY-AGEING PYRAMID

This may all seem a bit daunting and unfamiliar, but the healthy-ageing pyramid may make it a bit clearer and help you to think about making changes in stages. First, at the bottom is a basic broad-based change to the way you eat, using the principles of optimum nutrition; this is where our Anti-ageing Diet – a low-GL diet – fits in, along with lots of fruit and vegetables, and healthy omega-3 oils.

From there you can move up the pyramid, making more changes as and when you feel ready or to fit in with particular needs. Ideally though, you would combine optimum nutrition with the next one up – exercise, which benefits all aspects of ageing. Then there is sleep and relaxation and further up you will find the supplements of minerals, hormones and vitamins; our levels of all these decline as we get older. As you can see, the darker left-hand side of the pyramid shows what happens if you aren't getting these anti-ageing benefits: lack of nutrients, poor muscle mass, insomnia and so on.

The healthy-ageing pyramid

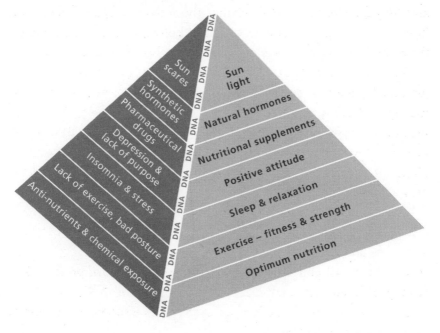

Ageing well shouldn't become a chore. The whole idea is that the changes you are making should make you feel better now. We want you to avoid the old joke that 'this doesn't actually make you live any longer – it just seems like it'. In fact, there is nothing like being stuck indoors on a dozen pills too ill to go out to make you feel that time is crawling by.

Ageing healthily is an active project. To start you'll need to discover which bits of you are ageing well by using a series of tests in the next chapter, the results of which you can enter online and then track your progress over time. The way you age is now a choice. What you do now will play a big part in what your life is going to be like in 10, 20 or 30 years' time. And that's not so far away. An average life span of 80 years is just 960 months. You may only have another 150 or 200 months left. Make the most of them.

Chapter 2

CHECK YOUR BIOLOGICAL AGE

We all know people who look older than their age, and envy those who look younger and seem to age more slowly. We hope you will become one of the latter. You may not reach championship levels, such as the 120 years achieved by male longevity record holder, Shigechiyo Izumi from Japan, or the female world champion, Madame Jeanne Calmant, who died aged 122, but the aim of this book is to make sure that, whatever your life span, you live healthily and avoid years of decrepitude.

There are also many other youthful centenarians who can be inspiring, such as 102-year-old Olive Patterson whose charm and indomitable spirit shows how active and alive you can be even after a century. She's also an example of the strange phenomenon that once you get into your nineties the process of ageing slows dramatically. Olive still lives in her own house in Gloucestershire with a collection of 280 dolls, which she lectures about, and a piano that she plays for two hours every evening, having once been a professional musician. Every morning, Olive does ten minutes of step-ups on her stairs followed by breathing exercises, and she believes that these have helped her to get off all but two of her prescription drugs. She also takes care to eat a balanced and varied diet with protein with each meal and vegetables with lunch and in soup in the evening.

Her tip for staying independent? 'The most important thing is not to give up. Even if you are feeling poorly you have to keep going.' As simple as it sounds, her diet and lifestyle include five of our healthy-ageing secrets.

WHAT'S YOUR bioage?

Although you can't change your chronological age, you *can* change your biological age. If you are ageing faster than you should be, following our ten Healthy-ageing Secrets in Part Two should slow down your rate of ageing. But how do you find out your biological age now? This chapter will tell you.

We give you a list of tests that you can do at home to measure how your body's essential functions are working. The results of those tests will give you a basic idea of your biological age. If you want to take it further, and we hope that you will, you can complete our free online **bioage check**, which will give you a much clearer picture. To complete the online check it helps to have the results from two other different sets of tests as well as the home test. The first – the home test – consists of a series of simple physical tests, which are listed immediately below. Then you'll need to go onto the Web and complete our comprehensive 100% Health Check, which is comprised of a set of questions designed to calculate how healthy you are right now, giving you information on how to become healthier. Finally, for the most accurate picture you will also need the results from some blood tests, which can be taken either by your GP or you can arrange to have them done privately. We explain later why they are important. Your **bioage check** will automatically calculate your biological age. (If you haven't done the blood tests, it will still calculate your bio-age.) Just follow the instructions on www. patrickholford.com/bioage.

To get your basic biological age so that you can work out where you are right now, start with the physical tests below.

Physical tests you can do at home

Add your scores beneath each section or record them in a notebook if you prefer.

Pulse

Sit quietly and calmly in a chair with your feet flat on the floor. Find your pulse and record the number of beats in 15 seconds. Continue to breathe normally throughout. Multiply by 4 – this is your pulse rate per minute.

A healthy level is around 60 beats per minute.

Score:

Blood pressure

You can do this at home if you have a machine, otherwise ask your GP, practice nurse or personal trainer to measure your blood pressure. It's most important that you are relaxed and sitting comfortably in a chair. A blood pressure reading is made up of two numbers: systolic (the top number) and diastolic (the bottom number). The first reflects the maximum pressure in the arteries when the heart has just beaten and blood courses through them, the second shows the minimum pressure, in the lull between heartbeats. If your arteries are narrowing, the bottom figure goes up. If the arteries are becoming less elastic, the top figure goes up.

The ideal reading is around 120/80, where 120 is the systolic and 80 is the diastolic.

Score:

BMI

Body mass index, or BMI, is a measure of your weight in relation to your height. It is calculated by taking your weight in kilograms and dividing it by your height in metres squared, so first, you need to know your weight and your height. BMI can be a useful measure, but its major shortcoming is that it doesn't tell you how much of your total weight is fat and how much is muscle, and this is probably of much greater importance than your weight and BMI. Other measures such as body-fat percentage and waist-to-hip ratio may be more useful, and these are discussed below.

To calculate your BMI, first calculate your height squared (which is your height in metres multiplied by that same figure) and then divide your weight by this number.

For example, if your weight is 65kg and your height is 1.72m, the calculation is:

$$1.70 \times 1.70 = 2.9, \text{ then } 65 \div 2.9 = 22.5$$
So that means your BMI is 22.5
A BMI of around 20–25 is ideal

If you complete the online **bioage check**, your BMI will be calculated for you and you can enter your weight in kilograms or pounds and your height in metres or feet and inches if you prefer. (There are also a number of BMI calculators on the internet.)

Score: ☐

WHR

Your waist-to-hip ratio, or WHR, is the ratio of your waist measurement to your hip measurement. The greater your waist-to-hip ratio the more 'apple-shaped' you are likely to be. Apple-shaped weight gain is thought to be the most concerning type of weight gain, because as fat accumulates around the middle, you are likely to be increasing the fat which is accumulating around your internal organs such as your liver, and this increases your risk of a number of age-related conditions including heart disease, diabetes and metabolic syndrome (we'll be explaining this later). Some authorities consider WHR much more useful than BMI.

To calculate your WHR, first take your measurements:

1. Your waist is midway between the top of your hips and the bottom of your ribcage.

2. Measure your hips at the widest point.

The ratio is calculated by dividing the waist measurement by the hip measurement.

For example, if your waist measures 105cm and your hips measure 116cm, the calculation is:

$$105 \div 116 = 0.91$$

A ratio below 1.0 is considered healthy for men and below 0.85 is considered healthy for women.

If you complete the online **bioage check**, your WHR will be calculated for you when you enter your waist and hip measurements, which can be in centimetres or inches. (There are also a number of WHR calculators on the internet.)

Score: ☐

Body-fat percentage

Your body-fat percentage tells you how much of your weight is made up of fat. You can find out your body-fat percentage in one of two ways. Get yourself weighed on a set of body composition scales (see Resources). You can also obtain this from a Zest4Life practitioner (see Resources), or if you're a member of a gym or have a personal trainer, they can usually calculate these measurements using skin-fold callipers, or they may also have body composition scales. (There are also a number of body-fat percentage calculators on the internet. Although they will not be as accurate as using scales, they will give you a rough idea.)

A healthy level for women over 40 is 23–35 per cent. Men should have a much lower body-fat percentage, with a healthy level for men over 40 being around 12–23 per cent.

Score: ☐

Visceral-fat percentage

Fat that accumulates around your internal organs in the area of your belly is called visceral fat and it is thought to be the most harmful type. If you have a high WHR and/or a high body-fat percentage, it's quite likely that you also have increasing levels of visceral fat. Like body-fat percentage, visceral-fat percentage can be measured on body composition scales as mentioned above. As before, you can visit a Zest4Life practitioner or if you are a member of a gym, they may have a similar type of scales. Without scales you could try to estimate your visceral fat, by tensing your tummy muscles and pinching the fat by your belly button. Although it seems counter-intuitive, if your belly definitely sticks out but there is little fat to pinch you are actually in a worse position; it means that most of the fat is the dangerous internal visceral fat.

The scales will grade your visceral fat into low risk and high risk
as follows:
1–12 = low risk
13–59 = high risk

Score: ☐

Muscle strength

Sit on a standard dining-room chair, ideally one where your feet are on the floor and your thighs are more or less at 90 degrees. Now, try to rise from the chair without using your arms. If you can stand easily in one swift movement without using your arms at all, score –2. If you need to shuffle forward in the chair and use both arms, score +2. You would score 0 if you could rise in one movement but perhaps had a bit of a wobble and needed to use one arm for a little assistance. Using this scale, score your muscle strength.

Easy, no arms, score –2
A little help from one arm, score –1
A little help from both arms, score 0
Quite a bit of help from both arms, score +1
Need to shuffle forward first and then use both arms, score +2

Score: ☐

Balance

Stand on one leg and put your hands on your hips. Note the time (in seconds) or set a stopwatch. How long can you keep your balance? Make a note of how long you lasted.

Excellent balance would be over a minute and is even better if you can do this with your eyes closed. This tests both your balance and strength, which tend to get worse with age. (If your balance is not good, practise each day and see how you progress – you can hold a finger against a wall to start with, if you are very wobbly.)

Score yourself as follows:

30 seconds to 1 minute or more, score –2
15–30 seconds, score –1
10–15 seconds, score 0
5 seconds, score +1
1–2 seconds, score +2

Score: ⬜

Flexibility

From standing, try to touch your toes with your legs straight (and your knees soft). If you can reach all the way to your toes, score –2, if you can only just reach your knees, score +2.

Score yourself as follows:

Touching toes without bending knees, score –2
Reaching ankles, score –1
Halfway down calves, score 0
Just past knees, score +1
Barely reaching knees, score +2

Score: ⬜

Lung capacity

Take a regular birthday or small candle, light it and hold it at arm's length. Try to blow it out. How many attempts does it take? If you were successful on the first attempt, score –2. If it took a couple of attempts, score 0. If you have to bend your arm to the equivalent of a hand's length closer, score +1; if you have to move your arm to the equivalent of two hand's lengths closer, score +2.

Score yourself as follows:

Successful first time, score –2
Successful second time, score –1
Took more attempts, score 0

Had to bend arm to bring candle closer, score +1
Had to bend arm more to bring the candle a lot closer, score +2

Score: ☐

Eye test

Eyesight tends to deteriorate with age. The important point is whether your eyesight is declining fast; you may wear glasses, but if your prescription doesn't change, then your eyesight is holding up well.

Think about how often you have to have a new (stronger) prescription for your glasses, if you wear them. If you don't wear glasses, score 0. If you do and you haven't had to increase your prescription for ten years, score –2. If you are having to increase your prescription (or you are buying your own over-the-counter reading glasses and having to buy new ones) every year or so, score +2.

Score yourself as follows:

No new prescription for 10 years, score –2
A stronger prescription every 5–10 years, score –1
A stronger prescription every 2–5 years, score 0
A stronger prescription every 2–3 years, score +1
A stronger prescription every year or so, score +2

Score: ☐

Libido

Give yourself a score from –2 to +2, with –2 being equivalent to a libido similar to your peak in your thirties and forties and +2 meaning you have no interest and great difficulty achieving orgasm or, if you're a man, maintaining an erection.

Score yourself as follows:

Usual desire and good performance, score –2
Slightly reduced desire and/or satisfactory performance, score –1
Less than half the desire and/or satisfactory performance, score 0
Little desire and much reduced satisfactory performance, score +1
No desire and absence of feeling or satisfactory performance, score +2

Score: ☐

Blood tests

To complete the picture you will also need to have some blood tests, which we describe below. However, we understand that few people will have these (at least at this stage) therefore the chart on page 26 will still enable you to get a good general idea of your bio-age score by looking at the results of your home tests so far.

BLOOD TESTS: THE BIOCHEMICAL MARKERS OF AGEING

The results that will probably still be missing from the chart overleaf are the ones for the blood tests. We think that the two of those tests that give you the most reliable information for working out your anti-ageing strategy are your blood sugar level, measured by what's called glycosylated haemoglobin (or HbA1c), and the amount of a potentially dangerous amino acid called homocysteine. Your doctor can measure both of these. Alternatively, you can buy a home-test kit (see Resources). If your GP does it for you, ask for a printout of the results so that you can ensure that you have the precise number and the units.

THE DANGERS OF SUGARY BLOOD

You may have heard about glycosylated haemoglobin in connection with people who have diabetes, who have to be very careful not to let their blood sugar get too high. But, as you will see in the sections about how the body ages, a gradual loss of blood sugar control is something that happens to all of us as we get older. For some, this leads to diabetes, but even for the rest of us the result is that we start producing more of a harmful by-product of the way the body makes energy from glucose.

It's called glycosylation and it results in what are known as advanced glycation end-products, or AGEs for short. These attach to, and damage, some of the proteins that your body is making all the time, such as the skin and the arteries, causing them to become stiffer and less flexible. This is one of the factors contributing to wrinkles and raised blood pressure. From a blood sample you can literally count how many red blood cells (haemoglobin) are sugar-coated (glycosylated), so you get a

INTERPRETING YOUR SCORES

First highlight your scores (or the closest equivalent) in the table below then, for a rough and ready bio-age score, take your actual age and add 2 years for every score in the '+2' column, add 1 year for every score in the '+1' column, take away 1 year for every score in the '–1' column and deduct 2 years for every score in the '–2' column. The more you have in the right-hand column the healthier and biologically younger you are. But don't worry if your scores are more towards the left, by following the advice in this book you should see an improvement when you retake the tests in a few months' time. Do note, however, that you'll get a much more accurate estimate by completing the online **bioage check** at www.patrickholford.com/bioage.

Your test results

	+2	+1	0	–1	–2
Home tests					
Pulse	80	75	70	65	60
Blood pressure	140/100+	135/95+	120/80–130/85	120/80	120/80–110/75
BMI	> 28	26–28	22–25	20–21	18–19
WHR – male	1.1+	1.05	1	0.95	0.9
WHR – female	1+	0.95	0.85	0.8	0.75
Body-fat % – male	> 31	23–30	20–22	16–19	12–15
Body-fat % – female	> 42	36–41	30–35	27–29	23–26
Visceral-fat %	> 20	11–20	6–10	4–5	1–3
Muscle strength	+2	+1	0	–1	–2
Balance	+2	+1	0	–1	–2
Flexibility	+2	+1	0	–1	–2
Lung capacity	+2	+1	0	–1	–2
Eyesight	+2	+1	0	–1	–2
Libido	+2	+1	0	–1	–2
Blood tests					
Glycosylated haemoglobin	> 6.5	5.5–6.5	5.5	5.0–5.4	4.0–4.9
Homocysteine	11+	8–10	7	6	5
Vitamin D	< 50	50–74	75–100	101–125	> 125

Your Bio-age: ☐

score usually between 3 and 20 per cent. Ideally, you want to be below 5.5 per cent, but again this depends on your age to a degree.

In the graph below you can see the 'average' versus the 'ideal' score depending on your age.

Glycosylated haemoglobin by age – average and optimal

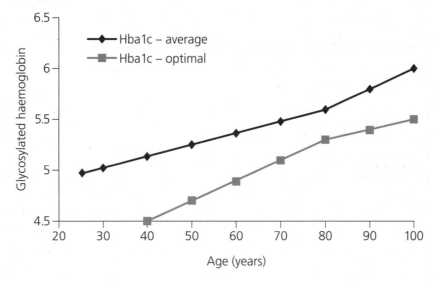

HOMOCYSTEINE – YOUR MOST VITAL STATISTIC

Knowing your blood level of homocysteine is important, because it tells you how well another fundamental process in your body is working. This process is called methylation and you'll find that it crops up again and again in this book. Methylation is a chemical process that is needed for just about everything in your body: making energy, making bones and joints, neurotransmitters and hormones, as well as detoxifying and, most importantly, repairing DNA and copying the correct information to make new cells. There are a billion methylation reactions taking place in nearly every cell in your body and brain every few seconds.

The best marker for how well your body is maintaining all these reactions is your blood homocysteine level, because homocysteine is needed to make the chemicals involved in the methylation process, and a high level means that it's not being converted properly. This can be measured by your doctor or health-care practitioner, or by using a home-test kit. The ideal level is below 7μmol/l (mcmol/l). (You will find more about this in Chapter 5.)

The graph below shows you what the 'average' level is, according to age, and also the optimal level for healthy ageing.

Homocysteine by age, average and optimal

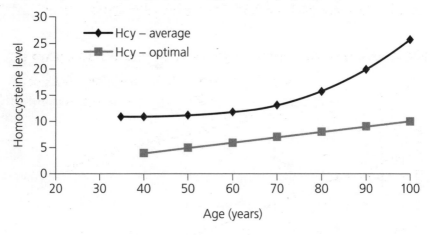

VITAL VITAMIN D – DO YOU HAVE ENOUGH?

Another useful test is your vitamin D status, which some GPs may be prepared to do for you, otherwise you can arrange to have one taken (see Resources). On its own it isn't really a predictor of your biological age, although people with higher vitamin D levels tend to live longer. Knowing your score is useful though, because it allows you to adjust your intake to achieve the healthy-ageing optimum of a blood level of above 100nmol/l. If you know your score, you'll be asked for this when you do your online **bio**age **check**.

There are other biochemical markers of ageing, but the three we've mentioned above are our favourites and the least expensive to be tested for.

THE 100% HEALTH CHECK

The final part of calculating your **bioage** score is taking the free 100% Health Check, which you complete online at www.patrickholford.com (the chart below summarises the results to date). It involves answering questions about your symptoms, diet and lifestyle along with your mental agility and memory. Allow yourself 20 minutes to complete the check. You will also get the chance to add your scores from the physical and blood tests you've already done. If you are missing any results, just go on to the next question. When you've put in as much information as you can (the more the better), you'll be given your **bioage** score.

100% Health score versus age, both average and optimal

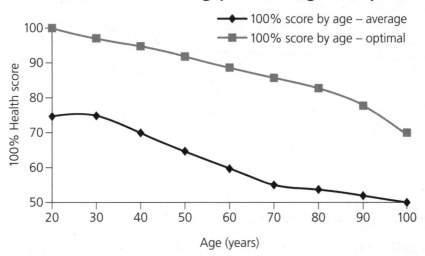

From those results we can then let you know what you can do to reduce your score, or at least reduce the speed by which you age biologically. The **bioage check** is free but you'll also have the option of receiving a personalised 100% Health Programme, with daily email prompts on key goals, adjusted every month, if you so choose. In this way you can monitor your **bioage**. (There's a fee for receiving the full 100% Health Programme, see Resources.)

We hope you will, at least, complete your free **bioage check** once a year. In this way you can help us to map what changes make the most difference and feed these findings back to you. Over 100,000 people have already completed the online questionnaire and, with your help, we can really find out what works best and help the whole process of learning the secrets of healthy ageing.

Chapter 3

THE SECRETS OF CELL REJUVENATION

As we get older, the cells in our bodies gradually become less efficient, leading to the symptoms, aches and pains we understand to be part-and-parcel of the process of ageing, but you'll discover in this book that you can slow down this decline by making particular nutritional and lifestyle choices. First, let's look at what happens to our cells as the years go by.

Imagine a factory in a town that has been hit by economic depression. The perimeter fence has developed a couple of gaps, output is down, but the smokestack is probably even more polluting than it used to be, and it's damaging the health of the workers. The toxic-waste storage unit is leaking, and with fewer competent managers in the boardroom, the response to falling sales and a demoralised workforce has been sporadic and ineffective.

It's not too fanciful to suggest that as we age something similar is happening to the cells in our body. Each cell is microscopic – about 50 micrometers across (1 micrometre =1/1000th of a millimetre) and we are made up of about 100 trillion of them. They vary according to where they belong – heart, liver, guts, blood, and so on – but their basic floor plan is similar.

They may be tiny but they are miracles of complexity. Like the factory, they really do have polluting power plants, garbage disposal units, assembly centres for building proteins, and much more. But as we age they begin to function less efficiently, just like the factory above. It's not unreasonable to suggest that an injection of new 'funds' (in the form of nutrients, proteins and enzymes) should help to lift our 'micro-factories' out of the slump; they will cut the pollution, clear away some of the garbage and improve the efficiency of the production line.

RENOVATING OUR 'FACTORIES'

The idea that the symptoms of ageing – the aching joints, thinning hair, stiffening arteries and raised risk of disease – is due to the gradual decline of cell function is known as the 'disposable soma theory'. It works like this:

Maintaining any factory is expensive. There have to be quality checks, machinery has to be upgraded, rubbish cleared away, damage repaired, and so on. So we have evolved to invest less in repair and renewal as we age and to devote our resources to reproduction, growth and defence when we're young, giving us a better chance of getting our genes into the next generation. Genes that encourage people to produce healthy kids early are more likely to be out there in the general population than ones that are brilliant at keeping your micro-factories pristine and keep you ageing well. When you stop being able to have children your body (soma) becomes disposable.

What this means is that as we get older our systems for repair and renewal become less effective and very gradually begin to silt up. In the days when 40 was a reasonable life span and 60 was a triumph (not so long ago) that didn't matter very much. But with the average life span pushing 80 (and rising) 20 or 30 years is a long time to put up with substandard maintenance, errors in protein production and their increasingly obvious effects. So, what we are looking for is a biological DIY shop that will allow us to conduct running repairs on our own factory population.

CALL FOR REINFORCEMENTS

The simplest solution is to replace what's missing. Hormones, for example, are involved in all sorts of vital functions – growing muscles and bones, providing energy, making you feel sexy – but by the time you are in your sixties, levels of various hormones will have halved. So, not surprisingly, hormone replacement therapy has been popular for years as a rejuvenation option in various forms. It's been especially controversial since the links with cancer and heart disease were recognised with conventional HRT, but there is another option and new ideas about how men can benefit too, as we discuss in Secret 10.

As we saw in the last chapter, there is also a decline in the levels of many of the minerals and vitamins that our cellular 'factories' need to function efficiently. So it makes sense that, if necessary, those supplies should be topped up. But this approach is also controversial: just how effective is it to 'top up' these levels, and can you get all the nutrients you need from your diet? We cover the latest research later.

INTRODUCING THE KEY PLAYERS FOR GOOD HEALTH

There's a fundamental difference between the nutritional approach to health and the pharmaceutical one, which is thrown into sharp relief by the problem of ageing. Nutritional therapy aims to support the body in a number of ways so that problems resolve themselves. Drugs, on the other hand, are designed, usually, to block or boost a single compound that is causing a problem – such as too much cholesterol or stomach acid, or not enough serotonin or insulin. This makes nutrition and other lifestyle changes particularly suitable for encouraging healthy ageing, because ageing never involves just one thing going wrong at a time.

What's happening in our micro-factories is that a number of processes are running down, but exercise and nutritional supplements can help all of them to perk up at once. As we've seen, drugs – at least the way they are developed and licensed at the moment – can only target one declining component at a time.

What is more, most of the key players for good health in our micro-factories are still pretty unfamiliar to us – you are unlikely to hear much discussion of them in the doctor's surgery, for example. Yet they are central to the decline that comes with getting older. They will keep popping up in this book, so here's a quick overview to introduce them.

The important components of a cell

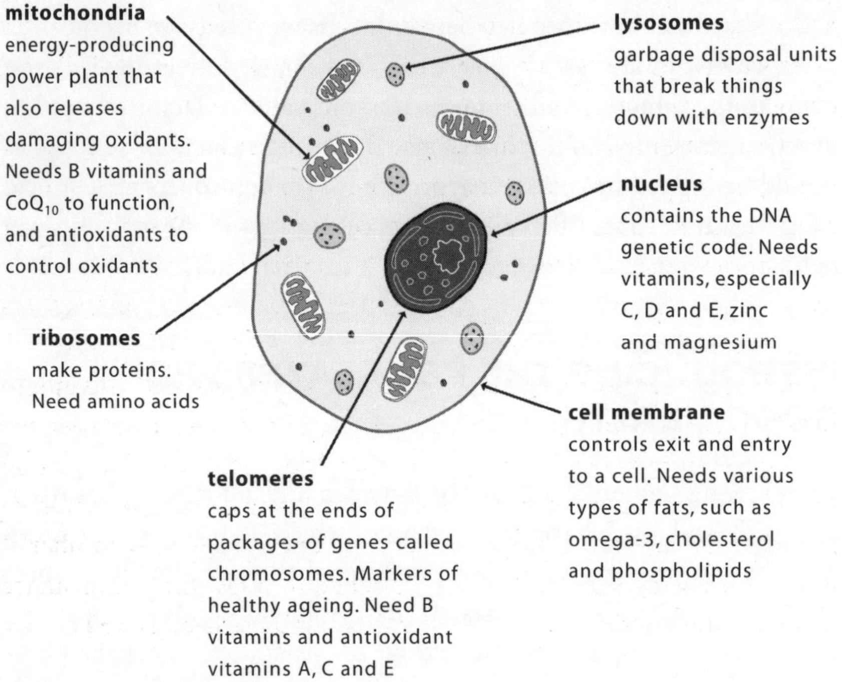

mitochondria
energy-producing
power plant that
also releases
damaging oxidants.
Needs B vitamins and
CoQ$_{10}$ to function,
and antioxidants to
control oxidants

lysosomes
garbage disposal units
that break things
down with enzymes

nucleus
contains the DNA
genetic code. Needs
vitamins, especially
C, D and E, zinc
and magnesium

ribosomes
make proteins.
Need amino acids

telomeres
caps at the ends of
packages of genes called
chromosomes. Markers of
healthy ageing. Need B
vitamins and antioxidant
vitamins A, C and E

cell membrane
controls exit and entry
to a cell. Needs various
types of fats, such as
omega-3, cholesterol
and phospholipids

These are some of the important players in a cell, what they do and what each
needs to function efficiently.

THE POWER STATION

Energy is generated in the body in the mitochondria: microscopic tube-
like structures in cells. It's here that oxygen (from the lungs) is used to
break down sugars and other carbohydrates from our diet to make the
energy molecule, ATP. It's ATP that powers nearly all the processes in
the body, from fuelling our muscles to providing the energy the liver
needs for detoxification (a process of cleansing inside the body).

The process that produces ATP requires a range of vitamins (as
shown in the illustration above). But this process also produces carbon
dioxide along with a changed and potentially dangerous kind of oxygen
called an oxidant.

Mitochondria are central to ageing because making energy is often
a dirty business, whether inside the body using the raw material of
carbohydrate or, in the case of a real factory, using coal. The oxidants

that are by-products can damage tissue in the cells, so cells need a good supply of antioxidants to 'snuff' them out.

To keep the mitochondria working properly, we all produce an essential compound in the liver, called CoQ_{10}, which can also disarm dangerous oxidants, because it is an antioxidant as well.

As your ageing body starts to cut down its 'repair budget', one of the casualties is the wall of the mitochondria, which normally keeps most of the oxidants safely inside. It becomes leakier, thereby allowing oxidants to escape into the cell where they can cause damage, especially to the DNA. To make things worse, production of the antioxidants we make naturally slows down, too, as we age. For a long time, this combination of more dangerous oxidants and fewer antioxidants to handle them was thought to explain the decline that went with ageing. Now the picture has become more complicated after studies have found that supplementing with antioxidants hasn't been as effective as hoped. We cover the debate this has provoked in the next chapter. A number of other anti-ageing supplements are designed to boost the performance of your mitochondria, and we'll be discussing these later as well.

THE SOFTWARE CODE

Your software code is the DNA that is housed in the nucleus in the middle of each cell, and its genetic information is used to run every function in your body. Your DNA is constantly under attack from the oxidants, however, some of them coming from the mitochondria and others from external sources such as cigarette smoke, ultraviolet light and radiation.

Cells make protein using DNA as the blueprint. So, damage to DNA speeds up ageing because it means that instructions for protein manufacture by the ribosome (see the illustration opposite) can become garbled. Much of our body is made up of proteins – from our muscles to the enzymes that speed up chemical reactions. But the chains of amino acids that make up proteins have to be folded very precisely. A faulty blueprint can mess that up, resulting in oddly shaped ones that don't work properly. By the time we are 80, our cells will have lost between 40 and 90 per cent of their ability to make new proteins.

DNA damage (in the form of mutations) can also have another very harmful effect – it makes cancer more likely by knocking out genes that are designed to kill off cells before they start growing out of control. Without a good supply of a range of minerals and vitamins, your risk of faulty proteins and cancer goes up. We'll be covering this in detail in Secret 6.

YOUR VERY OWN AGEING COUNTER

Inside the nucleus of every cell you have something connected to your chromosomes that can show how you have aged; it's called a telomere. Only a couple of years ago telomeres were an obscure part of the packaging of our genes, known only to gene researchers. But now they are prime targets for turning back your biological clock. You can even have an expensive test that claims to be able to tell you how fast you are ageing by measuring them. So what are they?

Among the many amazing tricks that cells pull off is regularly dividing into two. Some, like those in your blood or guts, do it very often, because they are constantly being renewed. Others, like those in the brain or the lens of the eye, do it very occasionally. Each time this happens, the telomere comes into action.

Telomeres are located inside the cell's nucleus where our strings of DNA are stuffed into sausage-shaped bundles known as chromosomes. The telomeres sit right at either end of each chromosome where, rather like the plastic caps that protect the ends of shoelaces from fraying, they prevent the chromosomes from damage when the cell pulls apart down the middle to divide into two.

Each time this happens, the telomeres unwind a little, so they shrink. What this means is that they give scientists a measure of how many times a cell has split: the shorter our telomeres, the more we have aged. The big discovery is that a number of healthy habits – such as exercise – are linked with having longer telomeres. There's a drug that increases length too, as well as an enzyme that can repair them. You'll find more on this in Chapter 5.

WHEN THE CLEAN UP OF WASTE BREAKS DOWN

Lysosomes are roving garbage disposal and recycling units found all around a cell. One of their jobs is to break down any of those damaged proteins created by faulty blueprints before they start to accumulate. Our micro-factories are very green, so the proteins are broken down into their amino acids, which are then reused. Lysosomes are also designed to get rid of harmful chemicals – both those we consume and those our body makes as 'exhaust fumes' from its normal metabolism – by 'eating' them up with enzymes. Lysosomes are part of the system that encourages unhealthy cells to commit suicide if they seem to be growing out of control. Left unchecked this leads to cancer.

If this clean-up process doesn't go smoothly, waste starts to build up until very little in the body is working properly – this is sometimes called the 'garbage catastrophe' theory of ageing. Damaged mitochondria are among the cell components that sometimes have to be recycled before they do further damage.

In a double whammy, the clean-up system is also built from proteins, so it becomes less effective too. Among the processes damaged by the rising tide of junk proteins are antioxidant production, DNA repair and the protein-making machinery itself. The challenge is how to reactivate them.

Unfortunately, there are many chemicals that lysosomes cannot break down. Once inside a lysosome, that junk is there to stay and can build up to a dangerous level. A proposed high-tech solution to lysosome failure is described in Chapter 5.

THE MEMBRANE – THE REAL CONTROLLER OF EACH CELL

Textbook biology usually describes the nucleus at the centre of the cell where the DNA genetic material is housed as the controller, or brain. But, if it were, the cell would immediately die without it. Cells whose nuclei have been removed in the lab can live for several months, however, although they can't divide. But a cell with its membrane – the surrounding wall – removed dies almost immediately. This shows that the nucleus is not the 'brain' but the cell's 'balls'– confusing the two is understandable, since science is dominated by men who often get the two mixed up!

A powerful factor controlling a cell is what is going on in the cells around it, and information about this has to come in through the membrane. So, the membrane acts partly like our senses, constantly responding to what's going on outside and feeding it back inside. It's made up of a mix of fats and proteins arranged so that certain molecules are allowed in but others are not. Drugs and other chemicals, along with nutrients, can enter through channels built of proteins.

Essentially, this wall is made up of what we choose to eat; so not getting enough of the right ingredients can therefore mean that your cell membranes will function less efficiently. Along with the protein, the cell membrane is composed of phospholipids and essential fats, which can be found, among other sources, in eggs and fish respectively.

THE BIG NUTRITION DEBATE: TO SUPPLEMENT OR NOT

No one disagrees that these key players in our micro-factories need vitamins, minerals and other nutrients for optimum performance and that one of the best ways to keep them in good shape is with those classic keys to ageing well: healthy food and exercise. Recent anti-ageing research has given new insights into exactly why the right sort of exercise and certain diets are so effective and how to get the maximum benefit from them, as we explain in Chapter 6.

It therefore seems sensible to take various nutrient supplements, especially as you are getting older and likely to be deficient, to keep yourself supple and energetic into your eighties and beyond. Not nearly enough controlled trials have been done to show for certain that improving our intake of minerals and vitamins will make you age more healthily. But simply stating that in theory you can get all the nutrients you need from a healthy balanced diet is of no help to those who aren't. Older people are among the most at risk of a poorer diet and even if they were eating in the best possible way, their diet couldn't supply the high level of B vitamins needed to stave off memory loss, or an adequate amount of vitamin D in the winter. This is where personal choice comes in.

It is true, however, that several large randomised trials have failed to show that taking regular amounts of the antioxidant vitamins – specifically C and E – turns back the clock. But even though those trials are regularly quoted, it seems likely that the failures have more to do with difficulties in conducting nutritional research coupled with misunderstandings about the way vitamins work. What's more, new information suggests that many of the drugs regularly given to older people actually reduce the supply of micronutrients (see below).

WHY THE TRIALS MAY HAVE FAILED

To start with, trials of vitamins are often carried out on older patients who are fairly sick, and on a cocktail of drugs that most likely interfere with the nutrients doing their job. Trials of new drugs, however, designed to obtain a licence, usually involve younger patients who aren't taking any other drug – purposely to avoid any such interferences.

Leading micronutrient researcher Bruce Ames, Professor of Biochemistry and Molecular Biology at the University of California, Berkeley, has a theory to explain why giving basic doses of vitamins to older people with a chronic disease is very unlikely to be effective; they, like many in the population, have been deficient in various vitamins for much of their lives.

The body has evolved to handle a nutrient shortage in a particular way. Like surgeons on the battlefield, it applies a 'triage' approach: operate immediately on those whose life might be saved as a result, and leave for later those who will probably die anyway as well as those who are likely to survive anyway. In vitamin terms, this means directing what supplies there are to the vital organs and skimping on the rest.[15] So, by the time you come to supplement, the damage may have already been done. As with the 'disposable soma' theory (explained on page 32), our systems are designed to maximise survival and reproduction now, even if it makes for sickness and disease further down the line. (There is more on the triage theory in the next chapter.)

And there are other objections to the claim that trials show that supplements don't work. Very few of them make any attempt to discover what people's nutrient levels were to begin with. Researchers at Rush University Medical Centre in Chicago point out that if you are already at an optimum level, supplements are unlikely to have an effect.[16]

A good example of the way your baseline for a nutrient affects how much benefit you get shows up in a study on the role of high doses of vitamin B in reducing 'mild cognitive impairment' in older patients. The details are covered in Part Three, Chapter 7, but the important point is that it was only those with dangerously raised levels of the toxic amino acid homocysteine who actually benefited from taking B vitamins.[17] We recommend getting tested for homocysteine, not only to help calculate your accurate bio-age (page 26) but also to find out what nutrients you need and what you don't.

ARE DRUGS MUGGING YOUR VITAMIN SUPPLIES?

Another reason why some supplement trials may have not been positive, especially those on older people taking a number of medical drugs, is that drugs can lower vitamin and mineral levels. You may have heard that cholesterol-lowering statins also cut the production of a powerful antioxidant called CoQ_{10}, which you may remember is also needed by your mitochondria to produce energy. That's why so many people on statins feel tired. And there are plenty more examples. Diuretics to lower blood pressure rush various minerals and vitamins out of the body, including vitamin C, calcium, potassium and magnesium – all of which, ironically, are involved in controlling blood pressure! Ace inhibitors, also used for hypertension, cut available zinc, which is needed by the immune system and to make testosterone – so bang goes your sex drive!

Details of these largely unknown interactions are contained in a book by a leading US pharmacist, Suzy Cohen, called *Drug Muggers: Which Medications are Robbing Your Body of Essential Nutrients.*

Another example of a drug blocking a natural process that provides the same benefit is SSRI antidepressants, which lower thyroid hormones, but these same hormones are involved in regulating energy and mood! As a consequence, most people on antidepressants find they work less well over time, but when they try to quit, many feel absolutely awful, with seriously depleted serotonin levels and thyroid problems to boot. Of course, this keeps people taking the drugs.

A BETTER WAY TO KEEP YOUR CELLS IN SHAPE

At the moment, changes in the efficiency of your mitochondria, the quality of your protein folding, or the flexibility of your cell membranes, are not on the medical radar. And even when the cumulative effects start showing up as cancer or creaky joints the focus is on the immediate problem rather than on how you got there.

One reason for this, as we saw in the introduction, is that prevention has always come rather low down on the medical agenda, and efforts are largely limited to general advice on smoking (fairly successful), the famous five-a-day (poor results), keeping the weight down (very poor results) and the low-fat diet (a disaster – see Secret 7 on heart disease). If these were A-level results they would rate an F. If we are going to age more healthily and avoid a nasty decline, we need to become a lot more sophisticated about, and committed to, prevention.

In fact, prevention shouldn't be left to doctors; they don't have the time or the training to do it properly. Ideally it should be outsourced to teams that might comprise a nutritionist, an exercise trainer, maybe a counsellor and others who can give patients the tools and the motivation to make the lifestyle changes that can nip health problems in the bud. It's a radical approach and cost effectiveness is unclear, but one of the hopes for GP commissioning is that it might make this approach more attractive. When a GP's budget involves paying for all the costs sick patients rack up, taking prevention seriously starts to make an awful lot more sense. In the meantime, you have to make healthy ageing a personal project.

You are going to age, so you might as well get good at it. That could mean treating your doctor like a midwife – someone who has valuable skills that might help you through a natural life event.

Keeping your mitochondria, DNA and the rest of the key players in your micro-factories working as well as possible is an essential part of that. Right now, the best ways of doing this are with certain types of exercise and a diet that is specifically designed to help with the changes that come with ageing, along with supplements where necessary.

Chapters 5 and 6 go into more detail about how to do this and cover new findings about genes that suggest that they aren't necessarily our destiny. In the next chapter we look at why trying to keep your micro-factories in good shape by relying on drugs is unlikely to work, and how to keep drugs to a minimum as you get older.

Chapter 4

STAYING DRUG-FREE AS YOU AGE

Long ago, as teenagers, some of us baby boomers flaunted our use of illegal drugs as a badge of rebellion and cheerfully ignored warnings of the harm they could do. Now we are encouraged to take drugs – to bring down the likes of cholesterol and blood pressure – in far greater quantities than even we ever did as youngsters, and I (Jerome) for one find that I spend a lot of time advising people to 'just say no' to drugs unless your doctor says one is absolutely necessary Why? The chances you personally will benefit from taking a drug to stop you getting ill in the future are pretty small and the more drugs you take, the more your chances of damaging side effects go up.

It's not because I've got anything against altering your mind or body with chemicals, and there are obviously times when a prescription is just what you need – neither my wife nor my two daughters would be alive today without having had access to antibiotics, for example. It's just that, after spending more hours than is sensible monitoring the latest research on the risks and benefits of pharmaceuticals, it has become very clear to me that as a way of cutting your risk of chronic disease when you are healthy, they are remarkably ineffective and not very safe.

There is no shortage of evidence about these shortcomings, but unless you have a rather geeky and obsessive interest in monitoring them you may not know the details. However, I'm not alone in having serious reservations.

DIABETES DRUGS RAISE THE RISK OF HEART DISEASE

In summer 2011, just as the manuscript for this book was being delivered, the *British Medical Journal* ran an article by the dogged Australian medical journalist and lecturer at the University of Newcastle, Australia, Daniel Moynihan, which raised serious concerns about current prescribing of drugs for diabetes. He gives the example of treatments for type-2 diabetes: 'Heavily promoted drug strategies to aggressively reduce blood sugar in people who have diabetes have raised people's risks of heart disease and death rather than lowered them, despite evidence that lifestyle changes are cheap and effective.'[18]

Moynihan is also critical of the massive use of 'preventive' medicines, such as statins and blood pressure pills for those at lower risk of disease. 'A rational assessment reveals many people must be treated to prevent one adverse event,' he writes, 'so most users gain no direct benefit despite years of treatment.' It's a point we make later in this chapter.

Such carefully considered reservations rarely get the widespread publicity devoted to the latest breakthrough drug, however. An example of the way serious problems with a drug can simply be ignored occurred in 2009 with aspirin that was prescribed to cut your risk of heart disease, if you haven't had a heart attack – this is so-called primary care. You've probably heard this is a good idea; you may even be taking one daily.

THE PROBLEMS WITH ASPIRIN AS A PREVENTIVE MEASURE

What you are far less likely to have heard is that the British Heart Foundation no longer recommends taking preventative doses of aspirin, following a number of major analyses which found that the benefit you were likely to get was more or less the same as your risk of having serious internal bleeding – one of the well-known side effects of aspirin. In both cases, about 350–400 people had to be treated for one to benefit, or for one to be harmed. Not exactly the sort of odds you'd go for at the betting shop.

The first paper was a little hesitant, saying that 'aspirin is of uncertain net value as the reduction in occlusive events [i.e. blocked arteries]'.[19] The second didn't beat about the bush. Its title said it all: 'Don't use aspirin for primary prevention of cardiovascular disease'.[20] And the third was just as clear: 'Use of aspirin in primary prevention of cardiovascular disease … is not supported by the current evidence'.[21]

All this is fairly unambiguous, but not only was the British Heart Foundation's reversal of a long-standing recommendation announced in the equivalent of a whisper but it has barely had any effect on prescribing. Before those papers came out, prescribing of low-dose aspirin in England was around 32 million per year; the following year it was 31 million. So it's always worth asking your GP some tough questions before taking drugs for prevention.

THE DOWNSIDE OF DRUGS

Our parents' generation trusted the doctor. He (it was usually a he) told you what was wrong and what to do about it. If you were given pills you took them and you didn't complain. We're more sceptical of authority figures today and some of you will already be taking very active steps to look after your own health, which probably involves a sparing use of drugs. Even so, you may find some of the information below surprising.

DRUGS CAN DOUBLE YOUR RISK OF DYING

Usually when you get a prescription for a drug it's because there are guidelines saying that, based on the evidence, the best way to treat your condition is with this drug. As you get older you are likely to have more things going wrong which means more prescriptions. And that means more chance that the drugs may interact in dangerous ways. The risk of this was highlighted in a study published in 2011, which found that elderly people, in particular, had a significantly raised chance of dying if they were on two or more of a widely used type of drug known as 'anticholinergic'.

These drugs lower the amount of a stimulating chemical messenger, called acetylcholine. Because acetylcholine is used by the brain and nervous system, it is active all over the body.[22] It can be tricky to recognise if you are being given one of these drugs because they are found in a large number of both prescription and over-the-counter drugs – about 100 in all. They are used for a wide range of usually relatively mild conditions such as pain, insomnia, anxiety, depression, allergy, leaky bladder and gut cramps. They are also known to increase your risk of poorer brain function.

Treating an elderly person who suffers from the sort of complaints often linked with ageing, such as difficulty sleeping, aching joints and bladder problems, with drugs that significantly raise their risk of dying seems a scary option. Remarkably, the head of the Royal College of General Practitioners was quoted as saying that the study was a wake-up call. 'We have to start looking not just at the drugs we are prescribing but also how they work in combination with other drugs.'[23] It's astonishing and alarming that it's not done already!

Why should these drugs reduce your cognitive functioning? The clue comes from the fact that drugs, such as Aricept given to Alzheimer's patients to improve memory and thinking, work by *increasing* the amount of acetylcholine in the brain. You can see how multiple drug use multiplies problems. One small Romanian study of 105 people with Alzheimer's found that while most of them were taking acetylcholine-boosting drugs, as many as a third were also taking the anticholinergic drugs to bring it down.[24]

DRUGS STEAL YOUR VITAMINS

There is another even less well-recognised drawback to relying on regular drug use which is that many of those widely used on older people can seriously bring down your levels of various essential vitamins and minerals, creating a whole new set of side effects. It's a problem we first raised in Chapter 3.

The diabetes drug metformin, for example, brings down vitamin B_{12} (needed for effective DNA repair, among many other things), while the heartburn drugs known as proton pump inhibitors can reduce magnesium and make it harder to absorb B_{12}, iron and a wide variety of other essential nutrients.[25]

The problem can be reversed with supplements, but it may be difficult to persuade your doctor to do this, although you probably have the best chance with statins. For years it has been widely known that cholesterol-lowering statins also cut production of a very important antioxidant called CoQ_{10} (as we previously mentioned in Chapter 3). Among other things it's needed for proper functioning of your mitochondria – the power plants in each cell that work less well as we get older. If you are taking statins it would be well worth raising this with your doctor; you might point out that in Canada packets of statins have to carry a warning that they deplete CoQ_{10}. Drugs can also cause some of the problems that older people are more likely to suffer from anyway, such as a greater risk of falls or cognitive decline, which, once again, vitamins can help to reduce.

The jigsaw of drugs for the different parts of your body

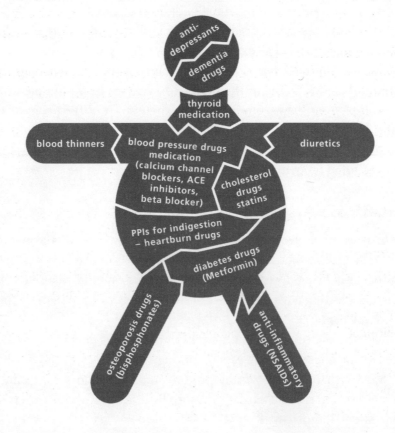

FIVE DRUG TYPES YOU SHOULD BE CAREFUL OF TAKING

You'll find below the risks with some frequently prescribed drugs that you may not have been warned about. Your doctor is likely to tell you that all drugs come with some risk and in the case of these drugs the judgement is that the benefits outweigh the risk. However, this information will enable you to have an informed discussion about what is right for you.

Proton pump inhibitors (PPI) Prescribed to reduce stomach-acid production.
Vitamin and mineral loss: all vitamins and minerals, but especially magnesium and vitamin B_{12}.
Symptoms of vitamin and mineral loss: magnesium – cognitive decline and muscle spasms; B_{12} – cognitive decline, irritable bowel, raised blood pressure, brittle nails and tiredness.
Recognised side effects: increased risk of pneumonia, osteoporosis and broken bones; and an increased chance of infection by superbug *Clostridium difficile* and kidney problems.
Additional information: PPIs are widely and unnecessarily prescribed to prevent gastric bleeding in hospital patents – over 700 people have to be treated for one person to benefit.[26]

Bisphosphonates Prescribed to treat osteoporosis and prevent bone loss.
Mineral loss: iron.
Recognised side effects: A range of side effects, including heartburn. PPIs (see above) are prescribed to deal with the heartburn, but they may seriously lower the drug's effectiveness.[27]
Additional information: 667 people need to be treated for one person to benefit. Although bisphosphonates are widely prescribed to people over 50, the trials done on these drugs have involved only a very small subset of people: younger women with osteoporosis.[28] (We discuss bisphosphonates further in Secret 2.)

NSAIDS (non-steroidal anti-inflammatory drugs such as aspirin) Widely used for pain and to lower inflammation.

Vitamin and mineral loss: vitamin C, folic acid and iron.

Symptoms of vitamin and mineral loss: depression, diarrhoea and mouth sores.

Recognised side effects: a raised risk of death from heart disease in patients with cardiovascular disease.[29] Aspirin seriously aggravates stomach and kidney problems in elderly patients.[30] PPIs are prescribed to deal with the side effects (see above). (For more on these drugs see Secret 8.)

Benzodiazepines Prescribed for insomnia and anxiety.

Mineral and vitamin reduction: folate, vitamins B_6, C and D.

Recognised side effects: poor balance after waking and a raised risk of falls and cognitive impairment.[31] (For more on sleeping pills see Secret 4.)

Anticholinergic drugs Included in many types of drugs, both over-the-counter and prescription, including: painkillers, sleeping pills, beta-blockers, antidepressants, and medication for allergies, leaky bladder and gastrointestinal cramps. These drugs block the nervous-system chemical acetylcholine.

Recognised side effects: increased risk of death when two or more taken together. The more you take the worse your cognitive functioning.[32] Also dry mouth, dizziness and blurred vision.

Additional information: Alzheimer's patients are prescribed drugs such as Aricept to boost their acetylcholine levels. It is very likely that many dementia patients will also be taking anticholinergic drugs at the same time.

And statins, see below.

DO THE BENEFITS ALWAYS OUTWEIGH THE RISKS?

As we've seen, striking the balance of benefit and risk for you personally can be tricky and it's particularly difficult in the case of statins, which are so widely prescribed to people over 50.

Official bodies recommend taking cholesterol-lowering statins to cut the risk of a heart attack, but if you haven't had an attack you might want to think twice about taking them. If you are discussing it with your doctor it would be useful to be aware of the findings of several recent large studies.

According to a recent report by the prestigious Cochrane Collaboration, statins have to be given to large numbers of people for just one person to benefit.[33] Around 1,000 healthy people who haven't had a heart attack but who do have some risk factors, such as being overweight or raised cholesterol, have to take statins for just one death from heart attack to be avoided.

There's strong disagreement over what your chances are of suffering adverse side effects from statins, but some clinicians say that they affect 10 per cent of patients. Accurate figures are hard to find, though, because many trials don't even report on the side effects,[34] and no one has any good data on the risk of potentially serious ones such as cognitive impairment or diabetes.[35]

Sometimes drugs can be prescribed to a large number of patients even though the evidence of benefit outweighing risk isn't there. One of the worst examples occurred with the heavy tranquillisers known as anti-psychotics, which were given to 200,000 elderly patients with Alzheimer's in England and Wales as a 'chemical cosh' for years, even though study after study had showed they were dangerous and ineffective.

Only after an official report in 2009 showed the drugs had been killing 1,800 patients a year[36] were prescriptions cut back.

SWALLOWING A SPIDER TO CATCH A FLY

Something else to consider when making a decision about prescription drugs is what might be called the swallowed-a-spider-to-catch-a-fly syndrome. You go on one drug to stop inflammation, but that causes headaches, so you are given another to stop the headache, but that puts your blood pressure up, and so on.

As with most drug-related problems, this is much more likely to happen the older you get. A good example is the prescription creep that begins with taking aspirin long term for something like arthritis. The drug is linked with the risk of developing an ulcer or damage to the lining of your stomach, so it's often given with a proton pump inhibitor (PPI), such as Omeprazole, to reduce acid production.

Handed out in vast quantities – 36 million prescriptions were written for PPIs in the UK in 2010 – these drugs are being linked with an increasing number of nasty side effects, as we saw on page 47. One of the most serious could turn out to be causing a vitamin B_{12} deficiency, because good levels of B_{12} may cut the risk of Alzheimer's (see Secret 1). Another is infection with the superbug *Clostridium difficile*, which affects thousands of older hospital patients every year.

Given these risks and drawbacks it makes sense to consider the other ways of treating arthritis covered in Secret 2. And while PPIs can bring short-term relief from heartburn from various other causes, there's a good chance you can reduce or eliminate the need for them by effectively identifying food allergies, improving your diet and/or supplementing inexpensive and safe digestive enzymes and probiotics. (For more details about this see Secret 8.)

SIDE EFFECTS ARE IMPORTANT TO YOU, BUT NOT SO MUCH TO MANY DOCTORS

When discussing whether certain drugs are right for you it's worth being aware that research has found that the way you think about risks and benefits may not match up to the way your doctor does.

'In practice doctors don't say much about adverse effects and concentrate on the benefits,' says Dr Dee Mangin, Director of Primary Care Research at Christchurch School of Medicine in New Zealand. 'What's more, patients regularly say that when they complain about side effects such as nausea and dizziness, doctors often say it's unlikely the drug was responsible.'

What Dr Mangin has found is that, not surprisingly, patients are more worried about side effects than their doctor. Side effects for the patient are personal, and when they are told clearly what the risks of a drug are, many don't want to take it, whatever the benefits.

She asked 350 older patients what made them decide to take a drug. Was it the amount of benefit that was important, or the chance of suffering unpleasant side effects? It turned out that the patients' priorities were the exact reverse of those of most doctors, whose natural tendencies are to play up the benefits.

Initially, nearly all the patients said they would take a statin whether one in ten benefited or just three people in a hundred. What did have a big impact on their decision, though, were the chances of suffering side effects. When told the statin would also cause mild fatigue, nausea or fuzzy thinking, over 50 per cent said they wouldn't take it, and if they were then told the side effects could prevent normal functioning, only 3 per cent said they would take it.[37] So, for patients, the benefit of taking a statin isn't as important as avoiding the side effects that come with it. The tendency to gloss over side effects by doctors, however, means that it is much more likely you will end up with an impressive range of pill boxes – and that is unlikely to be good for you.

'Following official guidelines which results in multiple drug taking (polypharmacy)', writes Dr Mangin, 'is probably one of the greatest but most invisible threats to health in the ageing population.'

WHEN DRUG SIDE EFFECTS LOOK LIKE AGEING

Once you start looking at drugs' side effects, a pattern emerges that will become increasingly important the older you get and the more drugs you take. Many of them cause side effects that are exactly the same as the problems that come with getting older anyway, such as falls, mental fogginess, joint pains and insomnia, as mentioned in our list of the drugs you should be careful about taking on page 47.

As we have seen, if you complain about a particular side effect you may be told that 'the benefits outweigh the risks' as if this were a precise scientific calculation. Doctors can say this because the drugs will have gone through several 'randomised controlled trials' and been tested against a placebo. But do these trials really tell you if a particular drug is going to benefit you, or even people like you? This is a question that becomes increasingly more important as you grow older.

Clinical trials are designed to treat a single condition, such as high cholesterol or blood pressure. That means they don't include people who already have a couple of other disorders, let alone those who are also swallowing a dozen other drugs at the same time.[38]

CLINICAL TRIALS THAT ARE OUT OF THIS WORLD

In fact, these trials are highly artificial situations and research is discovering that the risk–benefit ratio they claim – and this is the one your doctor relies on – are far more optimistic than actual results in the real world. This is because they usually involve much younger people (because they are less likely to have other illnesses), who have been given the correct diagnosis and who are carefully monitored to make sure they take the drugs. Compliance in most trials is around 90 per cent.

Things aren't at all like that in GPs' surgeries, hospitals and care homes where the drugs are actually used. What this shows is that it's well worthwhile getting as much information as you can from your doctor about just how much benefit you can expect from a drug and what the risks are. And the more drugs you are taking the more important this is, because of the way that they interact. In your forties and fifties you are unlikely to be taking more than one or two but, as we've seen, that number is very likely to rise the older you get.

So, just how relevant are those clinical trials to a new drug being offered to you? It was tested on people who weren't taking anything else, but you could be on six other drugs, which you are less likely to be so conscientious about taking – your compliance would probably be about 50 per cent.

The drug was initially tested on people whose system for handling toxins and absorbing nutrients was working pretty well; an older person's system, however, is becoming less efficient, which makes him or her more likely to suffer side effects. How does this new drug interact with those already being taken? No one knows for sure. So, just how good is the evidence that you are getting a treatment where the benefits outweigh the risks, especially when you are taking several drugs? That's hard to say too.

According to research published in the *British Medical Journal* in 2011 a drug that looked worthwhile based on trial results was five times less effective when it was being handed out in GPs' surgeries to real people than when it had be trialled.[39]

In the snakes-and-ladders illustration overleaf you can see just how easy it is to worsen your health the more drugs you take, but you can equally easily improve your health when you choose a nutrition-based solution.

FIND A DOCTOR WHO IS ON YOUR SIDE

It's quite likely that you've found some of this information about drugs alarming, after all we all want to believe that the drugs we are getting, especially when we are essentially healthy, are always safe and effective. The idea is not to scare you but to allow you to make more informed choices. Your doctor is a valuable resource with a huge amount of knowledge but if you are going to have a sensible discussion about the best way to stay healthy as you age it's worth being as well informed as possible. You also need a doctor who is interested in what you are doing and doesn't just dismiss it out of hand.

When my (Patrick's) father-in-law, healthy at 76, was asked by his doctor, 'What drugs are you on?' he replied, 'None, I just take a bunch of nutritional and herbal supplements and have acupuncture.' The doctor replied, 'You're in better nick than I am. What are you taking?' That's the kind of doctor you want.

You may have a doctor who tells you that you can't slow down ageing, that supplements are largely a waste of time and that you can get all the nutrients you need from a healthy balanced diet. We don't believe that this is true especially not as you are getting older. The last part of this chapter sets out a quite different view. It may not change his or her mind but it could form the basis for a stimulating discussion!

WHY REPLACING NUTRIENTS MAKES SENSE

An easy and effective first move to ensure you, and anyone older you are caring for, have a good chance of ageing well is to check your levels

Pharmaceutical snakes and nutritional ladders

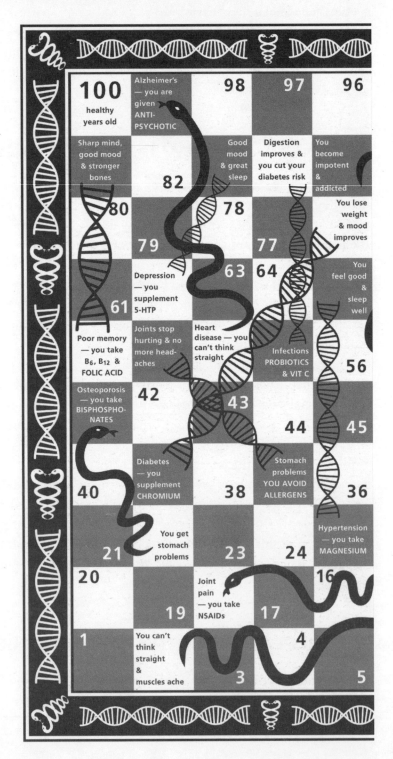

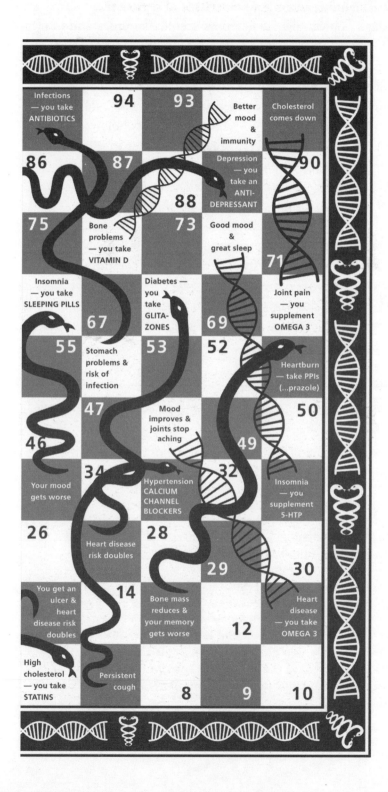

of minerals, vitamins and other nutrients, and replace them if they are low. Although you can debate just how useful vitamins are in healthy people, there is no serious disagreement that you are likely to become deficient in some of them as you get older.

A recent paper found a clear link between vitamin D deficiency and the development of cognitive problems that come with Alzheimer's. A study of 850 people aged over 65 whose health was followed for eight years found that those who were severely deficient in vitamin D, as many people are, were 60 per cent more likely to suffer with serious general cognitive decline than those who had healthy levels.[40]

Another common problem in older people, osteoporosis, can be significantly helped by a much less familiar vitamin – K2. It's been found to play a vital role in bone formation, but most people don't get enough from their diet. In one study, a supplement completely reversed bone loss in people with osteoporosis and even increased bone mass in some of them.[41] K2 supplements reduced fractures by between 60 and 80 per cent in an analysis of several trials.[42] (We discuss osteoporosis further in Secret 2.)

DISCUSSING DRUGS AND VITAMINS WITH THE DOCTOR

It can be very difficult talking about vitamins and supplements with your doctor. Suppose you suspect that you would do better without certain drugs – perhaps the anticholinergic ones mentioned above – and would like to supplement with some vitamins, perhaps CoQ_{10} because you are on statins, and B vitamins because you are taking PPIs? How do you go about raising that without infuriating the doctor?

'You need to ask for a medicines review,' says Nina Barnet, a pharmacist with the Royal Pharmaceutical Society. 'Sometimes patients can be put on repeat prescriptions that no one checks are still necessary.' If you are lucky you'll be able to establish a relationship with your doctor that encourages that kind of discussion. 'Ideally you can both work out if each drug is really what [you need],' says Barnet, 'but some doctors can still be very paternalistic.' This approach particularly applies if you are

CONTINUED...

trying to support an elderly parent who's on a number of drugs and suffering from a range of symptoms. Repeat prescriptions that haven't been checked can be even more of a problem then, but you need to tread carefully. If you go in too aggressively and your parent comes from a generation that believes doctor knows best, he or she may find it uncomfortable and you may offend the doctor. 'It needs to be done in a very respectful way,' says Barnet, 'and if your [parent] says [he/she] doesn't want to question the doctor, then you mustn't try to force the issue.'

FIVE SUPPLEMENTS WORTH TAKING AS YOU GET OLDER

Always make sure you are getting a good supply of nutrients from your food, whatever your age, but as you start moving into your sixties and beyond your levels of various minerals and vitamins can start declining. A deficiency of vitamins and minerals at any age is not good for health, and achieving sufficient from your diet may be harder as you get older, because we become less efficient at absorbing them from food. Studies regularly find that after about 65, the older you become the more likely you are to be deficient in the vital nutrients listed below.

(If you are worried about particular conditions, Part Two will tell you about the micronutrients you could benefit from supplementing.)

VITAMIN D

This is the only supplement that is officially recommended for older people.[43] Having a low level is linked with an increased risk of cognitive decline when you're over 65,[44] as well as a raised risk of diabetes and a pre-diabetic state known as metabolic syndrome.[45] A deficiency in vitamin D has also been linked with autoimmune diseases, such as rheumatoid arthritis, lupus and inflammatory bowel disease, as well as lower back pain, joint problems and cancer.

In 2011 a large analysis of 50 trials found that taking a vitamin D supplement for two years cut mortality in older women by 6 per cent.[46]

That's a small effect: 200 people would have to take it for one person to benefit, but it's still a larger effect than achieved by some preventative drugs. Side effects included raised levels of calcium, which is probably beneficial.

Supplementing vitamin D, along with taking exercise, cuts the chances of damaging your bones caused by falling,[47] but, as we've seen, some drugs regularly given to the over 65s increase the risk of both falls and cognitive decline. It's important to get your vitamin D status tested whatever your age, and if you are below 70nmol/ml you either need more sun, or three or four servings of oily fish a week or a supplement.

So how much should you take? The conservative view is about 20mcg a day for people over 70 but, increasingly, some experts are saying that 100 or even 200mcg are linked with a lower risk of various killer diseases such as heart disease and cancer. It's worth having your vitamin D level checked, because people vary hugely in how much they absorb from a supplement.

ZINC

Too little zinc is not good at any age, but as you get older it is worth being aware that being deficient becomes more likely. A study of 600 people in nursing homes found that those with a healthy amount in their blood were half as likely to develop pneumonia, and that they needed fewer antibiotic prescriptions and lived longer.[48] Correcting a deficiency in zinc has a clear benefit.

VITAMIN E

Over 600 people in care homes getting 200iu daily for three years in a controlled trial were 20 per cent less likely to suffer with upper respiratory tract infections than those on a placebo.[49] Healthy levels have been linked with a lower incidence of cancer.[50]

MAGNESIUM

The mineral magnesium is vital for a number of body systems, and a serious deficiency makes various ageing problems more likely, such as diabetes and cognitive decline, as well as muscle spasm, irregular heartbeat and convulsions. One survey has found that 81 per cent of elderly Americans are deficient[51] and levels in the UK are likely to be similar. The study also connected a deficiency to allergies, hypertension and osteoporosis.

B VITAMINS

This family of eight distinct vitamins, including niacin (vitamin B_3), B_6 and B_{12}, helps enzymes to do their job and is vital for healthy skin, muscle and the nervous system. The B vitamins are essential for maintaining healthy levels of the amino acid called homocysteine, which we met briefly in Chapter 2. High levels of homocysteine have been linked with a raised risk of age-related cognitive decline, but lowering homocysteine slows the decline.[52] Older people often have low levels of B_{12}, because they make less of a protein in the stomach that is produced along with stomach acid. There is now research to show that two in five people aged over 60 have insufficient B_{12} to stop brain shrinkage.[53] (The research hasn't been done on younger people.)

Acid-lowering PPI drugs can reduce absorption rates of B_{12} as can the diabetes drug metformin.

PROTECTING YOUR BOWEL AND BLADDER

Another way to ensure you can remain drug-free is to pamper your guts by nurturing the good bacteria that live there. Many people, especially as they get older, could benefit from taking probiotics – the 'friendly' bacteria that live in the gut and which are vital for all kinds of healthy functions, including how well we absorb nutrients, the working of our immune system and how effectively we break down drugs. They are particularly worth considering if you, or an older person you are caring for, has to go into hospital.

While in hospital, many people, especially older ones, are routinely put on antibiotics. Unfortunately, these can make diarrhoea more likely and you are also more vulnerable to superbug infections in the hospital. Taking probiotics cuts the diarrhoea risk from 17 to 5 per cent and the risk of *Clostridium difficile* infection from 17 per cent to zero.[54]

What is more, 70 per cent of long-stay hospital patients are regularly given laxatives, but in one trial, probiotics cut the number who needed them by two-thirds.[55] Probiotics can also help to boost the immune system.[56]

Antibiotics are also commonly used to treat urinary tract infections like cystitis, but as their side effects include killing off beneficial bacteria as well, they often cause a vaginal yeast infection. A side-effect-free alternative is the active ingredient in cranberry juice, a sugar called D-mannose. Because we can't digest it, about 90 per cent of it comes out in the urine within 30–60 minutes, which is why it can clear out the *E. coli* that resides in the urinary tract and which can be a cause of cystitis.

The *E. coli* bug sticks to the urinary tract by attaching itself to receptors on the walls that just happen to contain D-mannose. So, when the tract becomes filled with D-mannose molecules, the bugs latch on to them too and are pulled off the wall as your pee goes swirling past. No proper trials exist, but you'll know quickly if it's working (see Resources).

In Part Two there's a lot more detail about how a nutritional approach can help cut the risk of many more of the problems that come with ageing, such as creaking joints, poor blood sugar control and inflamed arteries.

FOOD AND NUTRITIONAL CHOICES WHEN IN HOSPITAL

There are a number of relatively straightforward things you can do about your food and nutritional choices that can make a big difference if you need to go into hospital even if you've never been very interested in 'healthy living' before. And they are also worth considering if you are caring for an elderly parent who has to go into hospital.

Being well fed means that you will recover more quickly from an operation and be less likely to develop infections. Rather shockingly, however, about 30 per cent of people who go into hospital are already at risk of malnutrition, but not enough is done either in the hospitals or out in the community to spot the problem and deal with it. And yet checking for malnutrition couldn't be easier. A three-point questionnaire, known as MUST, has recently been developed by the professional body responsible for medical nutrition, BAPEN (British Association of Parental and Enteral Nutrition), which campaigns to have malnutrition taken seriously. MUST is a simple and effective way of saving lives. 'If everybody coming into hospital was checked for malnutrition and then treated, that could save as many as 10,000 lives a year,' says Dr Mike Stroud, consultant gastroenterologist and chairman of BAPEN.[57] The test has been approved by NICE (the National Institute for Health and Clinical Excellence), which recommended that all hospitals use it.

So what can you do about this? Supplements have a role here. Patients will be lucky to receive even a calorie-dense supplement with only the most basic nutrients, yet there is evidence that nutritional supplements can produce dramatic results. Research has found that they improve your recovery from a stroke, if you are deficient,[58] and that giving an immune-boosting supplement to patients having surgery for gastric cancer can cut their chances of having infections afterwards by a quarter.[59] In fact, recovering from operations and serious disorders in general can be helped by careful attention to micronutrients at the beginning of treatment.[60]

THE IMPORTANCE OF PROTEIN

You might also want to check that while in hospital you (or your parent) are eating enough protein. Official figures in both the US and the UK suggest that about a third of patients over 65 eat a diet that is both calorie and protein deficient, but improving their diet or giving them the amino acids needed to make protein could protect their bones. American researchers put mice on a low-protein diet, which should have made their bones weaker, but they also gave the mice an amino acid supplement and found that their bones stayed strong. The team suggest giving an amino acid supplement to all hospitalised patients who might be deficient. See more on this in Secret 2.

CONSUMER CHOICE

As we said at the beginning of the book, how you choose to age is really a lifestyle consumer choice. Relying on the drug approach to do it is like trying to weed and prune your garden using chain saws and a turbo-driven plough. We are recommending more of an organic approach that encourages the body's own recovery and repair systems to do the work.

Using diet, lifestyle choices and supplements is not an exact science, but you are unlikely to do much harm to your body as you work out what's best for you. And the very process of working on it, rather than relying on increasing numbers of drugs, means that you will become familiar with what your body responds to and discover what works and what doesn't.

In the next chapter we look at some radical ideas for sprucing up the 'micro-factories' in your cells and the ways that diet and lifestyle can begin to tackle the underlying changes that are going on with ageing.

Chapter 5

THE LATEST TOOLS FOR TURNING BACK YOUR BIOLOGICAL CLOCK

The baby boomers' Silver Tsunami means that everyone is faced with an unprecedented problem: how to keep so many elderly people healthy. The conventional way of dealing with a medical crisis – which is to spend money developing new drugs – doesn't look like a very promising solution, as the previous chapter illustrated. So, what is the way forward when drugs get the bulk of research money and non-drug approaches, however promising, are not readily funded?

As we approach our fifties and sixties, we are all aware that the clock is ticking, and, even if vast sums magically became available tomorrow to run big trials of all the variations in anti-ageing lifestyles, you'd still have a long wait before the results were in, and even then they almost certainly wouldn't be definitive.

Once you start becoming aware that you are ageing, though, and you realise it doesn't have to all be downhill, you want to get started right away. In this chapter we look at some of the new research that *is* being undertaken and look further into other ways that may help us to live a healthier old age – and what we can start doing *now*. You will see that there are some interesting ideas being studied in these few small trials, although some are perhaps rather extreme! As we'll explain later in the chapter some of these new developments can be incorporated into the tried-and-tested lifestyle and diet choices that I (Patrick) have recommended over the years to improve health and well-being to make them even more appropriate for our bodies as we age.

CAN DRUG RESEARCH PROVIDE THE ANSWERS?

Let's take just one example of a health issue that is directly relevant to ageing: weight loss. Despite a growing obesity crisis and billions of dollars spent on research, what is on offer from the mainstream for someone who's on the overweight/obese border? There are effectively two options: pills (actually, only one type of pill, since two brands have been withdrawn in recent years because of their dangerous side effects) and the low-fat diet. The one remaining pill works by speeding fat – healthy and unhealthy alike – through your guts, taking the fat-soluble vitamins with it; all for the sake of losing about 5kg (11lb) in a year. Weight that comes off while following a low-fat diet is very likely to come back on again.

Even so, experts assume that the new focus on ageing will turn it into a medical speciality. In his recent book on ageing[61] Professor Wolpert asked a senior geneticist who specialises in ageing how she thought the field would develop. 'It will probably be introduced with some medical speciality like endocrinology, cardiology or neurology,' she said. 'Pharmaceutical companies will make the connection – drugs will be the way in.' That's probably a realistic assessment, but if that does happen, there is a good chance that research into the kind of DIY approach we are advocating here will be even more starved of funds and side-lined. We believe the effect on your long-term health could be disastrous and it would massively increase NHS costs.

AGEING WELL – A NEW LIFE SKILL

What about if we considered ageing as just the reverse of growing up? Like ageing, growing up is something we do naturally, but there are all kinds of systems that try, albeit not always successfully, to ensure that it goes well. There are many theories, as well as advice and help about the best way to bring up children, but randomised controlled trials are rare. The reason why is because not only would such trials be almost impossible to set up but parenting is not the kind of activity that is appropriate to test in that way. You can do studies to try to decide between alternatives, but you can never trial the whole package. Ageing is much the same. Like parenting, you are not interested in it until it hits you, but when it hits you it's fascinating and you want to know more. Both need medical help at times, but more important are the everyday things that you have to do.

This chapter aims to give you an overview of some of the 'new tools' for ageing thrown up by the latest research that you might want to consider for your own package. Much of it concentrates on what's going on in your cells and the key players we introduced in Chapter 3.

Remember the Healthy Ageing Pyramid on page 15? We explained how you start off with basic changes to your diet plus exercise and then build up and refine your personal healthy-ageing package according to your needs or personal inclination. In the same way that some people like gardening whereas others like running ultra-marathons, so people pursue healthy ageing with a greater or lesser intensity. At the base is the need to have the best nutrition, and avoid anti-nutrients as much as possible, and to keep fit. But some people – the 'ultra-anti-agers' – will be aiming to push the boundaries with combinations of power exercises, specialised food choices and lots more nutritional and hormone supplements a day.

THE MAGIC OF CALORIE CUTTING

There is one sure-fire way to live longer and to become much healthier in the process. It's a method supported by hundreds of trials involving animals, and scientists have known about it for over 70 years. It's the calorie restricted (CR) diet, which simply involves eating no more than 1,200–1,500 calories a day.

Many diets work by cutting calories, and you will certainly lose weight if you go on one of them. But these are not CR. Calorie-counting diets last for only a few weeks or months at the most, and they nearly always come up against the problem that your body's metabolism slows down to compensate. Once you stop the diet, the pounds pile rapidly back on. If you are a 'CRONie', however – someone who is serious about CR – you are doing it for life.

Animals live for 50 per cent longer than usual when put on an equivalent CR diet, during which time any of the players inside their cells that may have been failing – such as mitochondria, protein production and telomeres – function better. On top of that, there is also improvement in the various markers of how well your metabolism is working – blood pressure, blood sugar, weight, and so on.

The only drawback to this magical transformation is that it's almost impossible for us humans to follow. You have to be a fanatic, ready to put up with feeling cold because you are not taking in many calories, and prepared for feeling hungry most of the time. And even then it's not absolutely certain that you will actually live any longer, because we don't have a group of people who have been doing this for long enough to find out; although, recently, a long-running study found that primates benefited substantially from the diet, making it even more likely that humans would too.

GAIN WITHOUT THE PAIN – CALORIE 'MIMETICS'

Even so, CR has been the driver for a lot of anti-ageing research aimed at finding compounds made by the body or by plants that have a similar effect. Known as CR mimetics, they promise similar gains without the pain. The best-known CR mimetic is resveratrol. This antioxidant, famously found in grape skins – and so proposed as an explanation for the health benefits of wine – is believed to increase animals' life spans, and is also anti-inflammatory and lowers their blood sugar.

Other CR mimetics include carnosine (an antioxidant made in the body, especially in the muscles), L-carnitine, which carries fat into mitochondria, and two other antioxidants: lipoic acid, and CoQ_{10} (see Chapter 4). Some ultra-anti-agers take supplements of some or all of these. Although the logic is good, and the supplements benefit animals, there are no large clinical trials to support their use. We consider them to be optional extras. Drug companies are heavily investing in finding patentable versions of them, however.

There may be another way to get the remarkable benefits of CR with little of the pain, however, but its main benefits are in turning off genes for certain illnesses, such as diabetes, and turning genes on for good health. It's known as the Alternate Day Diet and we will be covering it in the next chapter. Exercise is the only other lifestyle change that has nearly as wide-ranging an effect as CR. It can also turn genes on and off, tune up mitochondria and spruce up your metabolism. The nutrition and exercise approach has a wide range of tools that, in combination, can make a difference to how well you deal with ageing. It's 'systems based', attempting to tune up your biology in the way that an organic farmer improves the soil, recycles and rotates crops so that plants can grow in as healthy a way as possible. Pharmaceuticals follow the agrichemical approach that knocks out weeds and bugs with pesticides, boosts growth with chemical fertilisers and directly manipulates plants' genes. So what are some of the ways that you can tune up those key players in your bio-factories?

MITOCHONDRIA – BOOSTING ENERGY OUTPUT

The power plants in our cells, called mitochondria, become less efficient as we get older: at age 90 they can be 90 per cent less productive than when we were children. Poor mitochondrial performance has been linked to chronic conditions such as congestive heart failure, muscle weakness, fatigue and neurological disease. So healthy ageing involves getting them up and running again. Efficient mitochondria have been linked to living longer, certainly in animals.[62]

Even though mitochondria are pretty unfamiliar (until very recently doctors generally only encountered them in rare genetic diseases), they are emerging as crucial to ageing well. Interestingly, they have been found to be responsive to something as mundane as beetroot; recently researchers found that beetroot can boost mitochondrial function – but so too could a compound known as PQQ (pyrroloquinoline quinone), found in most plants. PQQ is similar to the B vitamins – it has a range of beneficial effects, which are still being uncovered, including acting as an antioxidant and being needed for cell signalling, although with antioxidant properties. What's creating the buzz is that it can stimulate the body to make new mitochondria.[63]

The benefit from beetroot comes from the kind of nitrate it contains (also found in smaller amounts in lettuce and spinach) which the body converts to nitric oxide – well known for its role in relaxing blood vessels. Recent research found that when healthy volunteers ate the equivalent of 200–300g of beetroot a day (a hefty serving), their mitochondria worked much more efficiently, producing more of the energy-carrying molecule ATP, and using up less oxygen.[64]

Other compounds that have been reported to give mitochondria a boost are some of the low-calorie mimetics mentioned above, such as resveratrol, carnosine and L-carnitine, which help the cell to handle those oxidant exhaust fumes within mitochondria that are released every time we make energy.

WILL BEETROOT HELP US TO AGE WELL?

The question that keeps coming up in this whole area is: what can we do with this information? The results come from small studies usually run in test tubes or on animals. You may remember Dr Lippman, discussed in the Introduction – an ultra-anti-ager who takes large quantities of minerals, vitamins, supplements and hormones. Dr Lippman, and others like him, seize on these small studies magpie-like and try them out. It's obviously not an evidence-based scientific approach though.

But no one is going to run big trials on cheap unpatentable compounds like beetroot. The hundreds of millions paid for a company researching resveratrol (see Chapter 6) is an exception – so nearly all are doomed to the limbo of 'promising but unproven'. So, who *is* benefiting? One reason given for warning people off using these compounds that don't have clear evidence for their effectiveness or safety in humans is that they might be dangerous. But the greater risks involved when drugs tested in clinical trials involving a few thousand are licensed and then made available to millions are thought to be acceptable.

What if you could get a bit of benefit from resveratrol, a little more by adding carnosine and more from beetroot? With our final months flying off the calendar we want a far more sophisticated way of finding an answer.

TELOMERES: WINDING BACK THE CLOCK OF AGEING

You may remember that in Chapter 3 we described telomeres as the protective 'caps' at the tips of chromosomes and explained that they have recently received a lot of attention as a possible way to slow down ageing and as a marker for good health. As we age, telomeres gradually get shorter and shorter, so by the time we are middle-aged some telomeres are no longer fully protecting the chromosomes, so errors start to creep in when the cells divide. In the same way that the printouts from a bad photocopier become more smudged, so poor cell division creates more of the errors that show up as signs of ageing.

Already some of the ultra-anti-agers have seized on the idea of increasing life span by focusing on ways to lengthen the telomeres, even though no one knows yet whether it's possible in humans or what the effects would be. Depending on your point of view, that's either irresponsible and foolish or a brave pioneering leap of faith – something we admire in other fields.

There's now a test, taken using a few cells swabbed from the inside of your cheek, that reveals how long your telomeres are compared with those of other people of a similar age. People with longer telomeres do show up as being healthier. A study of 780 people with heart disease, found that those with the shortest telomeres had twice the risk of early death and heart failure after four and a half years than those with the longest.[65]

So the test could be a simple marker of how healthy you are, much like our own **bioage check** (see Chapter 2). Certainly, healthy habits, such as exercise and having good levels of omega-3 and vitamin D[66] are linked with longer telomeres, whereas shorter versions are found in people who are in situations that are generally considered to be unhealthy, such as being under a lot of pressure, or having had childhood trauma or those who suffer with prolonged depression. Such findings, though, don't prove that trying to lengthen telomeres will actually make you healthier.

That's why Professor Dean Ornish, a diet guru at the University of California, San Francisco, is testing the idea that slowing down telomere shortening could actually make you healthier. He is giving a group of stressed men suffering from early prostate cancer a vegetarian regime that includes a low-fat diet, plus regular exercise and activities such as yoga. The results may be out by the time this book is published.

TURNING ELDERLY MICE YOUNG AGAIN

Knowing the length of your telomeres could predict how well you will respond to a drug. Research in Scotland found that people with high cholesterol have half the risk of a heart attack if they have longer telomeres. When a group being treated with cholesterol-lowering statins had their telomere length tested at the beginning and end of the trial, those with the shortest telomeres had the greatest benefit.[67] This is perhaps one way of targeting the drugs more effectively, rather than handing them out on such a large scale to many who, research suggests, won't benefit.

The aim of scientists in this field, however, is not just to slow the rate at which telomeres are unwinding but to actually make them longer again. We all have an enzyme in our bodies called telomerase that will do this, but nearly all of it is found in stem cells – the ones that can make other cells and so have to be able to keep dividing. Consequently, there was great excitement at the end of 2010 when scientists at the Dana-Farber Cancer Institute in Boston revealed that treating the telomeres in ageing mice with telomerase seemed to rewind their ageing clock.[68]

Not only that, but there was also a dramatic reversal in the signs and symptoms of ageing in the mice. Their brains, which had been shrinking, started growing, their coat hair developed a youthful healthy sheen and they became fertile again.

THE CANCER CONNECTION

Unfortunately, there is a catch. The other type of cell that produces telomerase is a tumour. Telomerase is what allows them to grow indefinitely. Like the magic potion in fairy stories, telomerase has its dark side. Now, of course, that is a worry – especially if you are an ultra-anti-ager seeking telomere growth – and no one knows how big the risk is.

It would seem a strong possibility that a drug version of telomerase might have such a side effect, but we already know many basic things that slow down telomere shortening, such as exercise, diet, yoga, vitamin D – and it's far less likely that they will cause cancer. In fact, probably the opposite.

A PROGRAMME TO REWIND YOUR TELOMERES

None of these potential problems have dissuaded American telomere enthusiasts. The authors of a book optimistically entitled *The Immortality Edge* claim that telomere maintenance 'will allow you to extend life span to 120 or more while leading an active robust and independent lifestyle'.[69]

It's an approach that combines exercise with heavyweight supplement intake: 20 minutes of high-intensity aerobics (90 seconds flat out followed by a slow 90 seconds to recover) plus 16 or 17 pills a day. The supplements on the regime include 6g of omega-3 fish oil, some of the mimetics (such as acetyl-L-carnitine) plus high-dose multivitamins, especially magnesium, potassium, vitamins C, D and E, and green tea and broccoli extracts. It would certainly make you healthier; no one knows what effect it would have on your telomeres, though.

For those with deep pockets, there is currently the option of an extract of the Chinese medical herb astralagus, known as TA65, which can boost your production of telomerase. Yours for $8,000 a year! Those taking it claim more energy and improved skin elasticity.

MINERALS AND VITAMINS – CELLS CAN'T WORK WITHOUT THEM

You may remember at the beginning of Chapter 3 we compared a cell to a factory, complete with power plants, garbage disposal and the rest. What many factories also need to function efficiently are templates, patterns or recipes for whatever they are producing. DNA supplies the templates for cells, but to make them available to the production line involves a vital process called methylation. It's the conductor of your body's chemical orchestra, and for it to work well you need a good supply of B vitamins.

You're probably not surprised by now to learn that as you get older methylation gradually becomes less efficient, and as a result you feel tired, slow and disconnected, as if your get up and go had got up and gone. To make matters worse, at the same time, your guts are becoming less effective at extracting B vitamins from your diet and so cell processes slow down even more.

CONDUCTING THE CELL'S ORCHESTRA

If everything is working well you'll rapidly convert toxic homocysteine into mood-boosting SAMe, a highly effective antidepressant, supplements of which are sold over the counter in the US but are only available on prescription in the UK. Homocysteine is just a stage on a biochemical production line – methionine from food becomes homocysteine, which should then be turned into several other compounds that are needed in the brain, among other places. Too much homocysteine suggests the production line isn't working so well.

To convert homocysteine into SAMe requires three particular B vitamins – B_6, B_{12} and folate – and also zinc and an amino acid called TMG (tri-methyl-glycine). So, making sure you're getting all of these is one of the most effective things you can do to make sure DNA damage is repaired so that your risk of chronic diseases such as Alzheimer's, stroke, and probably heart disease, will be reduced. As we've explained earlier, one of the best health checks you can do is to test the level of homocysteine in your blood (see Chapter 2).

A recent study in the *British Medical Journal* found that, among older people, their level of homocysteine was a much more accurate way of predicting if they were going to die from heart disease than more familiar markers such as blood pressure or cholesterol, EEG diagnosis and smoking.[70] It only showed that high homocysteine was a marker for cardiovascular death, though, not that it caused it.

The big breakthrough in showing that lowering homocysteine could actually lead to a dramatic improvement in your health came in a ground-breaking study carried out at Oxford University in 2010. The research found that it was possible to slow or even stop the brain shrinkage that comes with a kind of forgetfulness and increasing vagueness that's known as mild cognitive impairment by giving very high doses of B vitamins to patients with high homocysteine levels.[71] In 2011, the same team published more results showing that the patient's worsening memory also stopped declining.[72] The details are covered in Secret 1.

Methylation shows just how responsive our genes are to nutrition and a range of other events as well as influences from the outside world.

This idea is an important part of the new thinking about ageing, and we'll come back to it in the next chapter.

VITAMIN BENEFITS: THE EVIDENCE KEEPS MOUNTING

The Oxford homocysteine study, along with the growing evidence for a higher recommended daily allowance (RDA) for vitamin D, makes it harder to claim that you can get all the vitamins and minerals you need from diet, although the large amounts being taken by those keen to extend the length of their telomeres will need a lot more research before it is widely accepted.

In light of this, it is worth coming back to Professor Bruce Ames, Professor of Biochemistry and Molecular Biology at the University of California, Berkeley, whose 'triage' theory of vitamin deficiency was introduced in Chapter 3. This is the idea that when there is a nutrient shortage the body first directs supplies to the most vital functions, leaving others to manage as best they can.

The importance of this is that a deficiency can go unnoticed for a long time because it may take years for symptoms to emerge. In one study, for example, he looked at vitamin K (its importance in making bones was mentioned in Chapter 4 but it is also needed for blood to clot properly). Ames found that losing clotting ability was fatal, but not having enough to make bones was less of a problem in the short term, although in the long term it was linked with osteoporosis.[73] The same pattern has recently shown up with the mineral selenium, which has a role in building heart muscle and healthy sperm, among other important functions. Animal studies found that proteins involved in less essential tasks become less active when selenium is low.[74] The results of this kind of research have prompted Professor Ames to recommend that the RDA for selenium should be increased from 55 to 75mcg a day. This is consistent with the UK government's 'reference nutrient intake' of 75mcg; however, the amount people are actually getting in the UK, according to official figures, is around 50mcg. So, can you get all you need from a healthy balanced diet? Not according to the UK government's nutrition experts. We'd recommend you to supplement it. The richest source of selenium, by the way, is seafood.

Professor Ames's research team has also shown that giving supplements can reverse some of the problems that long-term deficiencies have created. He's restored failing mitochondria, the energy units, in elderly rats by feeding them with that anti-ageing favourite, acetyl carnitine, together with lipoic acid – an antioxidant and another essential part of the mitochondrial system. The old rats rapidly became a lot sprightlier and their scores on mental tests improved.[75] Giving the same combination to humans improved their hypertension.[76] Studies haven't yet been done to show the effects on human mitochondria.

Older and elderly people are very commonly found to have low levels of vitamins and minerals, and there are studies showing that giving supplements leads to a number of improvements, as you'll discover in Part Two. Given the enthusiasm for filling elderly patients with a dozen drugs or more, checking their nutritional status and correcting deficiencies seems a sensible thing to do first.

STOP SUGAR AGEING YOU

When people who have diabetes check their blood, they measure something called HbA1c, or glycosylated haemoglobin, which tells them the percentage of their blood cells (which are made of protein) that have become sugar-coated. This process, known as being 'glycosylated', damages cells, and it doesn't only affect people who have diabetes. It can affect all of us and is fundamental to all ageing. The lower your glycosylation level the better your body will be ageing.

The more glucose there is in your bloodstream, which is likely if you eat a lot of sugar and refined carbs, the more opportunities there are for glycosylation to take place. It is actually a rogue version of one of the essential processes – known as glycation – that goes on in the protein-manufacturing module of your micro-factories (the ribosome) where the added sugar gives strength and stability to the protein.

Sugar-coated proteins turn up throughout the body and are like handcuffs that stop a cell from working properly. They are known as advanced glycation end-products, or AGEs for short. The fewer you have, the longer you will live; the more you have, on the other hand, the worse your diabetes will be and the worse your risk for heart disease will be. Having more than 7 per cent of your red blood cells sugar-coated is, in itself, the basis for a diagnosis of diabetes. You want to have a score below 5 per cent. You can test yourself quite easily using a home-test kit (see Resources) and it's one of the tests we recommend for getting a good reflection of your biological age, so that you can do what is necessary to reverse it. (See Chapter 2 and Secret 3 for more details.)

BEWARE OF INSULIN

As we'll see in the next chapter, your blood levels of glucose and insulin are strong predictors not just of your diabetes risk but also of a shorter life span, as well as raising your risk of cancer.

Rogue glycation is most dangerous in long-lived cells such as those in the nerves and the lens of the eye. This is why people who have diabetes are at high risk of eye problems. Dementia is also a risk for those with diabetes, because the plaques found in the brain may be linked with glycation.[77] Glycation can also make the collagen in the arteries less flexible, leading to high blood pressure. Other effects include inflammation and DNA mutations.

So, given the widespread damage that can be caused by the AGEs, what is the way to keep rogue glycation at bay? The answer is one of the most effective ways of ageing healthily and one of the simplest: eat what's called a low-GL (low-glycemic load) diet, which essentially means one that has very little of the refined carbohydrates that are rapidly turned to glucose in the blood. It is a key part of avoiding diabetes and heart disease (see Secrets 3 and 7) and it's also got some very interesting links with the new genetic findings covered in the next chapter. CR and exercise both reduce glycation too. There are also claims that some of the calorie mimetics can do the same thing, such as resveratrol,[78] L-carnosine, an old drug called Benfotiamine (a synthetic version of vitamin B_1)[79] and the Indian spice turmeric.[80]

A PLAN TO BEEF UP GARBAGE DISPOSAL

One of the themes of this book is the contrast between the drug approach to ageing and one based on nutrition and lifestyle. We believe that because of the nature of ageing's system-wide effects, trying to do it healthily with drugs is doomed to failure. What's more it seems perverse to largely ignore a whole range of lifestyle options that we already know directly impact on many of the problems that ageing involves. The fact that many of them aren't yet supported by full-scale clinical trials should be a starting point for exploring them properly, rather than a reason to dismiss them out of hand.

Just in case you are still thinking that maybe there is a technical fix out there that could allow you to eat what you like, never take exercise and not even have to think about fish oil or beetroot, here is an example of the kind of high-tech 'blue-sky thinking' aimed at solving the difficult ageing problems of what to do about the decline in the effectiveness of your garbage disposal lysosome system described in Chapter 3. What do you think? Is this the kind of thing you'd like to buy into?

READY FOR BONE-MARROW TRANSPLANTS AND STEM CELL INJECTIONS?

It only exists in theory at the moment, although it is being actively researched at several labs in Europe and the US. The basic idea, known as SENS (strategies for engineered negligible senescence), proposes using very invasive procedures, such as genetic engineering, stem-cell infusions and bone-marrow transplants, to restore cells to peak performance.

It is the brainchild of one of the most enthusiastic high-tech anti-agers, Dr Aubrey Grey, a Biomedical Gerontologist from Cambridge University, who aims to reverse ageing in mice 'within ten years' and in humans 'rapidly thereafter'.

BACTERIAL ENZYME INJECTIONS ANYONE?

Grey's solution to the garbage problem is to replace the lysosomes with new powerful ones that he expects to find in soil bacteria. 'By the time we have identified the enzymes in bacteria capable of degrading lysomal junk,' he asserts confidently, 'gene therapy will be sufficiently advanced to allow their use in humans.'

We are not holding our breath, as no one has even found these soil bacteria, let alone put their enzymes in our bodies, and gene therapy is still experimental. Even more bizarrely, Grey plans to conquer cancer by genetically engineering telomerase out of the body on the grounds that it is required by cancer cells. No telomerase, no cancer.

· The fact that telomerase is used by stem cells in certain places like the blood and guts, which have a fast turnover, doesn't faze him. Bone-marrow transplants every ten years, he claims, would be the way to replace the ones that make blood. We'd take a bet that no baby boomer will ever benefit from this kind of sci-fi fantasy.

REVERSING 'INTERNAL GLOBAL WARMING'

What we can do right now, however, is to directly tackle signs your body's metabolism is becoming less efficient because of these processes linked with ageing – poorer methylation and glycation, and inflammation. Those signs constitute a kind of internal global warming, warning us that we need to act before they reach a crisis point.

Are you suffering from internal global warming?

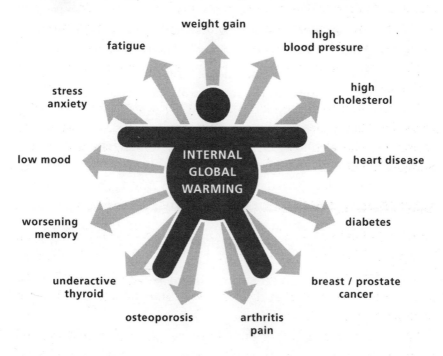

Many of the tools we suggest in this book – a low-GL diet, boosting B vitamins and minerals, eating healthy foods, taking exercise, and so on – form the human equivalents of a low-carbon lifestyle to halt the damaging effects that internal global warming has on your body.

THE NEED FOR A NEW DIRECTION

The science of ageing well is a new field with plenty of exciting possibilities, as this chapter shows, but not many certainties. So research needs to focus not just on new drugs but on how we can change our habits, and how to combine supplementation, exercise and food in sophisticated and informed ways. Based on what we know today, here are a few likely quick wins for turning back your biological ageing clock.

- Test your homocysteine level and reduce it to below 7 using high doses of specific B vitamins, especially B_{12} (see Secret 1).
- Supplement the basics every day – vitamins, minerals and essential fats – that reverse inflammation and balance your mood (see Secrets 2 and 4).
- Test your glycosylated haemoglobin and reduce it to below 5 by eating our Anti-ageing Diet, a low-GL diet (see Secret 3).
- Supplement the super-antioxidants that switch on your anti-ageing genes; for example, resveratrol, lipoic acid, glutathione and CoQ_{10} (see Secret 6).

In Part Two you'll find out exactly which of these secrets, and more, are most important for you to age healthily, and in Part Three we'll show you how to put it all together into your own Anti-ageing Action Plan. The big new discovery is that all these lifestyle approaches can directly change the activity of our genes, which opens up the opportunity to make them all far more precise. That's what we explore in the next chapter.

Chapter 6

HOW TO TURN ON THE ANTI-AGEING LONGEVITY GENES

Older baby boomers will remember Watergate – the failed attempt by the Nixon White House to cover up their bugging of the Democratic Party in the early 1970s. Like most other journalists I (Jerome) found it especially fascinating, because two journalists were the heroes, doggedly unravelling the conspiracy. One principle they used was that if two of their sources told them the same thing, there was a good chance that it was true. They were also advised by their mysterious, but reliable, informant, Deep Throat, to 'follow the money'. Both principles have proved useful in trying to understand ageing and how to do it well.

For a number of years, Patrick has been recommending that people who want to avoid heart disease and diabetes follow the low-GL diet mentioned previously, which involves cutting out the refined carbohydrates – especially white flour and sugar – that rapidly push up glucose levels in the blood (see Secrets 3 and 7, and Part Three). When he began, all dieticians and diabetic charities sang the praises of a low-fat, high-carb diet. Now, however, unable to ignore the success of low GL, they are slowly changing. So would low GL also show up as benefiting healthy ageing? It turns out that two key sources say that it does. One is that cornerstone of anti-ageing research, CR – the calorie-restricted diet – and the other is a remarkable genetic discovery.

CR is the only sure-fire way of extending life span, at least in animals, and years of research into its effects are clearly and comprehensively summarised in a new book on ageing called *The Youth Pill* by David Stipp. Time and again Stipp describes how the rats, mice, guinea pigs and monkeys on the diet showed up as having little fat in the blood, low cholesterol, low blood pressure and, crucially, low blood sugar and low insulin. The second source is new research into the genes that are linked with increasing life span – a story that forms a key part of this chapter. These genes seem to work by keeping insulin levels right down; but raised blood glucose, which has to be cleared away by increasing insulin, destroys their benefit. So, we're confident that keeping blood sugar down is a vital part of ageing well.

What has been the reaction to this consistent finding? It could have been something like: obviously, putting people on a proper CR diet isn't realistic, but what if we were to investigate diets that kept blood glucose and insulin low? It's true that a few mavericks did pick up on the benefit of low-glucose diets, Patrick among others, but the serious science response has been largely limited to finding a drug that has the same effect: ageing is a physical–medical problem, so the solution must be a new drug. In his book, after firmly establishing the CR–low-insulin link, Stipp spends several pages speculating about which drugs might do the same thing and he worries about side effects. There is never a mention of doing the same thing reliably, cheaply and safely with nutrition.

This is where following the money is revealing. Using these discoveries to develop a drug is perfectly legitimate. It may help some people – not everyone wants to follow a diet. The way money distorts the science is that here, as in most other areas of health research, investigating anything that might produce a pill swallows up the great bulk of funds. The division between the pharmaceutical approach and the non-drug approach is often caricatured as being the difference between evidence-based and evidence-free treatments. Actually, the difference is between well-funded and poorly funded research.

Is that really the best use of scarce research pounds? We reckon many baby boomers will be very interested in the non-drug approaches. It's time hard political questions were asked about how exactly it benefits our health to wait years for a drug that will inevitably come freighted with side effects, when funding research into uncovering the best way to present and apply the lifestyle approach might well rapidly produce safe and widespread benefits.

There has been a considerable shift towards the low-GL diet by the diabetes charities, according to an article in the *Daily Mail* in August 2011.[81] This revealed that Diabetes UK had 'quietly' issued new advice to those with diabetes that a diet of less than 45 per cent of calories from carbohydrates may be suitable – but only for a year. Why did we have to wait so long?

Genetics is also central to the other hugely optimistic finding about the possibility of healthy ageing – your genes are not a life sentence (see below). How often have you heard someone worrying about their risk of a heart attack because it runs in the family, or the centenarian who claims the secret of a long life is choosing your parents carefully? In other words, that our risk of disease and how well we age is down to the genetic hand we were dealt at birth. The truth is quite the opposite.

GENE ENGINEERING ON THE KITCHEN TABLE

It's now clear that our genes aren't the unchanging nuggets of information scientists used to think they were. Instead, they are remarkably porous; constantly responding to changes in your environment. Diet, micronutrients, toxins, love and affection, trauma and loss can all affect them. In fact, if you could see the genes in your body as points of light as they turned on and off, you would look like a firework display.

This has huge implications for anyone trying to improve their chances of a healthy old age by changing their lifestyle. No longer is genetic engineering something confined to research labs packed with millions of dollars of high-tech equipment, it is something that you can literally do on the kitchen table. The way to change the behaviour of your genes, even some of those inherited heart-attack ones, is with a good supply of omega-3 fats, healthy levels of vitamin D, eating a low-GL diet that keeps your blood sugar down and taking exercise.

THE METHUSELAH WORM

The gene–lifestyle link was first discovered when a top American geneticist became curious about exactly why CR had such a dramatic effect not just on life span but on ageing healthily. Professor Cynthia Kenyon of the University of California, San Francisco, wondered if the diet could be having a direct effect on gene activity, so she cut back on the calorie intake of a number of tiny roundworms just a millimetre long, known as *Caenorhabditis elegans*, which are the genetics researcher's 'lab rat'.

She found that one gene in particular was turned off by the CR diet. To her big surprise, it was one that normally made more insulin available. Even more of a surprise was the finding that turning the insulin gene off turned on another gene that controlled a cascade of extensive cell-repair processes. By tinkering with these genes she was able to breed some worms that lived for twice their normal 20-day life span.[82] Recently, with more sophisticated techniques, she's been able to genetically engineer a strain of *C. elegans* that lives healthily and actively for an astonishing 144 days. The human equivalent of 450 years!

Discovering this genetic mechanism opens the way to making healthy lifestyle changes in a much more focused way. It has also revolutionised ageing research, according to Jeff Holly, Professor of Clinical Sciences at Bristol University. 'Ten years ago we thought ageing was probably the result of a slow decay, a sort of rusting,' he says, 'but [Cynthia Kenyon] has shown that it's not about wear and tear but instead it is controlled by genes. That opens the possibility of slowing it down.'

INSULIN - THE SECRET AGEING HORMONE

The key to slowing ageing could be in keeping the amount of insulin in your bloodstream down. So, all those refined sugars and carbs that you just can't resist when you eat out could be speeding up the rate at which you are ageing. Dr Kenyon's discoveries about what the genes in her long-lived worms were doing suggests that too much insulin is crucial in not just diabetes but in other chronic diseases as well. 'We jokingly called the first gene the Grim Reaper,' says Kenyon, 'because when it's on, which is the normal state of affairs, [the worms'] life span is fairly short.' The second one had such a remarkable effect on the worms' health that it was quickly nicknamed 'Sweet Sixteen', because it reduced the worms' 'age' and turned them into teenagers. Kenyon had stumbled on a genetic Shangri la – the fictional valley where people barely aged.

Fortunately, humans have an equivalent to Sweet Sixteen called Foxo, and turning that gene on has a number of remarkable effects. 'Your supply of natural antioxidants goes up, damping down damaging oxidants,' says Kenyon. 'There's a boost to compounds that make sure the skin and muscle building proteins are working properly, the immune system becomes more active in fighting infection and genes that are active in cancer get turned off.'

What surprised many is that the research clearly implicated insulin as being a key player in ageing and very possibly in diabetes, heart disease and cancer as well. One clear message was that keeping your insulin levels to a minimum with a low-GL diet could be a recipe for healthy ageing. It is what we advocate and what Kenyon is already doing after she found that giving her super-centenarian worms just a drop of glucose rapidly made them wrinkly and dead. High blood sugar, which triggers insulin, means that DAF 3 (the Grim Reaper) stays on, and so Foxo never gets activated.

Professor Kenyon was happy to pass on some diet tips, saying that ever since these findings she had been keeping her carbohydrate intake really low. 'I've cut out all starch such as potatoes, noodles, rice, bread and pasta. Instead I have salads but no sweet dressing, lots of olive oil and nuts, tons of green vegetables along with cheese, chicken and eggs.'

CANCER AND THE DWARVES

What's even more remarkable is that an active Grim Reaper may also be linked to your chances of getting cancer. That's the message from a small remote community of dwarves living in north Ecuador who are cancer-free. They are missing the part of the Grim Reaper that controls a hormone called 'insulin-like growth factor 1' (IGF-1). The downside is that they only grow to 1.2m (4ft) because IGF-1 is needed for growth, but they are also less likely to suffer from heart disease or obesity.[83] The more dairy products you eat the more IGF-1 you make. You might grow taller but at what cost?

In fact, it looks as if our big chronic killers may have a common origin, linked by an excess of insulin. As well as controlling blood sugar, raised insulin triggers an increase in cholesterol production in the liver.

It also makes the walls of blood vessels contract so that blood pressure goes up and it stimulates the release of fats called triglycerides, which are linked with a raised risk of heart disease and diabetes.

Two years ago, in 2010, Harvard geneticist Dr Kevin Struhl made a surprising discovery when he found that 300 genes linked with tumour growth were also connected with obesity, heart disease and diabetes. Some of those genes affect insulin.[84] 'I was shocked when we found this,' he says. 'People had suspected there might be an underlying link between all these diseases but this puts it on molecular footing.'

THE PLEASURES OF CR WITHOUT THE PAIN

So, a low-GL diet looks like a powerful way of keeping insulin at a healthy level but, quite apart from the CR-mimetics mentioned in the last chapter, there is another way to get the benefits of CR without being condemned to a permanent state of semi-starvation. It is ridiculously simple. Eat every other day. That's it. You fast for one day and eat as much as you like the next. Fast for another day, then eat normally and so on. Of course there are variations and guidelines. Most people eat something on the 'down' day, as it is called: usually between 20 and 50 per cent of the calories you'd normally have, depending on how much or how quickly you want to lose weight. And it makes sense not to binge wildly on cakes and biscuits on the normal days.

In 2003 Dr Mark Mattson, a neuroscientist at the National Institute on Aging, discovered that rats put on the every-other-day schedule did just as well as their relatives on the gruelling CR diet.[85] Since then, it has become a popular 'underground' diet with websites devoted to schedules and possible variations for weight loss (see Resources).

It has a much wider health benefit, too. A number of researchers have discovered that its effect on genes can also help with various health problems. In one small study, asthma patients lost 8 per cent of their bodyweight but they also saw a dramatic drop in levels of inflammation and damaging oxidants; symptoms of wheezing and shortness of breath both greatly improved.[86]

In another study, overweight patients dropped pounds more easily than usual and produced more of a protein called adiponectin that reduces insulin resistance (so you need less of it) and damps down inflammation.[87] The same research team also found that getting patients to exercise, which is of course another cheap and not-patentable CR-mimetic, could produce a very similar effect.

WHY TESTING USING LAB RATS MAY BE RELEVANT TO HUMANS

Some scientists claim that because CR doesn't work on mice caught in the wild it's not really a true effect. But actually that seems further proof of its benefits. Mice from the wild will have been on a diet very like that anyway, whereas lab rats are a pretty good equivalent to Western humans. They have unlimited calories on tap, do very little exercise and quickly become obese. Alternate Day Dieting could be a real life-saver. We give you a simple way to do this in Part Three (and on page 298 you'll also find a case history for someone who is benefiting from following it).

The benefits of the Alternate Day Diet aren't limited to reducing weight and inflammation, however. There is still a lot of research needed, but from what we have so far, how well do other schedules, such as two days eating and one day not eating, work? It's likely that the diet can trigger the health-promoting gene Sweet Sixteen and possibly another one called SIRT1 (some studies have found that the latter is also activated by the compound resveratrol, found in grape skins, see Chapter 5). But as we've said several times, you are out on a frontier here – skiing off piste. Following our advice will help you age much more healthily, but there is still a lot more to be discovered.

Another question is, do some people benefit more from exercise than others? Undoubtedly, but there's no reliable way to spot who they are. The same goes for the different diets. The one thing we all know for sure, though, is that we are going to get older – if you are 65 now you may only have 170 months left! So, it's worth doing what you can to make that journey as enjoyable as you can, and that starts by staying well for as long as possible.

AGEING STOPS WHEN YOU ARE OVER 90

As an example of the mysteries of ageing that are still to be unravelled – which may be a signpost to another route to healthy ageing – take the curious fact, which we mentioned in Chapter 2, that when you get over 90 your rate of ageing slows dramatically. The magazine *New Scientist* recently explored the strange fact that once humans pass the age of 93 they are no more at risk of dying in the following year than they are at 100.[88] It's been investigated by Professor Michael Rose, an evolutionary biologist at the University of California, Irvine, who has shown that the same thing happens with large populations of fruit flies. When they reach a certain point in their life span, their rate of ageing seems to plateau.

Suppose you could make that plateau effect on ageing kick in earlier, at say 70? Professor Rose suggests the result could be a major increase in human life span. There's not room here to do justice to his theory about what is going on (more details can be found on his website, 555theses. org) but the basic idea is that when humans adopted agriculture about 10,000 years ago, some of the genes that had been valuable in hunter-gatherer groups began to cause problems in that new environment.

The major change was a large increase in foods that were based on grains and dairy products. Damaging gene reactions that kick in early in life are likely to be weeded out as the species evolves. Evolution is a numbers game: some people who are sick *do* reproduce, but not as many as those without the damaging gene, so on balance those with the damaging gene do less well. Rose suggests that humans are now reasonably well adapted to grains and dairy until about the age of 30, but after that they are more vulnerable to problems. So, to boost your chances of healthy ageing, he suggests that at 30-plus you adopt what's sometimes called the Stone Age Diet – a diet that is closer to the kind our hunter-gatherer ancestors would have been used to. Interestingly, it's a diet that shares a key feature with the low-GL diet: it keeps blood sugar and insulin levels right down.

ANTI-AGEING DRUGS – BEWARE

A couple of years ago it looked as though resveratrol would become the first anti-ageing drug, when the small company researching it was bought by GlaxoSmithKline (GSK) for 700 million dollars. GSK immediately began a clinical trial of resveratrol as a treatment for diabetes, but at the end of 2010 that was abandoned for reasons that haven't been made clear, although some recent studies have put a dampener on the idea of resveratrol as the universal panacea of ageing. Other synthetic versions, said to be more powerful and no doubt patentable and hence more profitable, are now being tested.

GSK's involvement prompted a striking change of attitude towards the possibility of slowing down, or even reversing, ageing. For years, companies and physicians selling or promoting compounds like resveratrol had been attacked in the US as hucksters and pseudoscientific, in a way similar to the attacks on supplement use in the UK. 'Products being sold that claim to be able to slow, stop or reverse human aging … have no scientifically demonstrated efficacy and in some cases they may be harmful,' wrote Professor Steven Olshanksy of the University of Illinois back in 2002.[89] For a few years he promoted the huckster charge by awarding – usually in their absence – the wittily named 'Silver Fleece' to the anti-ager whom he judged had made the most outrageous claim.

Following GSK's involvement, however, slowing human ageing didn't seem so fraudulent. In fact, Olshanksy was one of the authors of an article in the *British Medical Journal* in 2008 urging that anti-ageing be properly funded. He called for a programme to tackle chronic diseases such as diabetes and heart disease by modifying the 'key risk factor that underlies them all – ageing itself' by means of 'well validated interventions that slow ageing'.[90] So had there been a large study showing the benefits of promising compounds such as resveratrol since 2002 when such ideas had been dismissed as pseudoscientific? Hardly. The point is simply that by injecting such large sums into the field, with the promise of more to come, what had been seen as a fringe and rather disreputable area of research suddenly became respectable even though the evidence base had not changed.

COMMERCE MASQUERADING AS SCIENCE

So is anti-ageing research only scientific when it involves powerful synthetic versions of anti-ageing compounds? Or should the possible value of people using natural compounds for themselves be far better resourced and funded? Take a recent finding that resveratrol is even more effective against cancer in mice when combined with two other antioxidants also found in plants: quercetin (found in red onions) and catechin (the active ingredient in green tea).

A similar cocktail has been found to make the lining of blood vessels work in a more healthy way in human heart-disease patients.[91] But if no one is going to fund large clinical trials into such findings, does that automatically mean experimenting with them is a sign of scientific illiteracy? Might it not be a reasonable response to a situation that is heavily skewed towards a pharmaceutical approach that may not always benefit patients? Is this commercial interest masquerading as scientific principles? Are you happy to have your options limited in this way?

Perhaps, in the near future, as the number of sick, ageing people continues to mount, classifying one approach to maintaining our health as pseudoscience because there isn't adequate funding for research will be seen as a problem that needs a solution rather than making it an acceptable way to dismiss it.

VITAMINS THAT REPROGRAMME YOUR GENES

As we saw in Chapter 5, adequate levels of micronutrients are essential for the whole complex around the genes in every cell to work effectively; for example, a team working at Oxford in the UK and with the Multiple Sclerosis Society of Canada recently reported that vitamin D had a significant effect on the activity of 229 genes including some that have been associated with multiple sclerosis (MS), Crohn's disease and type-1 diabetes.[92]

'Our study shows quite dramatically the wide-ranging influence that vitamin D exerts over our health,' says Dr Andreas Heger from the MRC Functional Genomics Unit at Oxford, one of the lead authors of the study. Finding out if you are deficient, and a large proportion of the population is, and then bringing yourself up to a healthy level is the kind of direct action we can all take. It's a personal decision as to how long you want to wait for more research to come in.

The benefits of B vitamins for effective methylation have already been covered, especially in Chapters 2 and 5, and recently methylation's importance as a test of how well you are ageing was highlighted by scientists at the University of California, Los Angeles. They have patented a saliva test that can detect your biological age to within five years by measuring how much methylation has changed the activity of just two or three genes.[93] It's not known when the test will become available.

A LITTLE OF WHAT YOU *DON'T FANCY* DOES YOU GOOD

Another of the ageing mysteries that is still to be unravelled is exactly what role antioxidants are playing. There is no doubt that we need them: our bodies manufacture a wide range, and one of the health-giving actions of the Sweet Sixteen gene is to increase their production. But research also shows that there are times when *oxidants* have a beneficial effect, so damping them down at those times may not be a good idea.

The problem is that both CR and exercise, which have such health-giving benefits, also increase the production of oxidants. In fact, as far as the body is concerned they are both forms of stress. So, one of the ideas about how Sweet Sixteen and other healthy genes generate their benefits is that the oxidants trigger 'messages' that say, 'Help, we are under attack!', stimulating the repairing and housekeeping proteins to go into overdrive. Biologists talk about this effect as 'stress-proofing'. This idea, which might be called 'a little of what you don't fancy does you good', is known as hormesis; for example, some poisons used in very small doses can have a beneficial effect. Other stresses, such as raised or lowered temperature, radiation and hyper-gravity, can all have beneficial effects too. As yet, no one is sure what all the implications are. Should you, therefore, avoid taking antioxidants after exercise, as it could reduce the benefit? Unravelling what's going on will allow treatments to become more sophisticated.[94]

HOW STRESS CHANGES YOUR GENES

There are certainly times when stress isn't good for you, and definitely not in the long term. So, staying healthy and happy as we get older involves more than keeping your mitochondria in good shape and your micronutrient levels up. Older people often report feelings of loneliness and lack of purpose – negative emotions that can have as direct an influence on health as biological decline. A recent study found that good social connections – having friends, family, neighbours or colleagues – improve our odds of survival by 50 per cent. A lack of such connections was as harmful as smoking 15 cigarettes a day and twice as harmful as obesity.[95]

Because we have a medical system that concentrates largely on biochemistry, the psychological side of health is often ignored, and so insomnia is treated with sleeping pills, and depression is treated with SSRI antidepressants. Secret 4 looks at a number of different ways to deal with these and also gives a very useful technique for handling stress.

Stress can have a large impact on our genes in ways that researchers are only just beginning to understand. Studies on rats have found that good or bad early experiences can affect the gene methylation[96] and that the pups of attentive rat mothers are much better able to handle stress later in life; those with less nurturing mothers become more anxious. If rat social relationships can have an effect on their genes then it's a certainty that we intensely social humans will be directly affected too.

Stress may also increase the risk of cancer by changing genes, as scientists recently reported in *Nature*. Chronically stressed rats show increased DNA damage, an effect that includes turning off a gene called P53, which is known to protect against tumours. It may also affect normal brain function by causing nerve cells in the brain to make hormones and other signalling molecules they don't normally produce.[97]

The message that comes out of this very clearly is that we and our genes are affected in an almost minute-by-minute way by what is going on in our social environment: how people behave towards us, whether we are respected or rejected, whether we are valued or dismissed. Being rich usually comes with a sense of personal satisfaction while poverty is often demeaning – these differences are reflected in gene activity. One study has found that more than a hundred genes in the immune system behave differently depending on whether you were born rich or poor. Even if you are well off, you will have the gene patterns of poorer people if you were in a poor environment before the age of 15.[98]

YOUR INTERCONNECTED GENES, ENVIRONMENT, DIET AND STATE OF MIND

The picture that emerges from all this research is that our bodies are finely tuned ecological systems which are very sensitive to our physical environment: how good is the food we are eating; are we getting enough minerals and vitamins; is it easy to exercise? All these can directly affect the genes from birth onwards. And we are also very responsive to our psychological environment – how happy and loved we feel – which also changes our biological state. And given the right environment and support, we have enormous self-healing abilities.

Unfortunately, the current medical system isn't very interested in a sophisticated nutritional approach, nor in a patient's psychological state – antidepressants are the most common response to mental distress. More worrying in the longer term is that the system we have for researching health issues will have a minimal interest in teasing out the complexities of the interactions between nutrition, mental states and genes, because there is little product or profit there. So, the question for the baby boomers is do we say, 'That's the way it is – get over it!' or do we say 'That's not good enough – let's change it'?

ANTI-AGEING ACTION PLAN

However hard-nosed you are, it's hard to ignore the fact that our taxes are going to be paying to treat rising numbers of elderly sick people for years. So wouldn't it make sense to spend some of that money on discovering the best way to keep us healthy rather than simply relying on the remarkable resources of modern medicine when we are ill?

While that's being sorted out and incentives for health promotion put in place, there's a lot you can do to cut your risk of developing the chronic conditions – diabetes, cancer, heart disease, failing eyes and thinning bones – that lie in wait as you get older. That's what Part Two is all about. Then Part Three provides your Anti-ageing Action Plan.

Part Two

THE TEN SECRETS

The best way to live a long, healthy life is to avoid preventable diseases. In this Part we explore the most common health problems, the risks for which increase with age. You can keep your mind intact, your joints and bones strong, your energy good and your weight under control. You'll also find out how to sleep well, keep your skin young and your digestion good, as well as how to stop your eyesight from degenerating. You can also prevent cancer, diabetes and heart disease, and we give you advice on how to reverse your risk if you are already suffering.

Secret 1

STAY SMART AS YOU AGE – AND FORGET ABOUT ALZHEIMER'S

The greatest concern for many people as they age is fading memory and loss of mental agility. After all, what is the point of having a great life if you can't remember it? Some opinion polls show that Alzheimer's disease has overtaken cancer as the number-one fear. Too many people have watched their relatives' identity dissolve as Alzheimer's progresses, and they dread the same thing happening to themselves. In the UK, more than 500 people are diagnosed with dementia every day, most of which is Alzheimer's.

Fear not. Evidence is growing that there is more you can do to cut the risk of both Alzheimer's disease and fading memory than experts used to think, and the sooner you start doing the right things the better your chances. Contrary to popular belief, only one in a hundred cases of Alzheimer's is completely caused by genes, so if your parents have suffered it doesn't mean that you have to as well.

UNDERSTANDING MEMORY LOSS

There is a sequence of decline that starts with your memory getting a little worse as you age, which can progress to mild cognitive impairment (MCI) and then, for some, to dementia. Three-quarters of dementia is Alzheimer's disease. Much of the remaining quarter is vascular dementia, caused by narrowing arteries restricting the flow of oxygen and nutrients to the brain. Dementia is diagnosed on the basis of symptoms, although Alzheimer's is diagnosed using a more detailed examination and usually a brain scan.

Alzheimer's disease is not an inevitable part of the ageing process. As we age, our brains naturally shrink by as much as 0.5 per cent a year but, in Alzheimer's, that speeds up to 2.5 per cent, mostly in the medial temporal lobe (which is in the centre of the head, in from the ears). The figure below shows MRI scans of the brains of two elderly people of the same age, who have been scanned at a six-month interval. The black area in the one on the right shows where the brain cells have been lost. This is the hallmark of Alzheimer's, and the loss of brain tissue is irreversible.

Brain shrinkage – a hallmark of Alzheimer's associated with high homocysteine

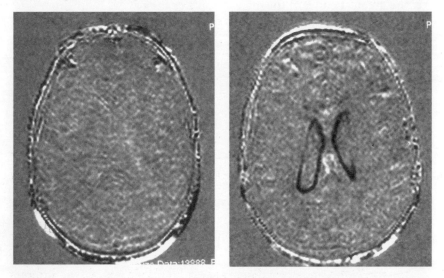

A high level of homocysteine is a marker for the beginnings of Alzheimer's. The brain scans above are of two elderly people of the same age. The one on the left has a healthy homocysteine level of 7.8. The one on the right has an unhealthy level of 13.1. Each had an initial MRI scan, and then another scan six months later, which was superimposed onto the first to reveal any changes during the six months. There were none in the person on the left. What you see in black, on the right, is the brain cells that have died in six months. This is Alzheimer's disease.

Used with the permission of Optima.

The question is: how do you make sure your brain stays like the one on the left, without accelerated brain shrinkage and declining memory?

The first step is to find out whether your cognitive function is showing any signs of worsening, and you can do this with a simple test.

TEST YOUR COGNITIVE FUNCTION

How's your memory and concentration? The charity www.foodforthe brain.org has a free, validated online Cognitive Function Test. It takes 15 minutes to complete and is validated for anyone over the age of 50. Depending on your score, it tells you what to do to improve your memory. The sooner you find out the better.

WHAT CAUSES BRAIN SHRINKAGE?

There's a heated debate about what causes damage to brain cells, called neurons, because knowing what it is would help to develop new drugs. At the moment, the most widely used type of drugs, such as Aricept, work by inhibiting the breakdown of the memory neurotransmitter acetylcholine, low levels of which are also associated with Alzheimer's; however, its effect is only temporary, helping some people slow down their rate of memory loss for two years. It does nothing to prevent neuronal decay, and once a brain cell is gone the drug has no effect. So, after a couple of years, those on Aricept are no better off than if they had never taken the drug. What is more, the drug doesn't deal with the underlying cause.

The most obvious immediate cause is the build up of two different sorts of damaged proteins that kill off neurons. So-called amyloid plaques are fragments of protein (beta amyloid) that fill up the spaces between the cells. In a healthy brain they are broken down and removed by lysosomes (which we met on page 36, Chapter 3), but in Alzheimer's they clump together to make hard, insoluble plaques. Another rogue protein that normally provides a framework for cells, called tau, collapses into insoluble twisted fibres inside cells. Billions of dollars of research has gone into searching for drugs that can stop these kinds of faulty proteins from forming, without any success.[1] As a result, some experts have suggested that they may not be the cause of Alzheimer's after all.[2] There is so much money behind the concept of amyloid protein, however, that you'll be hearing more and more about testing for it, and about miracle drugs around the corner.

There's no shortage of other possible candidates that might be damaging brain cells, which haven't received nearly so much attention. Here are just a few of them: a lack of antioxidants leading to oxidation damage; a lack of oxygen and a lowered blood supply due to thickening arteries; poor glycation[3] (which, you may remember, is what happens when cells get damaged by too much sugar); a type of damage to cells called excitotoxicity,[4] which involves the amino acid glutamate; faulty methylation (the chemical process explained in Chapter 2);[5] and a lack of the key building material for cell walls: omega-3 phospholipid fats. Although all these may be involved, however, there is evidence that most of them are linked with raised homocysteine (see the illustration below).

How homocysteine damages the brain

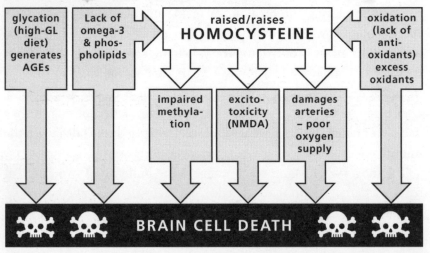

THE HOMOCYSTEINE CONNECTION

As we saw in Chapter 5, one of the most fundamental processes that keeps your brain and body 'connected' and firing on all cylinders is methylation. If the level of the amino acid homocysteine in your blood is high, it means that you aren't efficient at methylation.

The most reliable way to find out your risk for developing Alzheimer's is by a standardised test of various mental abilities such as memory and verbal expression together with a measure of your homocysteine.[6] To date, 70 out of 77 studies involving over 35,000 people have found that increased homocysteine levels predicts an increased risk of cognitive impairment and dementia or Alzheimer's.[7] Studies show the following:

- Homocysteine predicts cognitive decline.[8]
- The rate homocysteine increases or decreases over time predicts the rate of cognitive decline or improvement.[9]
- Both memory loss[10] and Alzheimer's are predicted by homocysteine.[11]
- Homocysteine predicts the rate of brain shrinkage and degeneration.[12]
- The rate of brain shrinkage predicts the rate of memory decline.[13]
- People with Alzheimer's have low blood levels of vitamin B_{12} and/or folate,[14] both of which are known causes of raised homocysteine.

DOES LOWERING HOMOCYSTEINE STOP MEMORY LOSS?

If high homocysteine is a critical indicator that brain cells are being killed off at a faster rate than usual, then does lowering it prevent, arrest or reverse the memory decline associated with Alzheimer's? That's the critical question. There must be a point of no return where the progression from age-related memory decline to Alzheimer's becomes irreversible. But if homocysteine has a causal link, then maybe there is a point where the damage can be slowed or even arrested.

Two studies are relevant here. One initially found no benefit from giving very high levels of B vitamins for 18 months to patients already diagnosed as suffering from mild to moderate Alzheimer's[15] (high levels of B vitamins is the only way to bring homocysteine down). When the researchers divided the patients into those with high and low cognitive test scores at the start, however, those who had milder Alzheimer's did respond significantly; those taking the B vitamins hardly got worse over 15 months, and those on the placebo showed a steady decline. So, it looks as though B vitamins may, at least, slow down Alzheimer's substantially in the early stages, but that when the disease has reached the moderately severe stage it may be too late.

Could B vitamins prevent Alzheimer's from ever developing in the first place? In order to test this, Professor David Smith and his colleagues from the University of Oxford gave high doses of B vitamins (folic acid 800mcg, B_{12} 500mcg and B_6 20mg) for two years to half a group of 270 people with age-related memory decline; a placebo tablet was given to the other half.[16] He also tested their homocysteine levels and gave most of them an MRI brain scan at the beginning and the end of the 24-month placebo-controlled trial.

The results strongly suggest that bringing down homocysteine has a beneficial effect, but only in patients who have quite a high homocysteine level already. Among older people with no memory loss, the total brain size normally shrinks at about 0.5 per cent a year. If you've got mild cognitive impairment, this increases to 1 per cent, and in those with Alzheimer's the brain is normally shrinking at 2.5 per cent a year. In the trial, those who took the placebo suffered more brain shrinkage the higher their homocysteine level was found to be. When their homocysteine was over 13mcmol/l their brains shrank at the rate of 1.5 per cent per year. But shrinkage in those with homocysteine below 9.5mcmol/l was only 0.8 per cent.

The effect of giving the B vitamins was remarkable, providing homocysteine levels were above 13mcmol/l. Shrinkage more than halved, compared with the placebo – a drop of 53 per cent (see the illustration opposite), down to almost normal levels for healthy ageing.

The effect of B vitamins on the rate of brain shrinkage

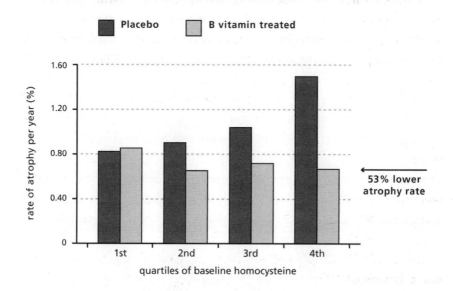

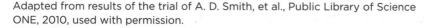

Adapted from results of the trial of A. D. Smith, et al., Public Library of Science ONE, 2010, used with permission.

The second part of this research, which looked at whether the vitamins also improved mental performance, found a similar pattern.[17] On the placebo, mental function got worse the higher the homocysteine, but where participants were given the vitamins, their mental performance stayed the same. The difference in cognitive decline between placebo and treatment was significant for those with a homocysteine level of over 11mcmol/l.

Since a shrinking brain and declining cognition is what shows up in people who go on to develop Alzheimer's disease, these results provide the strongest evidence yet that keeping your homocysteine low will protect you from both age-related memory decline and Alzheimer's disease. Unlike drugs such as Aricept there's no evidence that the effect of taking B vitamins and lowering your homocysteine level wears off after a couple of years.

> ### PROFESSOR DAVID SMITH'S PERSONAL HEALTH PLAN
>
> Professor Smith says, 'My diet is high in fruit and vegetables, with fish at least twice a week. I have one cup of coffee a day and a small amount of wine intake and I make sure I drink plenty of water. I have a daily multivitamin, high dose B vitamins and extra vitamin D_3. Every day I aim for two brisk 30-minute walks.' At the age of 73 he is as sharp as a razor, leading the field in scientific research on Alzheimer's prevention.

HOMOCYSTEINE-LOWERING B VITAMINS KEEP YOU SMART

Should we all be taking B vitamins? The answer is probably yes, but the amount you need depends very much on your homocysteine level, as well as how much you are getting from your diet. The three most critical B vitamins are folic acid, found in beans, lentils, nuts, seeds and greens; B_6, also high in those foods; and B_{12}, which is only found in animal produce – meat, fish, eggs and dairy products.

Folic acid A study by Jane Durga from Holland's Wageningen University gave people over 50 years old, without memory loss but with slightly raised homocysteine (greater than 13mcmol/l), a supplement of 800mcg of folic acid a day or a placebo for three years.[18] That's the equivalent of what you'd get in 1.2kg (2½lb) of strawberries, so it's more than you could reasonably eat. Those on the B vitamin supplement had a highly significant improvement in memory, information-processing speed and sensorimotor speed in the treatment group.

If you have a raised homocysteine level you may also benefit from supplementing 800mcg a day. The chart on page 105 shows you the ideal amount to supplement, depending on your homocysteine level.

Vitamin B_{12} The most critical nutrient as you age is vitamin B_{12}. This is because it becomes increasingly hard to absorb, probably due to decreasing levels of stomach acid. Some people lack, or produce insufficient amounts of, something called 'intrinsic factor' in the stomach, which is needed to absorb B_{12}. The result is a rare deficiency known as pernicious anaemia. Researchers from Oxford University measured blood levels of B_{12}, and rates of brain shrinkage in people over age 61. Two in five didn't have enough B_{12} in their blood to prevent accelerated brain shrinkage.[19] So the odds are quite high that you should be supplementing B_{12}. But how much do you need?

If your homocysteine level is high, or you have been tested and found to be low in B_{12}, you need mega-doses of B_{12} supplements, or an injection to bypass the poor absorption. Researchers in Holland found that only doses of over 500mcg of B_{12} were associated with correcting deficiency. In their words, 'the lowest dose of oral B_{12} required to normalize mild B_{12} deficiency is more than 200 times greater than the RDA', which is a paltry 2.5mcg in the US and 1mcg in the EU.[20] So much for a 'well-balanced diet' giving you all the nutrients you need!

The best food sources for B_{12} are fish, milk and eggs. A high intake cuts your risk of memory loss.

A good basic level of B_{12} for everybody in a multivitamin would be 10mcg per day. But it's really important to test your homocysteine level and then supplement according to the chart on page 105, including other key nutrients, such as vitamin B_6, zinc, TMG and the antioxidant N-acetyl-cysteine (NAC), which we'll be explaining more about shortly.

A COMBINATION OF HOMOCYSTEINE-LOWERING SUPPLEMENTS WORK BEST

Combined supplements are much more effective. One study found homocysteine scores were reduced by 17 per cent on high-dose folic acid alone, 19 per cent on vitamin B_{12} alone, 57 per cent on folic acid plus B_{12}, and 60 per cent on folic acid, B_{12} and B_6.[21] All this was achieved in three weeks! Adding TMG to the B-vitamin mix lowered homocysteine by a further 18 per cent, according to one New Zealand study.[22]

The moral of this story is, get your homocysteine level down at all costs, certainly to below 9.5mcmol/l, and ideally below 7mcmol/l. Your doctor can test your homocysteine level or you can buy an accurate home-test kit (see Resources).

TESTING AND INTERPRETING HOMOCYSTEINE LEVELS

Homocysteine is measured in the blood plasma, and it requires blood to be immediately centrifuged to separate out the plasma, then it is either immediately tested or frozen for later testing. GPs can refer you for testing, but tests must be carried out immediately in the laboratory. YorkTest devised a plasma separation device making it possible to 'home-test' homocysteine. The plasma, once separated, is fixed on a card and sent to the laboratory (see Resources for details of home-test kit). Both methods reliably measure homocysteine. Since homocysteine is made from protein, homocysteine levels may rise slightly after a protein meal. Therefore, homocysteine testing must always be done on an empty stomach, ideally first thing in the morning. Almost all data relating to reference ranges are derived on this basis.

The range of homocysteine scores that I (Patrick) have seen in clinical practice range from 4 to 119mcmol/l. The 'average' in most populations is between 9 and 13. In the UK it is 10.5. Levels rise with age. Alzheimer's disease risk roughly doubles if a person's homocysteine score is over 14 compared to an average of 9.[23] General guidelines are that an optimal level is below 7, with low risk of memory decline from 7 to 9, higher risk from 10, and exceedingly high risk above 15.

Lowering homocysteine with supplements

A number of nutrients are involved in lowering homocysteine (see animation at www.patrickholford.com/methylationcycle). The most critical are vitamin B_{12}, folic acid and B_6. Vitamin B_{12} and folic acid require a methyl group. Folate (in food) contains methyl groups. Alternatively, methylcobalamine or methylfolate can be used. Vitamin B_2 is also a co-factor in this process. There is an alternate way of processing homocysteine that requires tri-methyl-glycine (TMG) and zinc, and another that requires vitamin B_6 and N-acetyl cysteine or glutathione.

Therefore, the ideal diet and supplements for lowering homocysteine and improving methylation should contain B_2, B_6, B_{12}, folic acid, zinc and TMG. Methyl B_{12} and methylfolate are more bio-available and provide an additional methyl group. The amount you need depends on your homocysteine level and is shown in the chart below.

Supplement quantities

Nutrient	No risk	Low risk	At risk	High risk
Hcy score	Below 7	7–9	10–15	Above 15
Folic acid	200mcg	400mcg	800mcg	800mcg
B_{12}	10mcg	250mcg	500mcg	750mcg
B_6	10mg	20mg	25mg	50mg
B_2	5mg	10mg	15mg	25mg
Zinc	5mg	10mg	15mg	20mg
TMG	–	500mg	750mg	1500mg
NAC or Glutathione	–	250mg	500mg	750mg

CASE STUDY: CHRIS

Chris, 59, felt very unwell, with constant tiredness, worsening memory and concentration, and little zest for life. He was depressed, had no sex drive and felt brain dead. His homocysteine score was 119! He changed his diet and took the full combination of homocysteine-lowering nutrients and, within three months, his homocysteine level had dropped to 19. After six months it had dropped to 11, and after a year it was down to 9. He cannot believe how well he now feels. His memory and concentration are completely restored. In fact, he says it's as good as it's ever been. He has boundless energy from 6.00 am until 10.00 pm. He now exercises for an hour every day and has lost weight. 'You have saved my life, or at least made it worth living again. I'm a new man – and my love life has perked up,' says Chris.

OMEGA-3 FATS KEEP YOU BRAINY

Fish has many advantages over meat. It is high in vitamin B_{12} and phospholipids (see below) and high in omega-3 fats if it's oily – as in salmon, mackerel, herring, kippers and tuna. All these nutrients help to protect against memory loss. DHA and EPA are types of essential fat, both found in fish oils. EPA (eicosapentaenoic acid) helps the brain to function better, and is the more potent mood-boosting essential fat. DHA (docosahexaenoic acid) is used to build the brain, and may be more important in pregnancy and for young children, as well as later in life to prevent brain degeneration.

Eating fish once a week reduces your risk of developing Alzheimer's by a whopping 60 per cent, according to a study by Professor Martha Morris at Rush University Medical Center.[24] Prof. Morris studied 815 people, aged 65–94 years, over a seven-year period and found that the dietary intake of fish was strongly linked to Alzheimer's risk. She found that the strongest link was the amount of DHA in the diet: the higher the DHA intake the lower their risk of developing Alzheimer's. The lowest amount of DHA per day that offered some protection was 100mg.

EPA, in this study, didn't provide any extra protection; however, the highest intake of EPA consumed was 30mg a day, which is very low – less than what you'd get in half a sardine.

Does supplementing more of these essential fats protect your memory? In a placebo-controlled trial, older people with signs of cognitive impairment, but no diagnosis of Alzheimer's, were given 900mg of DHA a day for 24 weeks. Those on the supplements had clear improvements in learning and memory function compared to those on the placebos.[25] But when the group produced another 18-month controlled trial giving even more – this time 2,000mg of DHA – to 402 subjects who already had mild to moderate Alzheimer's, they found no measurable improvement.[26] Once again, the clear message is that you need to improve your nutrition as early as possible to protect your memory. We recommend supplementing omega-3 fish oils, for this and for many other reasons, on a daily basis. Chapter 7, Part Three tells you how much to take according to your age.

WHY EGGS AND FISH ARE GOOD FOR YOUR BRAIN

One of the most maligned foods are eggs. No, they don't raise your cholesterol level or increase your risk of heart disease. Eggs are an incredibly nutritious food, packed with many essential nutrients required for a chicken to grow. Among these are phospholipids.

The dry weight of the brain is 60 per cent fat and as much as this is either comprised of phospholipids or essential fats such as DHA. Phospholipids are not only a vital part of all brain cells (for example, the receptor sites for neurotransmitters are embedded in them), but one kind of phospholipid, called phosphatidylcholine (PC), is the raw material for building the neurotransmitter acetylcholine that is vital for memory. (You may remember from Chapter 4 that the drug Aricept works to raise acetylcholine levels in the brain.)

In animals given more choline, acetylcholine levels go up. In people who have had a stroke, giving more choline helps to repair the brain.[27] Choline, like so many other vital chemicals in the brain, requires methylation to be synthesised from food, and efficient methylation is linked to your homocysteine level. The lower your homocysteine level, in other words, the better you are at methylation; therefore the more able you are to make phospholipids and acetylcholine, and the fewer of those neurofibrilliary tangles you are likely to have.[28] So, make sure you have plenty of phosphatidylcholine in your diet from fish and eggs. You can also supplement it by taking lecithin capsules or granules, which you can sprinkle, for example, on cereal.

There are other important phospholipids, which are found in fish. Phosphatidylserine (PS) is highly concentrated in the brain. Sixteen clinical trials indicate that PS benefits measurable cognitive functions, which tend to decline with age; these include memory, learning, vocabulary skills and concentration, as well as mood, alertness and sociability.[29] A six-month placebo-controlled trial of PS (using 300mg per day) in 494 elderly people with moderate-to-severe cognitive decline found significant benefit.[30] Another small trial on eighteen people with memory impairment found improvement in 15 of them within six weeks.[31] Not all studies have been positive, however. A placebo-controlled trial on 120 elderly people with memory problems found no benefit.[32] It's in our 'optional extra' category, awaiting definitive proof.

There is a third beneficial phospholipid, called DMAE, found in the brains of fish and humans. It acts as an antioxidant and a building block for memory-enhancing acetylcholine. In animal studies, it is memory protective.[33]

The amount taken by participants in trials is way beyond what you can achieve by diet alone and so requires supplementation. You can buy supplements that provide a combination of phospholipids – the three most important being PC, PS and DMAE, or take a supplement of PS (100–300mg) plus two lecithin 1,200mg capsules, or a dessertspoonful of lecithin granules for PC. Being in my fifties (Patrick), but with no memory decline, I take a daily combination supplement. If I had memory decline I'd increase my intake PC and PS to these kinds of levels.

ANTIOXIDANTS PROTECT YOUR BRAIN

Since the brain is made of all these complex fats that can easily be damaged by oxidants, it makes sense that having a high intake of antioxidants would protect the brain from damage. Antioxidants disarm oxidants by teamwork: you need a combination of nutrients, not just vitamin C or E.

A study of 4,740 Cache County, Utah, elderly residents found that those supplementing both vitamins E and C cut their risk of developing Alzheimer's by two-thirds. A trend towards lower Alzheimer's risk was also evident in those who took vitamin E supplements together with multivitamins containing vitamin C, but there was no evidence of a protective effect in those taking only vitamin E or vitamin C supplements alone, with multivitamins alone, or with vitamin B-complex supplements. The lowest risk was reported in those supplementing at least 1,000mg a day of vitamin C together with at least 1,000iu a day of vitamin E.[34] Vitamin E on its own doesn't seem to work. In a double-blind study, people with mild cognitive impairment were randomly assigned to receive 2,000iu a day of vitamin E or a placebo for three years. There were no significant differences in the rate of progression to Alzheimer's between the vitamin E and placebo groups at any point.[35]

Your best bet is probably to eat a broad spectrum of antioxidants and also to supplement them. The older you are the more you are likely to need. Key antioxidants are:

- Vitamins A, C and E – associated with reducing Alzheimer's risk.

- Lipoic acid – protects acetylcholine and stops brain oxidation, and it is also anti-inflammatory.[36]
- Glutathione or N-acetyl-cysteine (NAC) – protects the brain and improves methylation.

Welsh GP, Dr Andrew McCaddon, has been piecing together the story of the links between homocysteine and Alzheimer's for the last decade and has been running small studies from the University of Wales. His clinical experience is that combining B vitamins with antioxidants is particularly effective.[37] According to McCaddon:

Patients presenting with mild cognitive impairment frequently have raised blood homocysteine levels; I routinely measure this in all such cases. There is now good evidence for lowering elevated levels with high dose B vitamins. I also prescribe the antioxidant NAC to further lower homocysteine. In my experience, I have found significant clinical improvement from this approach.

The reason for giving NAC is that it helps makes glutathione, the body's most essential antioxidant, which also improves methylation. Good homocysteine-lowering supplements include NAC.

Early on in Alzheimer's, patients suffer a heavy loss of synapses (the points where the brain cells connect). A recent study of 225 patients at the Massachusetts Institute of Technology found it might be possible to reverse that with a combination of supplements. Three of the ingredients are found in breast milk: uridine (a building block of the genetic messenger RNA); the B vitamin choline; and DHA omega-3. After three months on the patented mixture, which also contained B vitamins, phospholipids and antioxidants, 40 per cent of the patients improved their verbal memory compared with 24 per cent on the placebo.[38]

In terms of specific antioxidant-rich foods, these include:

- Onions, a rich source of quercetin.
- Beans, a rich source of isoflavones.
- Berries, a rich source of anthocyanidins and resveratrol.

- Green tea, a rich source of catechins.
- Chocolate (with high cocoa solids), a rich source of epicatechin.

People who either ate more fruit and vegetables, or drank more tea, or had some chocolate or red wine, tended to have better cognition, according to a study from Oxford University.[39] Generally, the higher your antioxidant intake the lower your risk of memory decline. See page 191 for a list of the most potent antioxidant-rich foods.

Resveratrol, although not yet proven to stop memory decline, is associated with reduced risk if your intake is high. An animal study has shown that supplementing resveratrol leads to less formation of plaques in the brain.[40] As we saw in Chapter 6, resveratrol switches genetic expression away from ageing. The more closely you follow a Mediterranean-style diet, rich in fish, wholefoods, fruits and vegetables, plus the odd glass of red wine, the less likely you are to suffer from the cognitive decline that can progress to Alzheimer's.[41]

CUT BACK ON COFFEE

The one antioxidant-rich food – or drink in this case – that may not be good is coffee. There is no question that it raises homocysteine levels quite substantially. Dr Verhoef, et al., at the Wageningen Centre for Food Sciences showed that two cups of regular coffee increased homocysteine by 11 per cent after only four hours, whereas caffeine tablets alone increased it by 5 per cent.[42] So, there's something other than caffeine in coffee that also raises homocysteine. Other studies have shown the same thing. One litre (1¾ pints) of unfiltered coffee a day – that's about four cups – for two weeks raised homocysteine from 12.8 to 14mcmol/l.[43] Coffee-drinking is associated with reduced circulating levels of folate, B_6 and B_2, possibly by increased excretion.[44] Having said this, there is no clear evidence that coffee-drinking raises your risk of dementia as such, just that it raises homocysteine.[45] So, if you drink more than one cup of coffee a day, it's doubly worth getting your homocysteine level checked. If it's too high, cut back on coffee, as well as taking a homocysteine-lowering supplement.

FOLLOW A LOW-GL DIET

One of the advantages of a Mediterranean-style diet is that it has a low glycemic load, in other words the carbohydrates contained therein are not the kind that are rapidly turned to glucose in the blood. Eating a low-GL diet, by keeping your intake of carbohydrates low and avoiding refined carbohydrates as much as possible, keeps your blood sugar level even, which means you need to make less of the hormone insulin. As discussed in Chapter 6, this not only switches off a key ageing gene but it also reduces your risk of age-related memory loss. In Part Three, Chapter 2, we explain the simple rules of low-GL eating in our Anti-ageing Diet.

Researchers at Columbia University in New York have found that twice as many people with high insulin levels developed dementia when compared to those with normal insulin.[46] Also, the people with high insulin levels had the greatest decline in memory. An Italian study of people free from dementia and diabetes showed that high insulin levels were strongly associated with poorer mental function.[47] A six-year Swedish study of 1,301 people aged 75 and over showed that those with diabetes were one and a half times more likely to develop dementia.[48]

So, staying free of diabetes, which we discuss in Secret 3, is a great way to keep your memory sharp.[49] In Secret 3 you'll learn that keeping your glycosylated haemoglobin level (the marker for high blood sugar and insulin) below 5.5 is a key factor in healthy ageing, because it cuts your chance of developing metabolic syndrome, which lies behind so many degenerative diseases, including dementia. Researchers at the University of California, San Francisco, studied 1,983 postmenopausal women and found those with glycosylated haemoglobin levels of 7 per cent or higher were four times more likely to develop mild cognitive impairment or dementia.[50]

SUMMARY

To keep your mind and memory as sharp as a razor:

- Eat greens and beans, lentils, nuts and seeds, which are rich in folate.
- Eat eggs and fish, which are rich in vitamin B_{12} and phospholipids.
- Eat oily fish, which is rich in omega-3 essential fats, three times a week.
- Eat strongly coloured fruit, vegetables and spices, which are rich in antioxidants.
- Drink (green) tea – not coffee – and red wine in moderation.
- Eat a low glycemic-load diet, such as our Anti-ageing Diet (see Part 3, Chapter 2).

In terms of supplements:

- Check your homocysteine level, and, if it's high, take a homocysteine-lowering supplement containing vitamins B_6, B_{12}, folic acid, TMG, zinc and NAC (see the chart on page 105).
- Take a daily omega-3 fish oil supplement.
- Optional extras are a phospholipid supplement containing phosphatidylcholine, serine and DMAE; and an all-round antioxidant supplement containing vitamins A or beta-carotene, lipoic acid, glutathione/NAC and resveratrol.

See Part Three, Chapter 7 for your general supplement programme. See also Recommended Reading for other helpful books on this topic.

Secret 2

KEEP YOUR JOINTS MOBILE AND YOUR BONES STRONG

The clear hallmarks of ageing are creaky and aching joints and reducing bone mass. For some people, decreasing bone mass leads to osteoporosis, which is usually discovered when a fracture occurs. Four-fifths of fractures occur after the age of 50 and the risk becomes quite significant from 70 onwards. Rates of arthritis are frighteningly high too.

There's an inevitable basic level of wear and tear on joints but, if you understand how this happens, and then do the right things to counteract it, you can avoid the discomfort of arthritic joints, back pain and osteoporosis, which plague older people. Although over half of people aged 55 and over have arthritis in the UK[51] and the US, other countries have a fraction of the incidence, notably some parts of Africa, Australia and Israel. There's every reason to believe that you can keep your joints mobile and your bones strong well into old age, avoiding aches and pains, and reversing arthritic pain if you have it already, by understanding what they need to stay healthy.

HOW TO KEEP YOUR BONES HEALTHY

Most people think of bones as something rather 'dead' – simply the scaffolding on which to hang the rest of the body. But there's a fascinating and, when you think about it, much more plausible theory emerging that suggests bones are a vital part of the metabolic system that controls our intake of energy, the amount of fat we store, how much insulin we produce, and so on. As we saw in Chapter 5, it's this system that is a major driver of our rising rate of chronic disease and it is also responsible for the changes that come with ageing.

Bones are made from a matrix of collagen, produced by vitamin C, into which bone-building minerals such as calcium, magnesium and potassium are deposited. Although they seem the strongest and most enduring part of us, our bones are in a constant flux, endlessly being destroyed and re-created. Cells called osteoclasts are the bone destroyers, whereas the osteoblasts create new bone – but age slows down this sequence of destruction and renewal.

Strategies for improving bone-mass density either focus on stimulating growth, helping to push minerals into the bone, or on preventing its breakdown. Weight-bearing exercise – such as walking – combined with eating sufficient protein, for example, stimulates bone growth. Getting enough vitamin D helps calcium to be absorbed into the bone, while the hormone oestrogen and drugs called bisphosphonates inhibit bone breakdown. B vitamins assist your body's methylation, and keep your homocysteine level ideal, which also helps to inhibit bone breakdown.

Most people who show up on a scan with osteoporosis or osteopenia (reduced bone mass), will be offered a bisphosphonate drug, so there are a few things that are worth knowing about them.

HOW EFFECTIVE ARE BISPHOSPHONATES?

The official figure given for the effectiveness of bisphosphonates in lowering the risk of having a hip fracture is 32 per cent, but although this sounds positive it's very misleading. A study undertaken in 2010 by researchers in Finland and published in the *British Medical Journal* concluded that if everyone in that country over the age of 50 had been put on a bisphosphonate – that would be 1.86 million people – just 343 hip fractures would have been avoided.[52] Meanwhile, the drug would have failed to prevent 7,068 of them. That is a long, long way from preventing 32 per cent, so how can the results be so poor and confusing?

The reason is that there is a big difference between how well drugs perform in clinical trials – the 32 per cent – and their results in the real world. Clinical trials are very artificial. As we have pointed out before, subjects are usually quite young, healthy and not taking any other drugs, and nurses will ensure that they take the drug for the trial. The patients who are given them on prescription, however, will very likely be older, frailer and starting to decline; usually they will have three or more other disorders and will be on several drugs for each of them. Furthermore, only about half the drugs prescribed are actually taken.

WHAT ARE YOUR CHANCES OF SUCCESS AGAINST THE SIDE EFFECTS?

How effective did bisphosphonates turn out to be when they became available on prescription? As a result of this mismatch between the trials and the real world, the Finnish researchers calculated that if everyone who had at least a 3 per cent risk of developing a fracture over the next ten years were treated with bisphosphonates, for every 667 people who took the drugs only one would avoid a fracture.

Side effects include upset stomach and inflammation of the oesophagus, if you don't remain sitting upright for 30–60 minutes daily after taking the drug. You might also develop cancer of the jaw bone (although this is rare), and what are called 'atypical' fractures of the thigh bone (femur) and a disturbed heart rhythm if you are female. So you need to weigh your chances of benefiting from the drug with that kind of rate of efficacy against the side effects.

What is more, we saw in Chapter 4 that if you are taking one of the proton pump inhibitor (PPI) drugs that suppress stomach acid – often given with bisphosphonates because heartburn can be a side effect – the benefit of the drug can drop to zero.[53] Both PPIs and bisphosphonates are on our list of drugs to avoid as you age (see Chapter 4), for these reasons.

The amount of vitamin D you have in your blood may also play a major role. Not only does research show that 75 per cent of people on bisphosphonates don't respond at all if they have the kind of low levels very common in the UK (below 50 nmol/l) but also getting double that amount would mean that you would be seven times more likely to have a favourable response to the drug.[54] It only costs your doctor a small amount – a fraction of the cost of a drug prescription– to have your vitamin D levels tested, but if your doctor doesn't want to test you, you can do it yourself (see Chapter 2 and Resources).

THE HIP-REPLACEMENT LOTTERY

It's worth knowing about how hip replacements, or indeed any other medical device, are tested. Hip replacements have brought relief to millions, but a shocking investigation by the *British Medical Journal* and the BBC news documentary *Panorama*, revealed a remarkable shortcoming in the regulation of all medical devices in Europe. The programme found that some models of hip used for replacement killed off bone and raised the levels of dangerous heavy metals in the blood, but although this was known by the regulatory bodies they were powerless to act, and the hip replacements in question are still being carried out. (The same problem appeared with regard to pacemakers as well.)

The problem is that the companies can introduce a new device to the market without being required to run any clinical trials, and if a company does conduct a trial, it can determine what the test consists of and then has no obligation to release the results to anyone, only to provide the regulator with a summary. If problems do arise, it is solely the responsibility of the company to look into them.[55]

This emphasises how important it is to look after your bones rather than relying on medical intervention.

VITAMIN D IS VITALLY IMPORTANT FOR BONE HEALTH

Osteoporosis becomes more common as you move north, suggesting a link between sunlight (which produces vitamin D in the body) and this condition. The vital role of vitamin D is well known. It helps deposit calcium and other minerals into the bones' collagen structure. Numerous studies have shown that the combination of vitamin D – at a daily intake of around 20–30mcg a day, along with 1,000mg-plus of calcium – improves bone mass density and reduces the risk of fractures.

It is certainly possible to make all the vitamin D you need from sun, depending on how near the equator you are, the season and your skin colour. In the UK, 20 to 30 minutes a day in the summer, with as much of your skin exposed as you are comfortable with, will keep you healthy. But between October and March the sun will provide very little and getting enough from your diet is challenging. Even eating three portions of oily fish a week and at least half a dozen eggs only gives you 15mcg. So to get around 30mcg that many experts now recommend as the minimum you will need supplements.

Vitamin D is a nutrient that we are going to keep recommending you supplement. It is essential for healthy muscles, joints and bones, and if you are already suffering from joint or muscle pain you might want to experiment with taking a higher dose. You can get vitamin D drops providing 25mcg per drop. One or two of these a day will really boost your vitamin D levels. They are well worth trying for a couple of months if you do have muscle or joint pain, or osteopenia or osteoporosis.

JUST TAKING CALCIUM ISN'T THE ANSWER

'Bones are made of calcium, and milk is rich in calcium, so drink milk to strengthen bones.' It's a good story, but it's very misleading. A recent review of studies giving calcium supplements finds that calcium alone doesn't significantly reduce risk of fractures in postmenopausal women[56] unless vitamin D is also given, and it doesn't increase bone mass density in children either. Marion Nestle, Professor of Nutrition at New York University, has long campaigned for good food and has also exposed the vested interests behind junk food. She is one of a growing number of experts who point out that there is no clear correlation between rates of osteoporosis and calcium intake from milk.[57] So, you and many medics may understandably be confused about calcium and bones.

Another recent study found that calcium alone, or even with vitamin D, slightly raised the risk of a heart attack,[58] while a third study found that getting more than 750mg was a waste of time. But such studies rarely consider the vitamin D levels of the patients, when low levels are linked with a greater risk of heart attack. What is more, giving a single mineral or vitamin is rarely effective.

In relation to calcium, your diet should provide around 800–1,000mg. The average intake is 900mg, because most people have a lot of dairy products. If you don't have dairy products but do eat seeds, nuts and beans on a regular basis you should still achieve 800mg calcium plus other bone-friendly minerals such as magnesium. To get the ideal 1,000mg intake means supplementing a further 100–200mg, which is what should be in your daily multivitamin–mineral.

Some nutritionists recommend getting 1,200–1,500mg of calcium later in life, which means supplementing a further 400–700mg of calcium in total. There's nothing wrong with this provided you also supplement the co-factor bone-building nutrients, which include magnesium, zinc, boron and vitamin D. A good multivitamin–mineral should provide these, plus at least 40mcg of vitamin K. This often-forgotten vitamin helps bone formation by stimulating a protein called osteocalcin, which also fixes calcium into the bone. Leafy green vegetables such as spinach, Swiss chard and Brussels sprouts are rich in vitamin K and are also good sources of calcium and magnesium. There are also bone-friendly formulas (see Resources) that might be worth taking as well to ensure you get the optimal levels for bone support.

MAKE SURE YOU EAT ENOUGH PROTEIN

The essential structure of your body and your bones is protein, which is found in meat, fish and eggs as well as beans, chickpeas, lentils, nuts and seeds. There's some disagreement about how much protein you need for healthy bones. Ongoing research by Dr Carlos Isales, an endocrinologist at the Georgia Health Sciences University in the US suggests that getting the correct amount and type of amino acids – which are the building blocks of protein – helps to stimulate bone building by affecting the stem cells. This also lowers fat production, high levels of which can be a problem when the diet is low in protein.

Official figures in both the US and the UK suggest that about a third of patients over 65 eat a diet that is both calorie and protein deficient. That, Isales explains, encourages the stem cells in your bone marrow to make fat rather than bone. 'Fat is the cheapest thing for your body to make,' he says, 'so making fat is the default.'

His team has already shown that the bones of mice put on a low-protein diet, which should have made them weaker, stayed strong when they were given an amino acid supplement. Together with vitamin D and calcium, the supplement triggers the signals that tell the body to make bone. 'Ultimately, we would like to give amino acid supplements to hospitalised patients,' says Isales, 'because that is where you see the highest rates of malnutrition.'[59]

The Anti-ageing Diet we'll be introducing to you in this book makes sure you get enough protein, but if you do have decreased bone-mass density or any joint degeneration disease, taking a good multivitamin–mineral twice a day, and an extra supplement that contains all the bone-building nutrients, is a good idea. Because collagen is made from vitamin C, we also recommend a daily intake of 1,800mg taken twice a day in divided doses. The most absorbable forms of calcium and magnesium are citrate, ascorbate and malate. These are always best taken twice with food. Also, avoid fizzy drinks, which contain phosphoric acid and caffeine, both of which leach calcium from bones. And don't drink lots of coffee – one cup a day is enough.

THE HOMOCYSTEINE CONNECTION

In Chapter 2 we mentioned that homocysteine would be appearing frequently throughout the book because a high level is connected to a number of health problems. One important discovery that few people are aware of is the link between homocysteine, low B_{12} levels and bone and joint health. High homocysteine, you may recall, is an indicator of poor methylation, which is one of the critical anti-ageing processes we discussed in Chapter 5. Over the last five years, there have been more and more studies linking high homocysteine and low B_{12} levels to an increased risk of fractures, osteoporosis and decreased bone-mass density. Your homocysteine level predicts both your risk of osteoporosis and bone-mass density, especially in women.[60]

Vitamin B_{12} levels, essential for keeping homocysteine down, decrease as you age, because it becomes increasingly poorly absorbed. A high homocysteine level means poor methylation, and both methylation and B_{12} are needed to build bone. In studies, lowering homocysteine by giving extra B_{12} plus folic acid to those over 65 reduced their risk of fractures.[61] It looks as if homocysteine actually damages bone by encouraging its breakdown and interfering with the collagen structure that holds bone together.[62]

BEWARE PPI 'PRAZOLE' DRUGS

One truly worrying trend is the widespread use of proton pump inhibitor (PPI) drugs. These stop you making stomach acid, which is required for the absorption of calcium, magnesium and vitamin B_{12}.[63] This is one of the 'drugs to avoid' we discussed in Chapter 4. These drugs are known to increase the risk of fracture, doubling the risk in those over 50 if taken long term, according to a study in the *Journal of the American Medical Association*.[64] If you are on these drugs, at the very least have your homocysteine level checked (see Resources) but, ideally, stop taking them (see Secret 8 for drug-free solutions to digestive problems).

DOES CONVENTIONAL HRT PROTECT YOUR BONES?

Until the results of a large trial that showed that HRT (hormone replacement therapy) raised the risk of breast cancer, it was widely prescribed to protect women's bones. Millions of women have now switched to the bisphosphonate drugs to maintain bone mass, although they have a range of side effects. Female hormones normally protect bones up to the menopause. Progesterone builds bone by stimulating the osteoblast,[65] while oestrogen slows the rate osteoclasts break down old bone. Perimenopausal women start losing bone mass faster as their hormone production becomes less regular.[66] After the menopause, women produce less oestrogen and virtually no progesterone.

If you take HRT, you get extra oestrogen plus synthetic progestins, which are progesterone-like chemicals. Although some studies, such as the Women's Health Initiative trial, have shown a small decreased risk of hip fracture,[67] it is no longer recommended as the first choice of therapy for prevention of osteoporosis[68] in the UK, as the risks outweigh the benefits. You have to take it for seven years or more to maintain bone mass[69] and even then, bone mineral density rapidly declines once you stop, and the longer you take it, the greater your risk of developing breast and womb cancer.

THE ALTERNATIVES TO BISPHOSPHONATES

If you don't want to start on bisphosphonates, what can you do? Not all women experience loss of bone mass around the menopause, so the first step is to get your diet and lifestyle as bone-friendly as possible, following the advice in this chapter. If your hormone levels have been tested and you haven't got enough to protect your bones, however, or if you are suffering symptoms from the menopause (or if you are a middle-aged man whose testosterone levels are too low), then there is certainly a case for supplementing with bio-identical hormones, rather than the synthetic ones used in HRT. One of the differences between bio-identical hormones and those used in HRT is that natural progesterone helps to build bone while the non-identical form used in HRT (progestin) can thin bones. Progesterone works by stimulating the bone-building osteoblasts while oestrogen damps down the demolition team of the osteoclasts. It's possible that progesterone plays a larger role in bone protection than oestrogen, although the results from trials are mixed. Testosterone is needed for bone building in men. We explain the role of bio-identical hormones in Secret 10 and in Part Three, Chapter 8.

BONES ARE METABOLICALLY ACTIVE

Eating a low-GL diet, as described in this book, and therefore keeping your insulin levels down, is another important key to bone health. (Secret 3 explains the importance of this way of eating for healthy ageing.)

The links between bone and metabolism are being explored by Professor Gerard Karsenty, Chair of Genetics and Development at

Columbia University, New York. His team have found that the insulin you produce after a meal doesn't only clear sugar but, among other things, it also triggers the 'clasts' in your bones to start building, because you've got the resources to do so – making bone uses up a lot of energy. That starts a whole sequence: the 'blasts' go to work as well, and that releases a hormone called osteocalcin into the bloodstream that stimulates insulin production from the B cells in the pancreas. Other metabolic players become involved, including the hormone leptin (which signals that you are full from eating) and serotonin from the brain.[70] This work hasn't had any practical effect yet, although osteocalcin is being looked at as a possible diabetes drug. But it does suggest that ensuring the natural rhythm of bone creation and destruction might also help to maintain a healthy metabolism.

THE FITNESS FACTOR

The importance of weight-bearing exercise for maintaining strong bones was brought vividly home when the first astronauts returned from space with seriously weakened bones after only a short period of weightlessness. Weight-bearing exercise can be as simple as walking, dancing or gardening. You can increase your bone mass by 5–10 per cent with just two or three weight-bearing exercise sessions a week.

Another option for bone health is the vibrating power plate – used by fitness celebs like Madonna – and now often found in gyms and rehabilitation clinics. A recent study with mice at an age equivalent to 55–60 human years, found that a 30-minute daily session on the vibrating plate kept their bones solid. The vibrations had a particular effect on the density of the hip and femur (in the thigh). 'It seems as if it would be a particularly good option for people with limited mobility,' commented the lead author, Dr Karl Wenger of the Medical College of Georgia in the US. The movement is transmitted into bone cells where it triggers the production of new bone-forming osteoblasts.[74]

The drawback to just relying on weight-bearing exercise is that it's usually concentrated on the lower part of the body. Therefore, it's best to add some resistance training that uses your upper body muscles too. Amazingly, you can maintain and build a significant amount of upper-body muscle in just five minutes three times a week. See Part 3, Chapter 4.

KEEPING YOUR JOINTS HEALTHY AND PAIN-FREE

There are few things more symbolic of growing old than the swollen finger joints and painful walk that come with the first signs of arthritic degeneration of joints. Diagnosed arthritis currently affects over 7.3 million people in the UK, and numbers are expected to increase, particularly relating to arthritis affecting the knees, if obesity rates continue to rise, because extra weight puts a lot of strain on them. By the age of 65, 80 per cent of us will have some evidence of arthritis.

Simple wear-and-tear on joints is a major cause, and sports such as football will increase your risk. But there may be something else going on that we don't understand yet, according to Phillip Conaghan, rheumatologist and spokesperson for the Arthritis Research Campaign. 'We start seeing signs of it in people in their thirties and forties, although that could be because they are more ready to visit the doctor.'

All of our joints have a protective layer of cartilage covering the end of each bone. This thins in arthritis and becomes pitted, or wears out completely, allowing the bones to rub together. This is what causes the pain and inflammation. Conventional treatment concentrates on treating the pain with over-the-counter painkillers and anti-inflammatories. Steroid injections are not a cure, although they can bring relief for several months. Over 150,000 people have knee and hip replacements in the UK each year when the pain becomes too severe, although losing weight and exercising can improve symptoms as much as joint replacements, according to the Arthritis Research Campaign.

We've already covered some of the problems inherent in long-term use of aspirin-like NSAID drugs in Chapter 4: damage to the stomach and gut lining and a cause of internal bleeding. A large study in 2011 of 22,000 patients with hypertension and heart disease found that these drugs double the risk of heart disease deaths in the elderly. The authors concluded that use of NSAIDs should be avoided 'wherever possible'.[72]

For every 100 patients taking NSAIDs for a year you would expect to see an extra 4.4 heart attacks, strokes or deaths.

Do NSAIDs work for arthritic pain? A review of 23 trials, including one involving 10,845 patients with arthritic knee pain, concludes: 'NSAIDs can reduce short term pain in osteoarthritis of the knee slightly better than placebo, but the current analysis does not support long term use of NSAIDs for this condition. As serious adverse effects are associated with oral NSAIDs, only limited use can be recommended.' What's particularly significant about this review is that it is the only trial that looked at the long-term effects of NSAIDs versus placebo on pain, and it showed 'no significant effect of NSAIDs compared with placebo at one to four years'.[73]

Obviously, when you are in pain you have to have something to reduce it, so what other options do you have?

KEEP YOUR CARTILAGE HEALTHY TOO

There are two sides to bone and joint health. The first is keeping bone and the cartilage that surrounds it strong and healthy, and the second is reducing the inflammation, which is the primary cause of the cartilage destruction that makes joints painful.

Cartilage is made up from collagen, which comes from vitamin C and a sugar protein compound called proteoglycans that is made from glucosamine. The only dietary source of glucosamine is prawn or shrimp shells, although crunching them up is not to everybody's taste!

Glucosamine is a basic building material of your joints, while the mineral sulphur acts like the nails that hold it together. Everyone knows about the link between glucosamine and healthy joints, although you'd do better with the more absorbable form, which is glucosamine hydrochloride. The best source of sulphur, found in onions, garlic and eggs, is MSM (see below). The combination of glucosamine hydrochloride and MSM has proven particularly effective.[74]

DOES GLUCOSAMINE WORK?

The popularity of glucosamine for joints dates to a 2001 study published in the *Lancet*, where Belgian investigators reported that it actually slowed the progression of osteoarthritis of the knee[75] while the knees of the patients taking the placebo steadily worsened. In another study, 1,500mg of glucosamine sulphate daily reduced knee pain as effectively as 1,200mg of ibuprofen and was better tolerated.[76] It's also been shown to be as good as NSAID painkillers for easing arthritic pain and inflammation, with less irritation to the stomach.

Not all studies have been positive, however. A placebo-controlled trial with 1,500mg a day for six months, given for back pain, found no benefit.[77] Recently, a combination of trials that involved a total of 3,800 patients found that neither glucosamine nor a type called chondroitin alone or together reduced joint pain or affected the narrowing of joint space. The authors recommended that neither product should be paid for on the NHS.[78]

Nevertheless, glucosamine may work better in combination with other anti-inflammatories, such as omega-3 fish oils for hip or knee osteoarthritis.[79] Almost half (44 per cent) of those on the combination had a greater than 80 per cent reduction in pain, compared to (32 per cent) taking glucosamine alone. Another trial found taking it with MSM was significantly more effective than glucosamine alone.[80]

MSM – A GOOD SOURCE OF SULPHUR

Methylsulfonylmethane (MSM) is a source of the essential mineral sulphur that is involved in a multitude of key body functions, including pain control, detoxification and tissue building. Extraordinary results have been reported for pain relief from arthritis.[81] Patients taking 2,250mg a day had an 80 per cent improvement in pain within six weeks, compared with 20 per cent for those who had taken dummy pills.[82] It's available both as a balm and in capsules. The therapeutic dose appears to be 1,500–3,000mg a day. Some people experience a worsening of symptoms in the first ten days, followed by an improvement.

B VITAMINS – THE NEGLECTED ARTHRITIS TREATMENT

Much less familiar than MSM and glucosamine are the B vitamins – a key element in the process of ageing. Inflammation is the root of the problem with arthritis, and inflammation is one of the symptoms found with the 'inner global warming' we explained on page 77, which is linked to high levels of homocysteine (explained in Chapter 2). These excessive levels promote the release of pro-inflammatory agents in the body.[83]

What is more, people with osteoarthritis often have other disorders marked by excess inflammation, such as diabetes, heart disease, hypertension, insulin resistance and excess weight. Homocysteine levels are frequently found to be much higher in rheumatoid arthritis sufferers[84] as well as those with ankylosing spondylitis, an inflammatory arthritic disease of the spine.[85]

Since rheumatoid arthritis is a 'systemic' disease – where the whole body's chemistry is out of balance and many tissues and organs other than the joints are affected – one would suspect that homocysteine plays a leading role. And it does. Research from the Department of Biochemistry at the University Hospital in Madrid, Spain, examined the homocysteine scores of women with rheumatoid arthritis versus those without. There was a massive difference. The average homocysteine score for those with rheumatoid arthritis was a sky-high 17.3, compared to 7.6 for those without![86]

Homocysteine is thought to directly damage joints[87] and other tissues. All of this suggests that reducing homocysteine may well help to keep your bones and joints healthy. Yet, disappointingly, very little research has yet been done to test the homocysteine theory of arthritis. A rare exception was a study nearly 20 years ago by researchers at the American College of Nutrition in Clearwater, Florida. They gave B_{12} and folate supplements to 26 people who had been taking non-steroidal anti-inflammatory, pain-relieving drugs (NSAIDs) for osteoarthritis of the hands for an average of more than five years.[88] The participants reported less tenderness in their hands and improved ability to grip objects but suffered *none* of the notorious NSAID side effects, which include premature death from kidney failure, ulcers and bleeding in the digestive tract.

As many as two in five people aged over 60 are B_{12} deficient, and supplementing 500mcg a day at least is needed to correct it. Although fish, meat, eggs and milk all contain B_{12}, only milk and fish increase blood B_{12} levels. Even so, you are unlikely to get more than 3mcg of B_{12} from your food. To prevent a deficiency we would recommend taking 10mcg a day.

Vitamin B_6, another homocysteine-lowering vitamin, has also proven helpful for arthritis sufferers. Back in the 1950s, an insightful physician from Mount Pleasant in Texas, Dr John Ellis, found that giving B_6 in higher daily doses of 50mg helped to control pain and restore joint mobility in his arthritic patients.[89] Vitamin B_6 shrinks inflamed membranes that line the weight-bearing surfaces of the joints, perhaps by helping decrease homocysteine and increasing SAMe and glutathione, both proven anti-inflammatory agents. B_6 also helps to regulate production of the prostaglandins, the body's own anti-inflammatory agents.

CASE STUDY: ED

Ed had always kept himself fit, by playing tennis and running, but he started to experience joint pain in his mid thirties and had operations on both knees to repair damage to the cartilage. By his mid forties he was suffering from severe arthritis, with ever-increasing pain, and he started taking a variety of anti-inflammatory drugs. But his knees just got worse, giving him excruciating pain after playing golf, his favourite leisure pursuit.

When I (Patrick) met him he was aged 57 and could barely walk without pain, let alone pursue his passion for golf. I told him to read and follow my book, *Say No to Arthritis*, and gave him a list of supplements to take; this included 1.5g of glucosamine, essential fats, high-dose niacinamide (500mg) and pantothenic acid (1,000mg), 3g of vitamin C, 250mg (400iu) of vitamin E and a high-potency multivitamin.

He followed the diet and took the supplements religiously every day. Although there was little improvement in the first two months, by the third month his knees were feeling better. By six months he was virtually pain-free.

'I would never have believed my pain could be reduced by such a large degree, and not return, no matter how much activity I do in a day or week.'

Five years on, Ed remains 95 per cent pain-free and has had no return or worsening of his symptoms – and he needs no medication. He regularly plays golf. I've switched him over to a daily nutrition supplement pack, which contains vitamins C and E, omega-3 and 6 oils, antioxidants and B vitamins. I am also giving him 1,500mg glucosamine hydrochloride with MSM and a combination of the herbs boswellia, hop extract and olive pulp extract, which is a superb antioxidant. I find these to be the most effective remedies for promoting comfortable joints, together with a healthy diet, low in meat and dairy produce, and high in fish, flax seeds, fruit and vegetables. Ed is living proof that the body can heal itself if you give it the right nutrients.

OIL YOUR JOINTS WITH OMEGA-3S

Omega-3 fish oils are one of the most potent natural anti-inflammatories, because they turn into type-3 prostaglandins, which switch off pain and swelling. There have been lots of positive studies proving benefit. A meta-analysis of 17 randomised, controlled trials assessing the pain-relieving effects of omega-3s in patients with rheumatoid arthritis or joint pain concluded, 'Supplementation with omega-3 PUFAs for 3–4 months reduces joint pain intensity by 26 per cent, the number of minutes of morning stiffness by 43 per cent, the number of painful and/or tender joints by 29 per cent, and NSAID consumption by 40 per cent.'[90]

We recommend both eating oily fish and supplementing omega-3 fish oils daily as part of your Healthy-ageing Action Plan.

STAY TRIM AND KEEP YOUR BODY MOVING

If the cartilage in the joints degenerates, the joints become painful when you move. Two major causes of cartilage degeneration are too much weight on the joints and poor postural alignment. Being overweight doesn't just stress the joints, it also switches the body into an inflammatory state. So, losing weight helps ease pressure on the joints and switches off the inflammatory process. Our low-GL Anti-ageing Diet is a highly suitable way to help to protect your joints.

Joints need space to move and that's why exercises that strengthen and stretch them are so important. Exercises need to aim for mobility in the back as well as the joints. Most people don't do these on a regular basis, however, and then suffer the consequences as they get older. That is why one of the hallmarks of unhealthy ageing is losing flexibility. Building in regular – and preferably daily – joint-stretching exercises is a vital part of keeping your joints healthy.

My (Patrick's) favourite exercises in this regard are yoga and Psychocalisthenics. What I like about Psychocalisthenics is that it really does work all your joints and muscles, and it develops back strength and keeps you supple, but it only takes 16 minutes a day. It's been the basis of my exercise routine for almost 30 years and now, in my fifties, I am as supple as I was as a teenager. You can learn Psychocalisthenics from a DVD but it's best to learn it in a half-day training session (see Resources for details). The only disadvantage is that if you are already significantly overweight or have back problems, the exercises may be a bit difficult to start with.

If you have arthritis in your knees, you need to strengthen your quadriceps – the main thigh muscles. You'd be better doing it with some non-weight-bearing exercise such as cycling or swimming, but don't make the joint pain worse. One point to remember is that if you are on cholesterol-lowering statin drugs and your muscles feel weak and painful you are advised to take a supplement of CoQ_{10}. Statins block this essential enzyme, which is needed for energy production.

Yoga is also excellent. You need to find a good teacher, but that shouldn't be hard, and it's important to join a beginner's or mixed-ability class if you're new to yoga. The teacher will advise you on how to tailor the postures the best way for you. Yoga, and also Pilates, are both good for flexibility and building strength, but the critical thing is finding something you enjoy and then doing it regularly.

NATURE'S PAINKILLERS

George Lewith, Professor of Health Research at the University of Southampton, has conducted a review of non-drug treatments for arthritis, and says, 'There's not enough research on them because they are not patentable … and they don't work for everyone but they are certainly worth trying so long as your weight is reasonable and you're exercising.'

The one that came out top was capsaicin gel, an extract of chilli available as a cream on prescription, which works by reducing 'substance P', a neurotransmitter that transmits pain signals in the brain. This is closely followed by Phytodolor – a herbal mixture of aspen, ash bark and golden rod, which cuts the production of inflammatory prostaglandins that cause pain. Equally effective is the amino acid SAMe, which is part of the methylation pathway affected by B vitamins.

Natural foods are full of potent anti-inflammatories, and our top six favourites are turmeric, containing curcumin; olives, rich in hydroxytyrosol;[91] onions (especially red) for their quercetin; and also lots of omega-3 fish oils. Eating an onion a day is associated with a 5 per cent increase in bone mass.[92] Turmeric, the yellow spice in curry, has anti-cancer[93] and anti-inflammatory properties.[94] Quercetin, found richly in red onions and cranberries, appears to be anti-allergenic and anti-inflammatory,[95] although there's a need for clinical trials.

Others with claims for anti-inflammatory qualities include:

- **Boswellia** Also known as boswellin or Indian frankincense.

- **Hyaluronic acid (HA)** is a key component of your cartilage, responsible for moving nutrients into your cells and moving waste out.

- **Astaxanthin** is one of the most powerful lipophilic antioxidants yet discovered and is the most abundant carotenoid pigment found in crabs, salmon, trout, shrimps, prawns and krill; it is now available in supplements. Studies have found that it can help support joint health and mobility.

- **Ginger** This spicy root is anti-inflammatory and offers pain relief and stomach-settling properties. Fresh ginger works well steeped in boiling water as a tea or grated into vegetable juice.

Of course, you can, and should, eat as many of these as possible, and they are included in our Healthy-ageing Diet in Part Three, but the real magic, if you are suffering from joint pain, comes when you supplement concentrates of these together. Nutritional therapists give 500mg of quercetin (the equivalent of 20 red onions). The combination of glucosamine, MSM and omega-3s, together with other natural anti-inflammatories, is a winning formula if you suffer from joint aches and pains. You can find combination supplements that combine many of these effective remedies. In Part Three we'll explain what's worth supplementing depending on your current health issues.

When you put all these factors together, miracles *can* happen, as in the case of Ruth:

CASE STUDY: RUTH

I had osteoarthritis most of my life. When I was 45, I was diagnosed with rheumatoid arthritis. I was going downhill. In fact my fingers were clawed. I really had to bend them open in the morning, like little twigs breaking. Then I heard about Patrick Holford, and I went to the Institute for Optimum Nutrition where I learnt about diet. I changed my whole diet and lifestyle, and started taking supplements. Everything got better very quickly and, after a few years, I was so much better. I am now 77 and I feel absolutely super – no pain of any description, all due to diet, supplements and a positive mental attitude.

SUMMARY

To keep your bones and your joints young:

- Eat more nuts, seeds and beans – high in bone-friendly minerals.
- Eat oily fish (salmon, mackerel, herring, sardines) at least three times a week for extra omega-3 and vitamin D.
- Exercise every day, including some weight-bearing, joint-stretching, back-strengthening and muscle-building exercises (see Part Three, Chapter 4).
- Make an effort to lose weight if you are overweight (see Secret 3).

In terms of supplements:

- Check your homocysteine level. If it is high (above 9mcmol/l) supplement high-dose B_6, B_{12} and folic acid (see Part Three, Chapter 7).
- Take a twice-daily multivitamin–mineral that provides at least 15mcg of vitamin D, 40mcg of vitamin K, 100–400mg of calcium, 150mg of magnesium and 1mg of boron; plus 1,000mg of vitamin C and an omega-3 supplement twice a day.

CONTINUED...

See Part Three, Chapter 7 for your supplement programme.

For people with osteoporosis

- Get outdoors for at least 30 minutes a day in the summer, to synthesise vitamin D, but for that time don't use sunscreen. Be sensible – watch you only go slightly pink and never burn (see Secret 5).
- Eat plenty of nuts, seeds, beans and greens, which are high in calcium, magnesium and other bone-friendly minerals.
- If you have decreasing bone-mass density, consider bio-identical hormones (see Secret 10).
- If you have joint problems or decreased bone-mass density, take a bone-mineral formula as well.

For people with arthritis

- Eat plenty of red onions, garlic, eggs and olives, and spice up your food with liberal quantities of turmeric.
- If you have joint aches and pains, make sure you are getting 500–1,000mg of the EPA omega-3 oil a day.
- If you have joint problems, supplement a natural anti-inflammatory formula providing glucosamine, MSM, turmeric, quercetin, olive and hop extracts.

See Part Three, Chapter 7 for your general supplement programme. See also Recommended Reading for other helpful books on these topics.

Secret 3

BEAT THE BULGE, PREVENT DIABETES AND BOOST YOUR ENERGY

Only a few years ago losing weight was, in theory, very straightforward. Being fat was just a matter of consuming more calories than you burnt up, so all you had to do to stay slim was either eat less or exercise more. Simple. As for cutting your risk of diabetes or heart disease, the answer was to make your low-calorie diet also low in fat – partly because fat blocked up your arteries and partly because fat was more calorie dense than carbohydrates.

Now, though, it is increasingly clear that every part of that official advice was wrong or misleading. The first mistake – known about for years but largely ignored – was that cutting back on calories continuously for days or weeks slowed down your metabolism, so as soon as your intake began to creep up as you started eating normally again, weight went back on even faster than before. So, you were set up for repeated diet failure. The second mistake – even more disastrous – was that cutting out fat meant it had to be replaced by something else, and that 'something else' has been sugar and more refined carbs, especially those based on white flour. As we've seen earlier in the book, though, sugar is a refined carbohydrate, and it is this, as well as a general tendency to 'fill up' on white flour products and starchy foods, that unbalances our blood sugar level, making us put on weight and, eventually, leading to diabetes.

The low-fat, added-sugar diet is hardly the way to keep diabetes at bay and there are now some experts who claim it is very likely that the low-fat diet has actually contributed to the diabetes epidemic. Researchers at Emory University have found that the sugar and carbs regularly added to low-fat foods affected two markers for heart disease risk: it pushed up fat in the blood (triglycerides) and reduced the 'good' HDL cholesterol, in contrast to saturated fat.[96] Exactly the opposite of the supposed benefits.

Meanwhile, the low-fat strategy has not had the promised effect on heart disease either. When Meir Stampfer, professor of nutrition and epidemiology at Harvard School of Public Health, compared the results of those on a low-fat or a low-carbohydrate diet he found that those who ate the most saturated fat ended up with the healthiest ratio of HDL to LDL (the 'bad' cholesterol) and lost twice as much weight.[97]

As a result of such upsets, the popularity of 'low-carb' diets has soared. The first of these was developed by Dr Atkins and outraged orthodoxy when people eating lots of protein and fats and very little carbs lost weight! Since then there have been popular variations, such as the South Beach Diet, the Dukan Diet, and so on. Now, this movement has gone one step further in Sweden where there's a wave of eating a low-carb, high-fat (LCHF) diet. Butter sales have gone up and, for the first time, Sweden is apparently reporting a small decrease, rather than an increase, in obesity! So, what's going on?

THE DIET THAT *DOES* WORK

If you are not a diet-and-nutrition fanatic, keeping up with the latest twists and turns gets very confusing. Some media experts fall back on advice to 'eat a healthy balanced diet' without any clear information about what that might involve. There is a way through the diet jungle, though. You may remember that in Chapter 6 we explained about how the American geneticist Professor Cynthia Kenyon described how she had found that giving glucose to her long-lived lab worms tipped them back into their normal 20-day life span. In other words, having extended their life span by adjusting their genes through their diet, she then completely destroyed this by giving them glucose. This emphasises the destructive role of glucose (through sugars and refined carbohydrates) on our efforts to stay fit, healthy and youthful. It also means that if we want to lose weight *and* cut the risk of diabetes and heart disease – and possibly live longer as well – we can do that quite easily if we reduce the quantity, but increase the quality, of the carbohydrates we eat.

There was another crucial piece of information in that chapter. Increased amounts of glucose (the substance carbohydrates are turned into in the body before the surplus becomes fat) trigger increased amounts of insulin, and some researchers now think that too much insulin is also linked with a raised risk of cancer. In 2011 a large review by the respected Cochrane Collaboration of over 50 studies on the heart-protection benefits of reducing the fat in your diet found that 'there was no clear benefit' if you replaced the fat with starchy foods.[98] This is precisely what the officially approved low-fat diet has been doing for decades. So, if you significantly reduce fat but then replace it with carbohydrate, you will have weight problems as well as potentially some serious health problems.

If want to eat to age well and stay healthy, here are the main things to look out for in a diet, whether it's a weight-loss diet or a diet to maintain optimum fitness:

- A diet that doesn't make the mistake of leaving you hungry all the time so that your metabolism slows down and any weight loss is rapidly replaced once you stop.
- It needs to contain the healthy fats, like omega-3s, that were often ignored by the old low-fat diets.
- You want to eat some carbohydrates, but not the ones that will push your glucose and insulin levels up.

The diet that fits the bill is called the low-glycemic (meaning low-glucose-producing) diet and it's what we recommend in this book. And we are not alone. Recently a large analysis of studies involving 350,000 patients concluded: 'There is no clear benefit of substituting carbohydrates for saturated fat, although there might be a benefit if the carbohydrate is unrefined and has a low glycemic index.'[99]

Essentially, following a low-glycemic diet means avoiding the kind of carbohydrates that rapidly push up your blood glucose levels – such as white bread, croissants, cakes, sugar, and so on, and replacing them with more complex carbohydrates that release their glucose more slowly. Some practical details follow. If you need to lose weight, it will certainly help with that, but the real benefit is the way that it can lower metabolic syndrome, or the 'internal global warming' we first mentioned on page 77.

WHY IT'S SO IMPORTANT TO AVOID METABOLIC SYNDROME

All kinds of markers for increasing ill health are raised if your insulin levels are too high and your body is heading for metabolic syndrome, as is illustrated below.

Conditions associated with metabolic syndrome

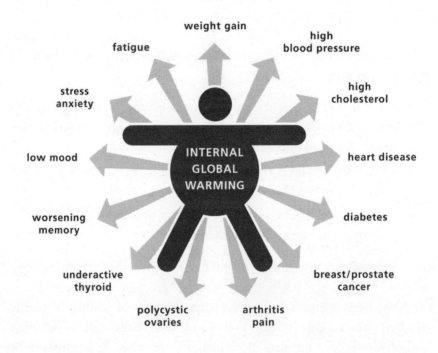

You can find out whether you have metabolic syndrome using this questionnaire. If you would prefer to fill this out online, and get your Metabolic Check score, visit www.patrickholford.com, as it is included in the online 100% Health Check.

Questionnaire: do you have metabolic syndrome?

	Yes	No
Part 1		
1. Are you aged 40 or over?	☐	☐
2. Are you or both your parents of African, South Asian, Hispanic or Native American origin?	☐	☐
3. Are you a woman with a waist circumference greater than 89cm (35in)?	☐	☐
4. Are you an Asian man with a waist circumference greater than 94cm (37in)?	☐	☐
5. Are you a white or black man with a waist greater than 102cm (40in)?	☐	☐
(To answer each of the next three questions see page 19 to calculate your BMI):		
6. Is your BMI 30 or more?	☐	☐
7. Is your BMI 27 or more?	☐	☐
8. Is your BMI 24 or more?	☐	☐
9. Have your parents or siblings been diagnosed with:		
a. diabetes?	☐	☐
b. heart disease?	☐	☐
c. high cholesterol?	☐	☐
d. high blood pressure?	☐	☐
10. Are you rarely wide awake within 20 minutes of rising?	☐	☐
11. Do you need tea, coffee, a cigarette or something sweet to get you going in the morning?	☐	☐
12. Do you crave chocolate, sweet foods, bread, cereal or pasta?	☐	☐
13. Do you often have energy slumps during the day or after meals?	☐	☐
14. Is your energy less than it used to be?	☐	☐

	Yes	No
15. Are you gaining weight and finding it hard to lose even though you're not eating more than usual or exercising less?	☐	☐
16. If you exercise for only a short period of time do your muscles feel tired?	☐	☐
17. Are you too tired to exercise?	☐	☐
18. Do you often forget things or have difficulty concentrating?	☐	☐
19. Do you quite often feel down or depressed, sad and defeated?	☐	☐
20. Have you been diagnosed with clinical depression?	☐	☐
21. Do you feel stressed or anxious and tend to overreact to unexpected situations?	☐	☐
22. Do you often feel angry, edgy and irritable?	☐	☐
23. Do you drink alcohol most days?	☐	☐
24. Do you smoke cigarettes every day?	☐	☐
25. Do you smoke at least ten cigarettes each day?	☐	☐
26. Do you eat less than one serving of vegetables each day?	☐	☐
27. Do you eat fewer than five pieces of fresh fruit each week?	☐	☐
28. Do you eat oily fish (salmon, tuna, herring, sardines, mackerel) less than twice a week?	☐	☐
29. Do you eat red meat (lamb, beef), fried foods or crisps?	☐	☐
30. Do you have aching or sore joints or arthritis?	☐	☐
31. Do you suffer from acne, dry flaky skin or eczema?	☐	☐
32. Has your sex drive decreased?	☐	☐
33. Have you been diagnosed with PCOS (women only)?	☐	☐
34. Do you have difficulty getting or maintaining an erection (men only)?	☐	☐

	Yes	No
35. Are you infertile or impotent, or have you been having trouble conceiving?	☐	☐
36. Do you find it hard to fall asleep (generally taking longer than 30 minutes)?	☐	☐
37. Do you wake frequently in the night or very early in the morning and find it hard to get back to sleep?	☐	☐
38. Do you wake up feeling tired and exhausted?	☐	☐
39. Do you feel sleepy during the day or nod off when being driven/in meetings/on the train/in front of the TV?	☐	☐

Score 2 for each 'yes' answer and 0 for each 'no'.

Total score: ☐

Part 2

	Yes	No	Don't know
1. Is your total cholesterol above 6mmol/l?	☐	☐	☐
2. Is your HDL cholesterol below 1.29 (women) or 1.04 (men)?	☐	☐	☐
3. Is your blood pressure greater than 130/85?	☐	☐	☐
4. Is your glycosylated haemoglobin (HbA1c) greater than 5.5 per cent but lower than 7 per cent?	☐	☐	☐
5. Is your glycosylated haemoglobin (HbA1c) greater than 7 per cent?	☐	☐	☐
6. Is your fasting blood sugar level greater than 5mmol/l (90mg/Dl) but lower than 7.0mmol/l (125mg/Dl)?	☐	☐	☐
7. Is your fasting blood sugar level greater than 7.0mmol/l (90mg/Dl)?	☐	☐	☐

Score 2 for each 'yes' answer, 1 for each 'don't know' and 0 for each 'no'.

Total score: ☐

RATING YOUR METABOLIC-SYNDROME RISK

Less than 20: very low risk

You have a very low metabolic-syndrome risk at present; however, modern living and a hectic lifestyle can easily take their toll on the body. Taking care over your diet, including regular exercise and finding time to relax and recharge your batteries, will keep your risk low and help to safeguard your physical and mental health.

21–40: low risk

You have a small metabolic-syndrome risk, so this is the time to make changes to reverse it. Start following a low-GL diet, and make some positive changes to your lifestyle, including regular exercise and finding time to relax and recharge your batteries. Together, these will keep your risk low and help to safeguard your physical and mental health.

41–60: medium risk

This score indicates a medium risk of metabolic syndrome and suggests you have started along the road to poor health. You may have developed a degree of insulin resistance, perhaps experiencing fluctuations in energy and mood on a daily basis. Addressing lifestyle factors, such as eating sugar and the GL level of your diet, as well as high degrees of stress, alcohol and cigarette use, where appropriate, are some of the changes that could have a significant impact on your overall state of well-being.

61 or more: high risk

You have a high risk of metabolic syndrome and may have already been diagnosed with any of the diseases associated with an advanced state of 'internal global warming', such as diabetes, cardiovascular disease or depression. As you start to make the dietary changes recommended in this book, however, you can greatly reduce your metabolic-syndrome risk, and the symptoms that you are currently experiencing should begin to improve, as you take your first steps on the path to better health.

If you are at risk, follow a low-GL diet, and also read the section on Alternate Day Dieting on page 297.

If you have now completed the metabolic syndrome checklist and noticed many of the symptoms of internal global warming, you may be at risk of insulin resistance. If you are concerned, you should ask your doctor to check your glycosylated haemoglobin level, which is the best early indicator of risk. This test is also available as a home-test kit (see Resources).

THE DANGERS OF TOO MUCH INSULIN

If your doctor runs a health check on you and the results are similar to the ones listed below, your internal global warming is rising and you are well on your way towards the catastrophe of diabetes.

- High average blood sugar, which is more precisely measured by something called glycosylated haemoglobin – written as HbA1c.
- High blood pressure (above 130/85).
- Increased waist circumference (above 102cm/40in in men or 89cm/35in in women).
- High blood fats, called triglycerides (above 3.9).
- Low HDL cholesterol (the 'good' cholesterol – below 1.03 in men and 1.3 in women).

So what is behind all this? When people are talking about diabetes, they often focus on the dangers of raised blood sugar and the importance of bringing it down, either with pills that boost insulin production or, at a more advanced stage, by injecting insulin directly. But the root of the problem is that your body has become insulin resistant; in other words the muscles and fat cells where insulin stores excess calories need more and more to respond to it. It's exactly the same sort of state you are in when you become an addict – you need more and more of the drug to have an effect.

What's put you in this state is simply eating too much sugar and refined carbohydrates. They push up your blood glucose level and you have to keep pumping out more insulin to send the excess amount in the blood to be stored as fat. Gradually, the receptors for insulin become blunted through overuse and start to shut down, so you have to make more and more insulin. The more insulin you make, in response to eating carbohydrates or something sweet, the more insulin insensitive you become, so you have to make even more.

Your blood sugar level now stays too high for too long, damaging your arteries, kidneys and brain, then, when the insulin finally kicks in, all that excess glucose is dumped into storage as fat, so you gain weight. Your blood sugar level then hits rock bottom, so you feel extremely tired, grumpy and hungry, and go hunting for more carbohydrates (or caffeine). Eventually, when you are so insulin resistant your body is unable to bring your blood sugar level down, you develop diabetes. This progression is shown in the figure below.

The progression of glucose and insulin towards diabetes

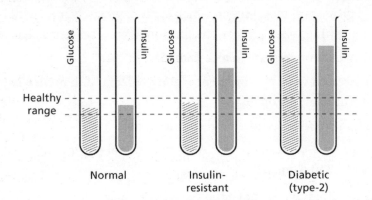

It's a vicious circle. Reversing insulin resistance – or preferably making sure you don't develop it in the first place – is a fundamental key to healthy ageing, because the implications of insulin resistance are not just that you will be overweight with high blood sugar. Raised blood pressure and more fat in the blood, as well as less of the good cholesterol, are also linked to insulin resistance and they lead to other health problems associated with ageing.

Constant high blood glucose leads to glycation (see Chapter 5) – a process that creates a sticky substance that clogs up the working of cells all over the body and brain. Glycation causes your brain to go foggy, your memory to get worse, your muscles to feel tired, your arteries to harden and your skin to look older, with more 'age' spots and darkened areas. Insulin resistance ends up damaging almost every cell in your body and is a fundamental cause of most Western 21st-century diseases. At the moment, nearly 10 per cent of the population in the UK is living with diabetes and/or heart disease but, combined with an ageing baby-boomer population and our increasing life span, that figure is set to climb steeply. Avoiding insulin resistance is possibly the single most important step you can take towards healthy ageing.

OUR LOW-GL DIET WORKS – THE PROOF

Acutely aware of the usual flight path of someone with metabolic syndrome and the medical costs involved, a group of GPs in Berkshire, UK, invited 21 people with the signs of metabolic syndrome to attend one of our Zest4Life groups. These groups involve attending a weekly meeting for 12 weeks, in which you learn Patrick's low-GL diet principles and put them into effect (no supplements are used).

All the patients had blood glucose levels that were too high. Their waist-to-hip ratio was greater than 1 for men or 0.85 for women, their blood pressure was up, and so were their triglycerides, and their cholesterol levels were upside down, with high LDL and low HDL. Not all were diabetic as such, but, with these statistics, they very soon would have been. A glycosylated haemoglobin (HbA1c) above 7 is indicative of diabetes, and the group's average was 6.9.

The doctors were hoping for a 10 per cent drop in glycosylated haemoglobin as the objective proof that these patients would be bucking the trend. Here's what happened:

Health markers	Before	After 12 weeks	% Reduction
Average weight	91.6kg (14st 6lb/202lb)	84.8kg (13st 5lb/187lb)	7.42%
Average HbA1c	6.9	5.9	14.5%
Average fasting glucose	6.3	5.6	11.1%
Average total cholesterol	5.27	4.59	12.9%
Cholesterol–HDL ratio	4.12	3.69	8.7%
Triglycerides	1.47	1.07	27%

These results are remarkable. Everyone taking part lost weight – 9 of the 21 participants lost over 6.3kg (1 stone/14lb). Drugs that lower HbA1c by 0.6 over several months are considered useful. In this short trial one person went from an exceedingly high 7.8 to a healthy 5.5 – a massive drop of 29 per cent. The average drop was half that, still very impressive. Most of the fasting glucose results had improved, as had cholesterol and blood pressure.

CASE STUDY: HENRY

Henry, one of those in the trial, is a great example of the kind of benefits the low-GL diet can produce. All of his metabolic markers came down dramatically. He said:

> *'My levels of energy were noticeably higher even after only a few weeks, and the health improvements in both my body and mind have given me the incentive to maintain these changes for life.'*

Others reported benefits such as improved energy levels, elevated mood, depression lifted, better sleep, less stress and anxiety, and even improved confidence and self-esteem. The GPs and practice nurses supporting the programme are going to use the low-GL diet and the Zest4Life approach to help similar patients.

HOW YOU CAN GET THE BENEFITS OF THE LOW-GL DIET

The rules are dead easy and explained in detail in Part Three, Chapter 2 in a practical way so that you can get started today. In a nutshell, they are as follows:

THE THREE RULES TO LOSE WEIGHT

Rule 1 Eat 40GLs a day (plus 5GLs for a dessert, drink or additional snack).

Rule 2 Always eat protein with carbohydrate.

Rule 3 Graze don't gorge – have three 10GL meals a day, and two 5GL snacks.

THE THREE RULES TO MAINTAIN A HEALTHY WEIGHT

Rule 1 For most people this would be eat no more than 50GLs a day (plus 10GLs for a dessert, drink or additional snack).

Rule 2 Always eat protein with carbohydrate.

Rule 3 Graze don't gorge – have three 10GL meals a day, and two 10GL snacks.

Of course, you need to become familiar with the GL scores of common foods, so that you can calculate your portion sizes to fit your GL total for each meal. The GL score is the measure of what a food does to your blood sugar level; for example, two servings of oat flakes (60g/2⅛oz), which is more than enough for a bowl of porridge, is 5GLs, whereas just *half* a serving of cornflakes (15g/½oz) is also 5GLs. A whole punnet of berries (300g/10½oz) is 5GLs, as is a *third* of a banana or *just 10* raisins. So, if you choose to eat porridge oats with berries for breakfast (as much as you can eat), you'll not exceed 10GLs. That's Rule 1 done.

For Rule 2 you need to increase the protein you eat. So, for breakfast, soya or cow's milk, or yoghurt, is protein, and so too are seeds or nuts. So, a dessertspoonful of pumpkin or chia seeds (the latter is our favourite, being high in omega-3 fats, soluble fibre and protein) added to your breakfast cereal sorts out Rule 2. Scrambled eggs on pumpernickel-style rye bread or oatcakes would be another suitable breakfast example. Adding a slice of smoked salmon, high in protein, to the eggs would further slow down the release of the carbohydrates.

For snacks, if you had an apple with some nuts, or some hummus plus a couple of oatcakes, that would be 5GLs. For lunch or dinner, if you had a piece of fish with a small serving of brown rice, or meat with about three small new potatoes, plus half a plate of veg, that would be 10GLs. You could have a low-GL dessert (from one of the books mentioned in Part Three Chapter 2) or a glass of wine for the remaining 5GLs. That's Rule 3 sorted. It's not that difficult.

BUT WHAT ABOUT DOING IT YOURSELF?

It may be easy to follow the diet if you are part of a support group like Zest4Life, but how easy is it to do it on your own, and do the effects last? Eamon, from Dublin, found it easy, and seven months afterwards he was in much better shape than he had been before.

CASE STUDY: EAMON

Eamon had retired from work in 2009 and was very overweight. His doctor had put him on drugs to lower his blood pressure.

'I overslept a lot and had very little energy, and I often felt depressed. In February 2010 I decided I had to do something about it, so I started going to the gym and walking more. I lost a few pounds in six weeks but I felt that I could do better.'

He discovered Patrick's book *The Low-GL Diet Bible* and began following the diet recommended in it.

'I was pleased by the weekly weight loss, but what really surprised me was that I seldom felt hungry. My mood has improved greatly and I would wake early every morning, clear headed and without the aid of an alarm clock.'

Seven months later, Eamon had lost 44.5kg (7 stone/100lb) and was able to give up the pills because his blood pressure was normal – and he started hill-walking.

'I now look forward to a healthier and happier future with the low-GL diet as the foundation of a healthy lifestyle.'

Eamon is just one of hundreds of people who have totally transformed their health, and lost all the weight they need by following the low-GL diet. Many had previously suffered with diabetes and have now reversed their condition.

TIPS TO MAKE THE LOW-GL DIET EVEN MORE EFFECTIVE

You can make further healthy choices when you follow the diet that will help you to keep your weight stable, or increase your weight loss if this is what you need.

A BIT LESS FAT

The average person eats up to 40 per cent of calories as fat, much of it as saturated fat, and that is probably too much and the wrong kind. But rather than trying to dramatically cut fat down, the important thing to do is to make sure the fats you eat are healthy. That means eating fish, nuts, seeds and their oils, and using spreads such as tahini, almond and pumpkin-seed butter, which are staples in a healthily stocked fridge. Also, use good-quality oils, including some cold-pressed virgin olive oil on salads.

THE FIBRE FACTOR

The fibre in complex carbohydrates is what slows down the release of sugars into the blood, so go for soluble fibres such as those found in oats, which are also present in chia seeds and flax seeds – you can sprinkle those onto a meal. But to get maximum fibre effect, try glucomannan fibre from the konjac plant. Add a heaped teaspoonful to a glass of water then take it at the start of a meal. Glucomannan taken this way will almost halve the blood sugar spike of that meal, therefore making the whole meal more slow-releasing and therefore healthier. In North America you can buy a similar super-fibre called PGX.

TAKE A SPOONFUL OF CINNAMON

The active ingredient in cinnamon, MCHP, mimics the action of the hormone insulin, so a teaspoonful a day helps to remove excess sugar from the bloodstream. It also seems to reduce levels of cholesterol and fat in the blood and to decrease blood pressure. The mineral chromium also makes you more sensitive to the effects of insulin, reversing insulin resistance and improving blood sugar control.[100] Some supplements combine chromium with a high-potency cinnamon extract if a teaspoon seems a lot.

YOU NEED TO EXERCISE TOO

As we saw in Chapter 5, exercise has a wide range of benefits that are linked to an anti-ageing effect. So its value here is that besides burning up calories it also lowers insulin, improves blood sugar levels and builds muscle. Muscle-building resistance exercise, such as using weights, makes your body more sensitive to insulin. Also, simply getting moving after a meal, such as taking a brisk 10-minute walk, actually helps get glucose out of the blood into the cells that need it, such as the brain and muscle cells.

A BIT OF BODY FAT WON'T HARM YOU

Provided you don't have any of the markers of metabolic syndrome, and you score low on our questionnaire on page 137, it doesn't matter if you have a little bit of extra body fat. Plenty of people stay healthy being a little overweight. 'As many as 20 per cent of people who are overweight or obese have no sign of metabolic problems,' explains Keith Frayn, Professor of Human Metabolism at Oxford University. 'They have low cholesterol, good blood sugar control and healthy blood pressure. Something else has to happen to tip them over into the dangerous state.'

Fat cells, called adipocytes, can be thought of as storage units for a rainy day. Having enough adipocytes, with available storage capacity, is important because they can store away sugars and fatty acids that would harm you if left floating around in the blood. The problem seems to come when you run out of storage space, then excess fatty acids leak into organs, getting stored in the wrong places, and into the bloodstream in excessive amounts. That's why you don't want to have a high blood level of triglycerides (fats). This is more predictive of your health than your cholesterol level. Having a low level of HDL cholesterol, and high triglycerides, is particularly bad news – much more so than a high total cholesterol.

In fact, losing *too much* weight when you are older may not be such a good idea, although keeping slim when you're younger is consistent with extending life span. A recent study of nearly 10,000 Australians aged between 70 and 75 and followed for ten years found that those who were overweight (but not obese) were less likely to die in the period than those with a so-called healthy BMI. But they didn't get the benefit if they took no exercise, which doubled the risk of death for women. Unfairly, couch potato men had only a 25 per cent increased risk.[101] Some research shows that being overweight and fit can give you a healthier set of metabolic markers – low blood sugar, low blood fats, and so on – than someone who stays at what appears to be a 'healthy' weight but who takes little exercise or who eats foods that are not nourishing. Exercising and keeping your insulin down, whatever your age, is probably more important than grimly keeping your weight within a 'one size fits all' range.

SUMMARY

To beat the bulge:

- Follow our low-GL Anti-ageing Diet (explained in Part Three, Chapter 2).
- Eat plenty of soluble fibre, found in especially high amounts in oats and chia seeds – and you can also take a fibre supplement such as glucomannan or PGX as a powder in water before meals, if you like.
- Have a teaspoonful of cinnamon a day or supplement chromium with cinnamon.
- Exercise, including a combination of aerobic and resistance training, which builds muscle and prevents muscle loss.

See Part Three, Chapter 7 for your supplement programme. See also Recommended Reading for other helpful books on this topic.

SWITCH OFF THE STRESS FACTOR, AND SLEEP FOR SEVEN HOURS STRAIGHT

Ageing well is a matter of making the most of all the natural repair-and-restore systems your body has access to. Exercise and diet are obviously major players, but so is sleep, which can take a knock in our 24/7 culture. Not only do busy lifestyles tend to encroach on the territory of sleep – 'I'll stay up late/get up early to finish it' – but the stress that many of us are under means that even when we get to bed, falling asleep can be a problem as we replay the day's events or construct scenarios for tomorrow. Then, not being able to fall asleep becomes something else to worry about.

Missing out on sleep, as well as making us feel lousy the next day, also directly impacts on our life span. One study of 21,000 twins followed for 22 years uncovered the optimum number of hours' sleep you should be getting. Less than seven, but more than eight, increased your chances of dying sooner.[102] Men did worse than women, if they got too much or too little. But, even more damaging than not getting the optimum seven and a half hours was the effect of the regular use of sleeping pills, which had a worse effect on women. Just the right amount of quality sleep predicts life satisfaction.

NOT SLEEPING MAKES YOU FAT

Not getting enough sleep can also make you put on weight. A large study looking at over 9,000 Americans found that the less sleep you have the more likely you are to put on weight.[103] Less than four hours makes you 73 per cent more likely to be obese than those getting between seven and eight hours; an average of five hours gives you a 50 per cent greater risk, and even six hours pushes your risk up by 23 per cent.

Disrupting our basic daily rhythm can have widespread harmful effects, according to studies on mice. After six weeks of being on a 20-hour instead of a 24-hour cycle, mice got fatter, showed less mental flexibility and were more impulsive.[104]

SLEEP IS ESSENTIAL FOR REGENERATING YOUR CELLS

Some of sleep's life-enhancing effects come because during the deep sleep phase, your body releases growth hormone, which stimulates the regeneration of cells. Most bone growth, for example, happens at night. Growth hormone also burns fat and builds muscle, and it also stimulates your immune system. Some people are so enamoured with the anti-ageing effects of growth hormone that they supplement it. We discuss the pros and cons of this in Secret 10. For now, the best way you can naturally promote your own growth hormone is to sleep well, reduce stress and also take resistance-type exercise, which builds muscle (see Part Three, Chapter 4). All these factors benefit younger as much as older people.

SAY NO TO THE DRUGS

If you're not getting enough sleep, you may have been tempted to try sleeping pills. Although insomnia can be very troubling, the good news is that there are many ways you can handle it. There are natural compounds that can make a big difference, and you can learn ways to deal with stress, so that you get the excitement out of life without the constantly racing heart and the anxiety; also, a form of therapy called cognitive behavioural therapy (CBT) is proven to be effective for sleep problems, and food nutrients can help too. Yet, the most common response to sleep problems is to be given a drug prescription.

Even though for years there have been worries about the benefits, safety and risks of addiction with sleeping pills, doctors still write prescriptions for over 10 million of them every year at a cost of over £30 million in the UK. Studies regularly find their benefits are small and that they should be used sparingly on older people, as the risks of falls and cognitive impairment may well outweigh the benefits.[105] However, GPs continue to believe, wrongly, that a relatively newer type, known as 'the Zs' are safer for older people and less likely to be addictive.[106] Like many drugs, they can be useful in an emergency, but we don't advise taking them on a regular basis without a good reason.

CALMING DOWN WITH GABA – THE START OF A GOOD NIGHT'S SLEEP

Whether you're working or you've retired, you can experience stress hotspots. The physical effects of these stresses show up in the bloodstream as the hormones our bodies produce when we're stressed: adrenalin and cortisol. When they are active, your energy reserves are channelled towards immediate survival, known as 'fight or flight'. So your body stops repairing itself and regenerating in favour of dealing with the perceived threat. The time when this physical and emotional self-healing is most effective is when you are asleep.

If you go to bed worried, the natural antidote to the extra adrenalin that may still be pumping around your body is an amino acid and neurotransmitter called GABA (gamma-aminobutyric acid) that switches the adrenalin off. Sleeping pills boost the production of GABA. There's an added bonus to bringing down adrenalin, because there is a strong connection between feeling emotionally het up, not sleeping well and feeling down and depressed.[107]

In the US and Ireland you can buy GABA itself over the counter in health-food stores and pharmacies, but in the UK it is classified as a medicine and is therefore available only on prescription. Whether that is an effective way of protecting consumers is a moot point. It is certainly a shame, because GABA is a natural antidote to anxiety and the inability to relax. The trouble with the drugs is that they either interfere with your body's own ability to make GABA or rapidly make you less responsive to it. The net result is that they are highly addictive, so when you try to stop taking sleeping pills you are likely to develop extreme anxiety and insomnia. Patrick's book, *How to Quit Without*

Feeling S**t, explains how to come off these drugs, but you do also need some professional guidance and support.

There is another ironic drawback to sleeping pills: they reduce the availability of the sleep hormone melatonin!

ALCOHOL AND COFFEE ARE NOT HELPFUL

Many people use alcohol to relax. Alcohol promotes GABA, and switches off adrenalin, but it only works for an hour or so. When the effects wear off, you want another drink. The danger lies in regularly drinking to get this effect, because more than one drink a night starts to be bad news, especially if it slips into half a bottle of wine a night. This amount of alcohol increases your risk of many diseases. Also, if you go to sleep under the influence of alcohol, it disturbs your normal sleep cycle, which can promote a low mood as well as increased stress and tiredness the next day. The net consequence of regular alcohol consumption is GABA depletion, which leads to more adrenalin, anxiety and emotional oversensitivity and less good-quality sleep.

There is something else you can do to keep adrenalin down: avoid the caffeine found in coffee and tea, and that includes green tea, after midday if you have difficulty getting to sleep, because it suppresses the sleep hormone melatonin for up to ten hours.[108]

THE OTHER KEYS TO GOOD SLEEP

Although bringing down adrenalin is one half of getting you ready for sleep, there are two other brain chemicals linked with mood and sleep: serotonin and melatonin. Sleeping pills focus on GABA, but there is a lot more to sleep's biochemistry; understanding it can help you get the right amount of good-quality sleep. It can also help to reduce your stress levels and get you out of the vicious cycle whereby a lack of sleep keeps making you more stressed, tired and low.

Biochemically speaking, mood and sleep have a lot in common. The amino acid tryptophan, which turns into 5-hydroxytryptophan (5-HTP), is not only the raw material for the mood-boosting neurotransmitter serotonin, but also for melatonin, the hormone that helps you sleep, controlling the sleep–wake cycle. It's the brain's neurotransmitter that keeps you in sync with the earth's day-and-night cycle.

Jet lag, for example, happens when the brain's chemistry takes time to catch up with a sudden shift in time zone. What's happening inside your brain is that melatonin, which should be released at night to make you sleep, gets released during the 'old' night time. Taking melatonin just before bed in the new time zone helps to reset your brain's chemistry so that it can recover from jet lag. (Take 1mg for every one hour's time-zone difference.) And melatonin not only helps you to sleep but is also a powerful antioxidant. Low levels are linked to an increased risk of cancer.[109]

How the brain makes melatonin

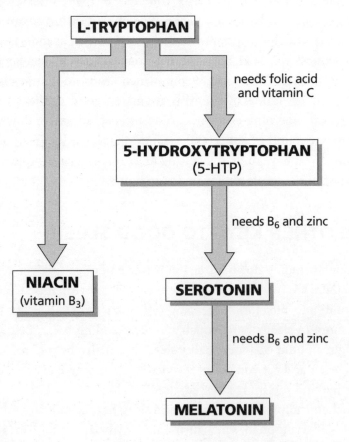

As you start to wind down in the evening, serotonin levels rise and adrenalin levels fall. As it gets darker, melatonin kicks in. Melatonin is an almost identical molecule to serotonin, from which it is made, and both are made from 5-HTP, which you can buy as a supplement, itself derived from the amino acid tryptophan, which is present in most protein foods.

SLEEP CHEMICALS ARE TEAM PLAYERS

As often happens with natural compounds, converting one to another needs the correct amounts of various minerals and vitamins for the process to work most efficiently. Turning tryptophan into melatonin requires folic acid, vitamins B_6 and C, and zinc; tryptophan is found in chicken, cheese, tuna, tofu, eggs, nuts, seeds and milk. Other foods associated with inducing sleep are lettuce and oats. So, if you are having sleeping problems, it makes sense to eat those foods and to supplement with a high-potency multivitamin–mineral that contains at least 200mcg of folic acid, 20mg of vitamin B_6, 10mg of zinc and 100mg of vitamin C.

Or you could take melatonin and the other natural chemicals directly. Melatonin, which is a neurotransmitter and not a nutrient, is proven to help you get to sleep, but it needs to be used much more cautiously than a nutrient. In controlled trials it's about a third as effective as the drugs, but it has a fraction of the side effects.[110] Even so, supplementing too much can have undesirable effects, such as diarrhoea, constipation, nausea, dizziness, reduced libido, headaches, depression and nightmares.

Nevertheless, if you do sleep badly, or if you can't get to sleep until late and are prone to low moods, it's particularly effective both for helping you sleep and for improving your mood.[111]

You may want to try between 3mg and 6mg before bedtime. In the UK, melatonin is classified as a medicine and is only available on prescription, so you will need to discuss this option with your doctor. It is available in other countries, such as the US, Canada and South Africa, over the counter, and on the internet from these countries too.

Another option is to supplement with 100–200mg of 5-HTP 30

minutes before you go to bed.[112] It's best taken on an empty stomach, or with a small amount of carbohydrate, such as an oatcake or a piece of fruit, one hour before sleep. But be careful if you are on SSRI antidepressants. These raise serotonin, so raising it further with 5-HTP could theoretically give you too much; we don't recommend combining the two.

The combination of GABA and 5-HTP is even better. In a placebo-controlled trial, it cut the time taken to fall asleep from 32 minutes to 19 minutes and extended sleep from five to almost seven hours.[113] Taking 1,000mg of GABA, plus 100mg of 5-HTP is a recipe for a good night's sleep.

If you are taking sleeping pills, supplementing 5-HTP or melatonin for a month can bring you back into balance, re-establishing proper sleep patterns. This will make it much easier for you to wean yourself off the pills. But don't swap one dependency for another. If you are on melatonin, then switch to 5-HTP after a month and then gradually tail off. By this time your brain chemistry should be back in balance and you should find you sleep just fine.

MAGNESIUM AND HERBAL PREPARATIONS THAT CHILL YOU OUT

Other nutrients that help are magnesium, which calms the nervous system, and the herbs valerian, hops and passionflower. Magnesium has been reported to help reduce restless legs as well as insomnia.[114] A deficiency is certainly a potential reason for feeling low or anxious. For this, and many other reasons, we recommend supplementing 150mg of magnesium every day and twice this, 300mg, if you have difficulty sleeping. One study in Italy gave people who suffer with insomnia 225mg of magnesium, together with 11.5mg zinc and 5mg of melatonin. Compared to those on placebo, those on the food supplements got to sleep much more easily, slept better through the night, and woke feeling refreshed and alert.[115] Combinations of these herbs, minerals and amino acids are particularly effective (see Resources).

Valerian is the most potent GABA-promoting herb and, as such, can also cause daytime drowsiness, so it's best to take it only in the evening if you have anxiety or insomnia and an inability to 'switch off'. Valerian is sometimes referred to as 'nature's valium'. As such, it can interact with alcohol and other sedative drugs and should therefore be taken in combination with them only under careful medical supervision. It seems to work in two ways: by promoting the body's release of GABA, and by providing the amino acid glutamine, from which the brain can make GABA. Neither of these mechanisms makes it addictive.[116] One double-blind study in which participants took 60mg of valerian 30 minutes before bedtime for 28 days found it to be as effective as oxazepam, a drug used to treat anxiety.[117] Another found it to be highly effective in reducing insomnia compared with placebos.[118] A review of studies to date cites six that show a significant benefit.[119] Our experience is that it works exceptionally well for many people. To help you get a good night's sleep, take 150–300mg about 45 minutes before bedtime.

REDUCE YOUR STRESS

As well as these natural ways of dealing with the biochemical effects of stress to ensure a good night's sleep, there is another approach that makes handling stress itself more effective. Dealing with stress poorly not only fills you up with negative emotions and makes you feel exhausted but it also stops you from sleeping. What is more, it is another block to ageing well, because it increases your risk of the chronic killers, including cancer and heart disease. Stress triggers a cascade of hormones that, over time, accelerate ageing, encourage inflammation and increase disease risk. Indeed, a study in the *Journal of the American Medical Association* found that too much stress can be as bad for your heart as smoking and high cholesterol.[120] And just in case you need any more proof of the damaging effects stress can have, research now shows that those of us who are regularly stressed have:

- A five-fold increased risk of dying from heart-related problems.[121]
- Double the risk of developing diabetes, in men.[122]
- A 65 per cent increased risk of developing dementia.[123]
- Double the chance of developing obesity.[124]
- An increased risk of breast cancer.[125]

If you are one of those who thrive on stress, seeing it as the spice of life, that's fine – just give yourself time to recuperate occasionally. But the majority of people aren't that lucky.

In our 100% Health Survey,[126] 68 per cent of the 55,000-plus participants reported feeling that they have too much to do, 66 per cent said they frequently felt anxious or tense, 82 per cent often became impatient and 55 per cent get angry easily.

Such stress symptoms are our body's way of warning us that something is out of balance. Your in-built survival kit – the 'fight or flight' response – is designed to be an emergency coping reaction. When it's activated many times a day by traffic jams, conflicts with colleagues or your family, or work overload, the results are unpleasant and can be overwhelming.

You can tell if you aren't handling stress well if you experience these on a regular basis:

- Difficulty in thinking straight
- A negative attitude
- Feeling out of control
- Anxiety
- Tension
- Irritation
- Feeling overwhelmed
- Heightened worries and concerns
- Frustration
- Hostility

Notice that these are all negative emotions. So, not only are you feeling bad but you are also tired out and not performing as effectively as you could. In a negative emotional state your options all narrow down. It's hard to think creatively or come up with fresh options. There seems to be no way out. What you want is a way to change the way you respond to stress so that you get the benefits of positive emotions. Fortunately we have one.

THE HEARTMATH APPROACH

HeartMath® gives you a way to transform the feelings of fury or anxiety you experience in a traffic jam, or while having yet another pointless discussion with your least favourite person at work, into something positive *right at the time it is happening*. This makes it quite different from the more familiar stress-relieving techniques, such as listening to music, having a warm bath, a massage, or a glass of wine, which all focus on relaxation *after* the event. With those techniques, by the time you do wind down, you've been feeling steamed up and angry for far too long. That's because the stress hormone cortisol stays in your system for hours rather than minutes once released.

HeartMath is a technique that combines slow rhythmic breathing with digital imagery that transforms the rhythms of your heart into a pattern on a computer screen via a sensor attached to your finger or earlobe. As you watch the screen you can see immediately how your breathing and emotions directly change the way your heart responds. The difference can be very dramatic as the printouts below show.

How a positive emotion affects your heart

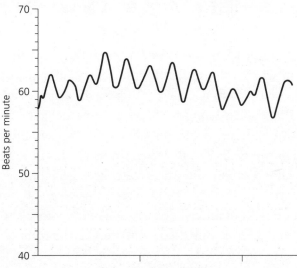

This graph shows the heart rhythm pattern typical of a positive feeling, such as appreciation. The smooth shape is what scientists call a 'highly ordered' or 'coherent' pattern and it is a sign of good health and emotional balance.

How a negative emotion affects your heart

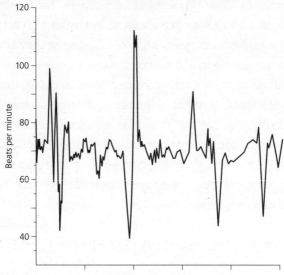

This graph shows the irregular jerky heart rhythm pattern typical of stressful feelings like anger, frustration, worry and anxiety. This is called an 'incoherent' pattern.

GETTING CHEMISTRY AND BRAIN WAVES IN SYNC

What HeartMath teaches you is how to turn the incoherent patterns that show up when you are faced with a stressful situation into the smooth, coherent pattern you have with feelings of appreciation. Inside your body, that shift is being made by a whole range of biochemical changes, as your adrenalin and cortisol levels drop and the amount of the relaxing hormone DHEA increases (more on this in Secret 10).

In most major diseases, and with accelerated ageing, what you would see on a HeartMath screen is an incoherent pattern with low DHEA. It is also found with brain-cell death, impaired memory and learning, decreased bone density, impaired immune function, increased blood sugar and increased fat accumulation around the waist and hips.[127]

The wild swings you can see on the screen tell you that your system is switching between the two parts of your nervous system: the active sympathetic side and the relaxing parasympathetic side. We shift between them all the time, but your aim is to move rhythmically between the two. The HeartMath scientists have been able to demonstrate that the messages about this switching that your heart sends to your brain can profoundly influence perception, emotions, behaviour, performance and health.[128]

When your heart rhythm is coherent, you are able to think more clearly and see more options, whether you are making decisions or playing sport.[129] But when your heart becomes incoherent under stress, your behaviour becomes much more limited and robotic. It's a hardwired response designed to focus all your energies on the narrow task of getting out of trouble. But, and this is the important bit, you *can* learn to change it.

BECOMING COHERENT WITH HEARTMATH

You do this by combining simple rhythmic breathing with creating positive feelings of love and affection while watching the effect they have on your heart's activity on the screen. The feedback the scrolling lines give you allows you to learn what works far more quickly than more traditional breathing methods, such as meditation. When practised regularly, research has found that the exercise can help you to feel better emotionally and improve your intuition, creativity and cognitive performance.[130]

You focus on your heart and imagine your breath flowing in and out while you breathe rhythmically. As your breathing becomes more steady, with the heart-centred visualisation, you recall a positive emotional experience – such as a magical place or time when you felt really good, until you can actually experience the positive emotion of that experience. Then you identify and hold on to that feeling while breathing into the heart.

When practised daily for five minutes it can help you learn how to de-stress, feel calmer and more content. Once you can see that you can quickly put yourself into a coherent state, you can then use it any time you encounter a stressful event: when you are tense in heavy traffic, overloaded at work or facing an emotional crisis. Tossing and turning as you rehash the day's crises at night will be a thing of the past.

Numerous studies have shown that regularly practising HeartMath can have hugely beneficial effects, emotionally and physically; for example:

- After just one month, cortisol (the stress hormone) was reduced by 23 per cent and DHEA (the anti-ageing vitality hormone) increased by 100 per cent.[131] A remarkable improvement.

- A small study with diabetics reported significant reductions in anxiety, negative emotions, and a reduction in HbA1c – a marker for sugar damage in the blood.[132]

- Hypertension patients found their blood pressure had dropped substantially after three months, along with improvements in emotional health.[133]

- Nearly all of 75 patients with abnormal heart rhythms (atrial fibrillation) said they were substantially improved after three months and 14 were able to discontinue medication altogether.[134]

There's also a great book written by HeartMath founder, Doc Childre, called *Transforming Stress*, which gives lots of useful information about using HeartMath and developing your practice. You can also attend workshops or work one-to-one with a HeartMath practitioner (see Part 3, Chapter 6).

MUSIC TO SWITCH OFF YOUR BRAIN

New York psychiatrist Dr Galina Mindlin, an assistant professor at Columbia University's College of Physicians and Surgeons, uses 'brain music' – rhythmic patterns of sounds derived from recordings of patients' own brainwaves – to help them overcome insomnia, anxiety and depression. A small double-blind study from 1998, conducted at Toronto University in Canada, found that 80 per cent of those undergoing this treatment reported benefits.[135]

Another study found that specially composed music induced a shift in brainwave patterns to alpha waves, associated with the deep relaxation before you go to sleep, and that this induced less anxiety in a study of patients going to the dentist.[136] This music, composed by John Levine, especially to induce a relaxation response, sounds something like very calming classical piano music and is specifically designed to switch the brain waves from beta waves, associated with adrenalin and excitation, to alpha waves, which is a prerequisite for going to sleep. Our favourite CDs are called *Silence of Peace* and *Orange Grove Siesta* (see Resources) and we have received a huge number of testimonials from people who have found almost immediate relief from insomnia by listening to them.

CASE STUDY: SUE

Sue had been suffering from post-traumatic stress disorder: sleeping for about three hours, then waking every 45 minutes or so. Here's what she says:

'I ordered, almost wearily, Orange Grove Siesta *CD for insomnia and* Silence of Peace. *The improvement happened from night one, and now, just one week later, I am sleeping for six to seven hours. If I wake, which is becoming rare, I simply tune in again! I haven't heard the end of the CD yet.'*

PRACTISE SLEEP HYGIENE

A piece of essentially commonsense advice, rather quaintly known as 'sleep hygiene', forms part of most sleep regimes:

1. Keep the bedroom quiet and at a temperature that's good for you.

2. Wear comfortable clothing, don't have a big meal in the evening, and avoid coffee and alcohol at least three hours before bed.

3. Your room should be as dark as possible; even a faint light can reduce the amount of melatonin you are producing.

4. Exercise regularly, but not within three hours of bedtime.

5. Be aware that certain prescription medications can cause insomnia, such as steroids, bronchodilators (used for asthma) and diuretics.

6. Keep your bedroom only for sleeping – no working or TV.

7. It is also a good idea to create regular sleep-promoting habits such as taking a bath before bed or reading a chapter of a book.

SUMMARY

To release the grip of stress and benefit from a good night's sleep:

- Practise 'sleep hygiene'.
- Exercise regularly, but not in the evening before sleep.
- Listen to alpha-wave-inducing music while in bed and practise relaxation techniques.
- Eat more green leafy vegetables, nuts and seeds to ensure you're getting enough magnesium, and supplement 150mg a day, and twice this if you have difficulty unwinding in the evening.
- Avoid sugar and caffeine, and minimise your intake of alcohol. Don't combine alcohol with sleeping pills or anti-anxiety medication.
- If you do often react stressfully, discover the sources of stress in your life and do what you can to reduce them.
- Practise HeartMath or other stress-reducing techniques, including mindfulness and meditation (more on this in Part Three, Chapter 6).

In terms of supplements:

- Supplement 100mg of 5-HTP and, if you live in a country where you can buy it, GABA 1,000mg an hour before bed. If you can't get GABA, taurine and glutamine are precursors. Some formulas provide this in combination with calming herbs.
- Alternatively try valerian – 150–300mg about 45 minutes before bedtime. Choose a standardised extract or tincture and follow the dosage instructions.
- If you feel the need for a sleeping pill, ask your doctor to prescribe melatonin, in which case don't take extra 5-HTP. Take 3–6mg an hour before sleep.

See Part Three, Chapter 7 for your general supplement programme and Recommended Reading for other helpful books on this topic.

KEEP YOUR SKIN YOUTHFUL

Your skin is a remarkable thing. Weighing in at around 5kg (11lb) and with a surface area of 2m² (22ft²) it is the largest organ of the body – and it is constantly renewing itself. The outermost layer of dead cells is sloughed off and replaced every month. Like all frontiers, it has to keep out invaders – such as micro-organisms and pollutants – and keep vital resources in. But at the same time it must allow warmth to flow in and water for cooling to be sweated out, while simultaneously working as a vast sensory organ for touch.

As we get older, another of the skin's special features becomes all too obvious. The skin is the external representation of the processes of ageing going on within. It reflects our gradual decline, starting at about the age of 25 when the replacement of old cells begins to slow down. By 45 the skin is thinning, partly due to hormonal changes, and so it becomes more fragile and vulnerable to damage.

YOUR SKIN UNDER ATTACK

Meanwhile, other processes of decline are going on in the skin's lower layers as water, fat and strength drain away. The coils of collagen and elastin that give skin its strength and elasticity begin to suffer cross-linking damage caused by glycation, the result of high levels of sugar in the blood (explained on page 74, Chapter 5), fat cells shrink and there are fewer of the large chains of sugar molecules that hold water. Your skin then becomes dryer and looser, and looks less plump and smooth. Finally, as the network of blood vessels shrink, skin loses its youthful colour and glow.

On top of this decline, which it shares with blood vessels and other organs, your skin has to cope with the relentless onslaught of the outside world: cuts and bruises and the damaging oxidants created by smoking, environmental pollution and, especially, by sunlight. Skin can really have a rough time.

Not so long ago, the general belief was that the sagging, wrinkling and loss of plumpness was an inevitable part of ageing and that there was little you could do about it. But now we know that, just as you can help interior processes to age more healthily, so you can slow down the visible signs of decline your skin reveals, by understanding its specific nutritional needs. As well as explaining how you can slow down natural ageing, we'll show you how to reduce the harmful external effects and how you can undo some of the damage that has already occurred.

UNDERSTANDING YOUR SKIN

First, a quick overview of the territory. The top layer, the epidermis, is extraordinarily thin – a millimetre at most; as thin as a pencil line.

A cross-section of the skin

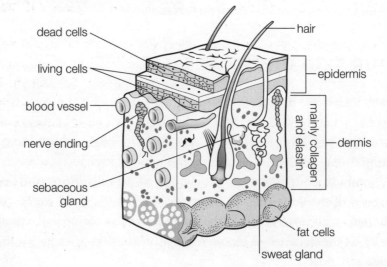

It's made up of three types of cell: those that make the tough protein keratin; the melanocytes that produce the pigment melanin, which is what gives you a tan; and a cell type that's part of the immune system. Below the epidermis is the much thicker dermis, composed of a dense network of the structural proteins collagen and elastin, interwoven with nerves, muscles, water carriers and sweat glands. It's here that anything that penetrates the skin gets absorbed.

WHAT YOU EAT TODAY YOU WEAR TOMORROW

It's possible to influence the way your skin ages, because you need the right sort of nutrition at every stage of your skin's lifecycle. In many ways, what you eat today affects what you wear tomorrow. To begin with, the collagen in the dermis is made when vitamin C converts the amino acid proline into hydroxyproline. So, if there is no vitamin C, you'll have no collagen. Then, one of the reasons collagen and elastin fibres become less flexible with age is because of the damage caused by free radicals, such as those generated by smoke and sunlight. But this damage can be greatly reduced by having a good supply of various antioxidants, especially vitamins A and C.

THE A TO Z OF SKINCARE – AN OVERVIEW

In fact, vitamin A is a vital part of any programme for encouraging your skin to age healthily; it helps to stop the build-up of old keratin cells, which can happen as replacement slows down. Dry, rough skin can be a sign that you aren't getting enough vitamin A. So, including it in your diet and supplementing it if necessary is a good starting point, but even more effective is using a vitamin A-rich skin cream, and we'll be explaining about this in more detail shortly.

Vitamin B_{12}, which is increasingly poorly absorbed with age, is vital for the process of methylation that protects DNA, and so it is likely to slow down skin ageing. You need sufficient B_{12} along with the other B vitamins to make sure your homocysteine is kept at a healthy level (see Secret 1).

Another vital nutrient for healthy ageing are the essential fats, which form part of most cell membranes and which are needed to hold water in – the better the skin cells carry out that task the plumper and younger-looking your skin will be. If you are not eating sufficient essential fats, the cells dry out too quickly and you'll find you need to keep moisturising. Essential fats also damp down the inflammatory processes that damage arteries and which can also harm skin cells.

Your skin is not going to look as good as it could without sufficient zinc, a mineral that is needed for the accurate production of new skin cells. Without it you are likely to have stretch marks and be poor at healing, as well as a wide variety of skin problems, ranging from acne to eczema.

AND THE D PARADOX

Finally, there is vitamin D, the vital anti-ageing vitamin that most of us don't get enough of. It's made by the action of sunlight on the skin and needs the cholesterol found there to do it. (Incidentally, there is almost no research on the effect aggressively lowering cholesterol with statins has on vitamin D production.) The need for sunlight brings up a contradiction, however, because standard advice to keep your skin looking young and to avoid skin cancer is to stay out of the sun. But vitamin D, as well as improving immunity and being a natural anti-inflammatory, may very well also cut the risk of cancer. We suggest a way round this contradiction in the next section.

STOP PHOTO-AGEING YOUR SKIN

Sunlight contains three kinds of ultra-violet rays: UV-A rays, which cause the skin to age more rapidly and can penetrate into the dermis where they damage collagen; UV-B rays, which cause sunburn if you stay out too long, but on the plus side they make vitamin D; and UV-C rays, which would fry us, but fortunately the planet's atmosphere blocks them.

UV-A rays can speed up ageing because the photons – the packages of energy – that they carry get into the dermis where they produce the same damaging oxidants or free radicals that leak out from the mitochondria found in all cells (explained in Chapter 3). One effect is to cause breaks in the skin cells' DNA, and many of the signs of ageing skin is the result: less elasticity, and more wrinkles and age spots. What is more, the UV-A rays get through to your skin even when the weather is cloudy.

The way the skin protects itself is with light-sensitive vitamins that act as antioxidants effectively soaking up the potentially damaging sun's rays. These are mainly vitamins A, C and E, and the carotenoids found in orange foods. If you sunbathe too long, smoke and live in a polluted atmosphere, your body is deluged, inside and out, with trillions of free oxidising radicals. Our bodies have to deal with, on average, about 10 trillion free radical hits a day.

VITAMIN A CAN HALT PHOTO-AGEING

The extent of damage depends almost entirely on the balance between antioxidants in the skin and exposure to oxidants, so the best way to protect your skin, as we have already noted, is to increase the amount of vitamin A held in skin cells. It absorbs the photons from UV-A rays, preventing it from damaging your skin, but it doesn't inhibit vitamin D production. Because of the way vitamin A works, however, relying on your diet to keep you topped up may not be enough. That's because it gets destroyed as it damps down the oxidants – within the first 20 minutes of sun exposure 80 per cent of the vitamin A in your skin has been lost. Replacing that just through your diet could take weeks.

So, the most effective way to stop photo-ageing is to apply vitamin A directly to the skin. Research by Dr Des Fernandes, a South African plastic surgeon and founder of the skincare company Environ, has found that with adequate doses of vitamin A cream, the outer horny layer of keratin becomes smoother, the skin maintains its moisture more efficiently, pigmented blemishes are reduced and melanin, which controls skin colour, is more evenly distributed. Vitamin A also promotes thick layers of normal collagen in the dermis, which keeps the skin's shape and elasticity.

Evidence for this comes from a small study published several years ago, which found that vitamin A could not only slow down photo-ageing but even reverse it.[137] When applied to the skin of 36 people in their eighties for six weeks, vitamin A reduced wrinkles and increased collagen production.

It also ensures that the keratinocytes (the cells that make keratin) stay healthy with effective DNA repair.

Bear in mind, however, that too much vitamin A applied to the skin, especially in the form of retinoic acid, can irritate the skin, therefore it is preferable to start with a lower dose in the skin cream and build up to a higher dose. The best results are achieved by combining skin-friendly nutrients from food and supplements,[138] alongside daily topical vitamin A and C. If you look at the results section of Environ's website (see Resources) you will see some extraordinary skin transformations achieved with transdermal vitamins.

TOPICAL VITAMIN A PLUS VITAMIN C: THE SKIN ESSENTIALS

The body's response to absorbing increased amounts of vitamin A is to start producing more vitamin A receptors, allowing you to store more. You can get vitamin A creams from the high street, but there are several things to watch out for. Few contain a high enough dose and most lack adequate protection from oxidation. Vitamin A oxidises easily, so any skin cream has to be in a light-proof container, with a shelf life of months, not years. You also need to check that it contains the most effective forms of vitamin A – retinyl palmitate, retinyl acetate and retinol. Environ's products tick all these boxes (see Resources).

Topical vitamin C is immensely helpful too. Not only does it help to produce collagen, which supports your skin's shape, reducing wrinkles and sagging skin, but also, like vitamin A, it protects DNA, reducing errors on the skin-cell production line. Look for a cream that contains the most absorbable form: ascorbyl tetraisopalmitate. Should you ever burn your skin, the result of applying vitamin C cream is almost miraculous.

YOUR VITAMIN D QUOTA FROM THE SUN, FOOD AND SUPPLEMENTS

By being sensible about your sun exposure (see box below) and using these vitamins, it is perfectly possible to get the vitamin D you need from sunlight (at least during the summer in the UK) without speeding up the rate that your skin is ageing.

Most vitamin D is made in the first 15 minutes of sun exposure, so we advise you not to apply sun cream during that time unless your skin is already sun damaged. On a hot summer's day in the UK, 30 minutes' sun exposure, when your shadow is shorter than your body, makes roughly the equivalent of the amount you'd get from 1,000iu of vitamin D, or over 3,000iu if you expose your legs and arms – and even more if you expose a large area of your skin. A good high-potency multivitamin can provide another 600iu (15mcg). A serving of oily fish such as mackerel or wild salmon might provide another 600iu, although most farmed salmon would provide a little more than half this amount. That's in the ballpark of 2,000iu, and probably enough.

HOW TO BENEFIT FROM THE SUN SAFELY

The ideal routine during the summer, when you are going to be exposed to reasonably intense sun, would be as follows:

1. Load up your skin with vitamin A in the morning, or before going out into the sun, by using a good skin cream with vitamin A added.

2. Don't put on sunscreen for the first 15 minutes, to really boost your vitamin D stores.

3. Then, put on an antioxidant-rich sunscreen that isn't a total block. Keep reapplying it depending on how long you are in the sun. My all-time favourite is Environ's RAD, which provides a range of antioxidants including beta-carotene, vitamins C and E. RAD is, technically, sun-protection factor (SPF) 15, but I find it acts more like SPF 30: you tan but you don't burn.

CONTINUED...

4. After sunbathing, reapply vitamin A to the skin. If you don't, it can take a week to restore normal skin levels. So, accumulating sunbathing without vitamin A application is bad news. Vitamin A also protects DNA.

5. If you spend too much time in the sun and have some redness or burning, apply transdermal vitamin C. You want something that contains ascorbyl tetraisopalmitate. Environ's C Boost is perfect. Some people put this on anyway, since vitamin C also protects DNA.

6. Also, make sure you drink sufficient water and eat, or supplement, enough omega-3 fats from oily fish, as well as chia, flax or pumpkin seeds and walnuts. You need essential fats, and water, to keep your skin hydrated.

IF YOU WANT TO GO ONE STEP FURTHER ...

For those really wanting to push the boat out on reversing skin ageing, the state-of-the-art treatments focus on how to allow the vitamins we've mentioned above to penetrate deeper into the skin. There are four effective ways of doing this.[139] One is light, repetitive peeling. When performed properly this helps to remove the thick, rough outer layer of sun-damaged skin.

The second method, called iontophoresis, uses a device to generate a small electrical charge in the skin, driving a water-based solution of vitamins A and C into the skin. This can increase the rate of penetration by four times.

The third method is sonophoresis, which uses sound waves of a particular frequency to open up channels in the fatty layers of the skin; this method claims a 40-fold improvement in absorption.

The last method is skin needling, where the skin is penetrated with tiny needles contained on a roller, then the transdermal vitamins are applied. (You can do this yourself with a specialised roller device, see Resources.)

There is a deeper skin-penetration technique that actually induces a tiny amount of bleeding, which is now known to stimulate collagen formation.[140] Apart from the skin-roller, all these techniques should only be done under the supervision of a well-qualified skin-care therapist.

ANTI-AGEING HORMONES

After the menopause, many women complain that their skin looks older, but a big plus for HRT for many was that their skin looked better while they were taking it. One reason could be that vitamin A levels in the skin decrease during the menopause. All the hormones we discuss in Secret 10 (progesterone, oestrogens, testosterone, DHEA, melatonin and thyroxine) have anti-ageing effects on the skin, and there's a good case, if you are deficient, for supplementing these. Bio-identical hormones are usually absorbed directly through the skin, and local application is claimed to have anti-ageing effects.

More contentious, however, is growth hormone. There is no doubt that it stimulates cell regeneration, but the flip side of this is its potential for increasing cancerous abnormal cell growth, so we don't recommend it; however, there is a case for using localised growth hormone on the skin. Some skincare products contain colostrum, which is found in the first milk of mammals, and which contains many growth factors. This might work locally, without the same level of risk, although there is little research on this to confirm either way.

Milk itself, on the other hand, is a major promoter of acne.[141] This is largely thought to be due to its excessive promotion of insulin-like growth factor (IGF-1).[142] We would not advise the use of any form of growth factor on the skin in those with acne or severe skin damage or who have a history of skin cancer.

HOW TO KEEP YOUR SKIN HYDRATED

Youthful skin cells are plumped up with water, so the more you can help them stay that way the better your skin will look. Vitamin A is important here too because it creates a thick healthy epidermis which will help keep moisture locked in. Each individual skin cell also contains water and will hold it for longer if the membrane that surrounds it has been built from a good supply of the essential fats, omega-3 and 6. As we have seen, omega-3 fats come from oily fish such as salmon, mackerel, sardines, herring, kippers and fresh (not canned) tuna. Also from cold-climate raw seeds and nuts, such as chia, flax, pumpkin, hemp and walnuts. Omega-6 fats are found in hot-climate nuts and seeds, such as sunflower and sesame seeds.

Most people are much more deficient in omega-3 than omega-6. Thus, when you supplement, it is best to have larger quantities of omega-3 fats. Gamma-linolenic acid (GLA) is the most potent omega-6 fat and, as you saw in Secret 1, EPA, DPA and DHA are the most potent omega-3 fats. You want ten times more of these omega-3s than GLA in a perfect supplement.

The best source of linoleic acid is olive oil. Moisturisers containing olive oil are therefore good news for dry skin. It is also good to eat olives, and use olive oil in salad dressings. Eating these foods and taking supplements makes a big difference to dry skin.[143]

AN EXTRA WATER LOCK-IN

There is also something else you can do that may be even more effective for keeping your skin moisturised. Commercial moisturising creams contain various combinations of oil and water, which slow down the loss of moisture from the skin, but only briefly. So, it may make sense to support the actual water stores in the skin. Special sugar and protein combinations, known as glycosaminoglycans (GAGs), hold water and link up into long chains called proteoglycans (PGs). The chains are part of the dense network of fibres, such as collagen, that pack the dermis. GAGs are very like the building blocks in the mucus that lines the nose and the guts. They are also found in the linings of joints and become damaged if affected with arthritis. So, for a longer-term solution, it makes sense to feed the GAGs with various glucosamine supplements such as N-acetyl-D-glucosamine and D-glucosamine hydrochloride, similar to the ones taken to help with arthritis. Evidence for this approach is skimpy, but lab studies look promising.[144] (A good supply of vitamin A also supports the GAGs.)

Drinking enough water is a healthy-ageing absolute essential – the equivalent of eight glasses of water a day – and bear in mind that alcohol dehydrates the skin.

THE FISH PROTEIN THAT FIRMS THE SKIN

DMAE is a phospholipid found principally in fish, mentioned in Secret 1 for its brain-boosting properties. It is needed to make the neurotransmitter acetylcholine that is lacking in people with Alzheimer's. It's not only important for brain cells – it also makes muscle cells tighten up, for reasons that are still unclear (although dermatologists have a number of theories). It would seem, though, that DMAE can benefit the skin, both as a supplement or when applied directly, although because DMAE is an antioxidant, it may work best in combination with other antioxidants.

One fan of the transdermal route is dermatologist and nutritionist Dr Nicholas Perricone, who has a range of skincare products based on DMAE. In studies, DMAE applied to the skin, thickened the epidermis, giving the skin more protection. It also increased collagen fibre thickness, which equates to firmer skin.[145] Vitamin A also has the same effects. It also improves wrinkles and has a general anti-ageing effect on the skin.[146]

One view is that DMAE swells cells but may also speed up their death.[147] Although this may sound bad, skin cells do move to the surface and die off as part of their natural cycle. Long-term users of DMAE skin creams report nothing but benefits, however. DMAE may be able to break down lipofuscin, the pigment granules that produce age spots. If you're happy to try some more risky approaches in the search for healthy-ageing solutions, DMAE is certainly a skin-cream ingredient to consider. I (Patrick) supplement DMAE on a daily basis.

SUMMARY

To slow down the ageing process in the skin:

- Drink the equivalent of eight glasses of water a day.
- Eat omega-3 rich fish, seeds and nuts – best are chia seeds and walnuts and minimal fried food. Also, eat olives and use olive oil in salad dressings. Follow our Anti-ageing Diet, to eat for optimum nutrition.
- Avoid sugar and high-GL foods – eat a low-GL diet, as above.

CONTINUED...

- Apply transdermal vitamin A and C to the skin, ideally twice a day.
- Use an antioxidant-rich sunscreen when you are outside.
- Don't overexpose yourself to direct, strong sunlight.

In terms of supplements:

- Make sure your daily supplements include vitamins A, C, zinc, essential omegas and other antioxidants.

See Part Three, Chapter 7 for your general supplement programme.

STAY FREE FROM CANCER

Winning the war on cancer is a bit like predictions of the end of the world – the date for it keeps moving forward. In spite of confident assertions made over 40 years ago that a cure would soon be found, the battle to cure cancer is still raging. Back in 1971 President Nixon declared war on cancer and set a victory date for 1976. Then, in 1984, the American National Cancer Institute asserted that the mortality rate from cancer would be halved by 2000. Finally, in 2003 the Institute announced that suffering and death from cancer would be eliminated by 2015 – a target that has been quietly forgotten.

It is precisely because cancer is so feared, and kills so many people, that there has always been a big gap between hope and reality. The stark reality today is that at the moment cancer kills over 150,000 people a year in the UK, making it the second biggest killer after heart disease, responsible for one in four deaths. Men are at a slightly higher risk – it's involved in 29 per cent of male deaths and 24 per cent of female deaths.

Despite the failed predictions, there is a widespread belief that the longed-for cure for cancer – the magic bullet – is on its way, and it will probably be some sort of drug. But media stories about the latest breakthrough rarely make it clear that the most effective cure for cancer is successful surgery to remove the tumour.

This was true over 40 years ago when President Nixon made his pledge, and it is still true today. The earlier your cancer is detected, the lower the chance that it has spread to other parts of the body (metastasised) and the greater the chance the operation will remove it completely. The new and expensive drugs that are often the subject of campaigns for wider access and availability are nearly all given to patients with advanced cancer, and the amount they extend life is usually measured in months. What makes this picture even worse is that in the industrialised world your lifetime risk of getting cancer has been steadily increasing and is now a scary one person in three.

THE POSSIBILITY OF PREVENTION

The statistics don't have to be like that, however. In some parts of the world the risk is less than one in a 100. In the UK, a woman's lifetime risk of developing breast cancer is one in eight, while in rural China, Thailand, much of Japan and parts of East Africa the risk is a tenth of this.[148]

This shows that cancer is not an inevitable part of growing old, but is a consequence of where and how you live. By looking at those other cultures we can learn that even in the West there are things that we can do to reduce our risk. The first step towards this is to understand some of the causes. Breast cancer incidence rates in the UK have increased by more than 50 per cent over the last 25 years, and prostate cancer rates have tripled over the last 30 years. Why?

WHAT CAUSES CANCER AND HOW CAN YOU CUT YOUR RISK?

Your genes have relatively little to do with your cancer risk. According to research with identical twins, if one developed cancer the other had no more than a 15 per cent chance of developing the same kind. Choices about diet, smoking and exercise accounted for between 58 and 82 per cent of cancers studied.[149] The massive increase in pesticides and carcinogenic chemicals in our environment also play a role, but there is a limit to how much you can realistically do about your exposure to them.

The first place to start looking at closely is the cells in your body. You may remember from Chapter 3 that our cells are the places where the factors responsible for our decline as we age are first apparent, and this happens in a number of ways.

- Damage to the DNA by oxidants is one cancer driver (although this damage can be repaired by a more effective methylation system).

- Many of the new chemicals in our external environment turn on genes that promote cell growth, leading to cancer. An ageing immune system means natural killer cells are not effectively eliminating cells that start to grow abnormally.

- Inflammation, which is part of the process that damages cancer cells, also increases as we age.

- Many people in the West have high levels of glucose and insulin in the bloodstream and, as we saw from the worm research described in Chapter 6, this is linked to both ageing and cancer.

These ageing processes can be improved through diet, supplements and lifestyle choices, strengthening our body against cancer. As always, a healthy diet is fundamental.

YOUR DIET AFFECTS YOUR CANCER RISK

An indication of the role that diet plays comes from the massive European Prospective Investigation into Cancer and Nutrition study, nicknamed EPIC, published in 2010.[150] The project has accumulated a large database of the health and eating habits of over half a million people, as well as retaining blood samples from participants, which scientists can then search to find which elements are linked with raising or lowering our risk of various cancers. Some examples are given below.

A RAISED RISK

Stomach cancer Eating red and processed meat.
Colon cancer Eating red and processed meat, drinking alcohol, being overweight, according to your BMI score, and having extra fat around the middle – the 'apple shape'.
Breast cancer Eating a lot of saturated fat and drinking more than the recommended amount of alcohol. Being overweight according to your BMI score, if you are postmenopausal.
Prostate cancer Eating lots of protein and calcium from dairy sources. A high level of insulin-growth factor in your blood.

A LOWERED RISK

Stomach cancer Eating a Mediterranean diet with plenty of carbohydrates that contain fibre. Having high levels of vitamin C in the blood, and good amounts of vitamins A and E.

Colon cancer Eating a high intake of dietary fibre, fish and calcium. Having good levels of vitamin D in the blood.

Lung cancer If you smoke, eating lots of fruit and vegetables.

Breast cancer Physical activity, if you are postmenopausal.

ARE DRUGS THE ANSWER – OR IS PREVENTION BETTER?

Cancer and its treatments are now highly complex, and cure rates – that is, surviving for more than five years – can be as high as 80 per cent for a few of them. But once a cancer has spread, the benefit you are likely to gain from a gruelling treatment is usually small, and the cost for a few months extra of life can be huge. For these reasons alone a far more serious focus on prevention makes a lot of sense.

How much benefit would you expect from a course of chemotherapy? One analysis of a large number of studies concluded, 'The contribution of chemotherapy to five year survival in adults was 2.3 per cent in Australia and 2.1 per cent in the USA.' Furthermore, the researchers emphasise that these figures 'should be regarded as the upper limit of effectiveness', in other words they are an optimistic rather than a pessimistic estimate.[151]

A recent American study of the cost and effectiveness of cancer drugs given to patients with colon cancer that had spread – so their survival chances were low – found that they increased survival by an average of 6.8 months at a cost of $37,000 (or £41,000) for one year.[152] With the Silver Tsunami underway, can we afford to keep paying such sums? Wouldn't it be better to spend much more on cutting the risk that people will develop cancer in the first place?

POSITIVE STEPS THAT WE CAN TAKE

The fact that the same features of a healthy lifestyle keep showing up whether you are looking at ageing, cancer, heart disease or diabetes is one of the central ideas of this book, and it tells us several important things. Firstly, it highlights the huge difference between the nutritional and the drug approach to health. One aims to improve the functioning of the whole system, whereas the other homes in on a narrow problem area. Specialists in any single area of health, such as cancer or heart disease, are often sceptical about the benefits of antioxidants, vitamin D or omega-3s to the diseases they work with, but studies regularly link these nutritional factors with promoting good health in *other* specialist areas; for example, if you take vitamin D for your bones, it reduces cancer risk, or if you take omega-3 for your heart, your joint pain reduces. This surely must suggest that relatively few nutritional changes in a person could make a big difference to their overall health. What's very encouraging about the research reported in this book is that the things that keep showing up as cutting your risk of chronic diseases are the same things that are repeatedly reported as slowing the broad-spectrum decline that comes with ageing. By following our DIY plan you get a two-for-one: a cut in your risk of specific diseases plus a slower rate of ageing.

The 'protection packages' for ageing well and avoiding cancer, for example, look very similar and include the following: ensure a good supply of antioxidants to slow DNA damage, plus B vitamins to promote methylation and repair, and vitamin D to slow cell division; eat anti-inflammatory foods – such as omega-3s found in fish, as well as herbs and spices; eat a low-glycemic diet; and go easy on pro-inflammatory meat and hormone-rich dairy products.

Twenty years ago a statement signed by 69 highly respected medical and scientific experts in the USA stated: 'Over the last decade, some five million Americans died of cancer and there is growing evidence that a substantial proportion of these deaths was avoidable.'[153] Their deaths were, of course, a tragic waste; what is different now is that soon we may not be able to afford the costs of cancer treatments.

So here are our top eight cancer-prevention steps.

1: INCREASE VITAMIN D

Over 30 years ago the brothers Drs Cedric and Frank Garland, both US scientists, noticed that the further north people lived the more likely they were to develop certain disorders, including colon cancer, diabetes and rheumatoid arthritis. They suggested that there was a link between sickness and a lack of exposure to sunshine. Several decades later, research is mounting that vitamin D can directly affect our DNA, the genetic material at the centre of almost every cell in our bodies.

The latest research has discovered that almost 3,000 genes have their activity boosted or damped down by the presence of vitamin D. Cedric Garland of Moores Cancer Center, University of California, San Diego, is still investigating vitamin D, and his recent research suggests that to reduce your risk of cancer you need to be getting between 27 and 100mcg of vitamin D a day, giving you between 150 and 200 nmol/l in your blood.[154]

There seems no doubt, however, that the majority of the population in the UK, or anywhere else with relatively low levels of sun exposure, are deficient. By deficient we mean having a blood level below 80nmol/l. A level of between 100 and 125nmol/l, according to some, equates with the lowest quantity needed to reduce cancer risk.

Others are more sceptical, however. A review in the *New England Journal of Medicine* concluded that 'evidence that vitamin D reduces cancer incidence and related mortality was inconsistent and inconclusive'.[155] Other reports, which have been heavily criticised, have recommended no more than 20mcg a day.

VITAMIN D: HOW MUCH DO YOU NEED AND HOW MUCH TO SUPPLEMENT?

Working out how much vitamin D you need can be confusing, because there are two different ways your intake is measured and two different measures for the amount in your blood, and it is almost impossible to find out how much you need to take to raise your blood level.

Vitamin D intake from sun or food, or on supplement packs, is measured in two ways: either as iu (international units) or

CONTINUED...

mcg (micrograms). One mcg is equal to 40iu. The daily amount officially recommended in the UK is 200iu or 5mcg. The amount found in your blood is measured either as ng/ml (nannograms per millilitre – US) or nmol/l (nanomoles per litre – UK), which is what we are using in the book. In case you need to convert one to the other, 1 ng/ml = 2.5 nmol/l.

How much will your intake push up your blood levels? The basic 5mcg (200iu) of vitamin D per day can raise the vitamin D in your blood by 5nmol/l (2ng/ml) in two to three months. Bear in mind, though, that this is an average; people vary considerably in how much of their intake gets into their blood.

Most people in the UK have a blood level, depending on the time of year, of between about 52 and 72 nmol/l, which is only just enough to protect your bones. Scientists arguing for much more say we need at least 75nmol/l and probably nearer 125nmol/l. They therefore recommend at least 25mcg to push you from 50 to 75nmol/l and possibly another 50mcg to get you to 125nmo/l. So, it really is worth getting your level tested to find out what you need.

In the summer, you should aim to expose as much of your skin as possible to the sun for about 15 to 20 minutes a day – enough time for your skin to go pink but not red. Even the cancer charities have recently had a change of heart on this and they now recommend 10–15 minutes exposure to the sun at midday during the summer months.

There is disagreement how much of a supplement could be dangerous. A recent review article recommended no more than 100mcg, whereas several experts claim that up to 250mcg is safe.

Calcium *and* vitamin D are important

Joan Lappe, professor of medicine at Creighton University in the US, has been looking at the effect of combining vitamin D with calcium. She tested vitamin D levels in a group of 1,179 postmenopausal women and found 80 per cent were below 80nmol/l, and 15 per cent were very deficient, with levels below 50nmol/l. She gave them 27mcg of vitamin D, more than double the RDA. Their average blood level went up from 76 to 96nmol/l, so even this amount wasn't what many experts recommend. But what difference did this make to cancer risk?

Four years later, those on the calcium plus vitamin D had a 40 per cent lower relative risk of getting cancer compared to the placebo group. Those taking calcium had a non-significant trend towards slightly lower cancer risk.[156]

Vitamin D researcher William Grant estimates that you can cut your risk of breast, prostate and colorectal cancer by about a third by increasing your vitamin D levels from 50 to 100nmol/l. We think that the small amount of cost for taking one drop of 25mcg (1,000iu) of vitamin D per day would be well worthwhile.

It is certainly an attractive proposition when you look at some of the benefits the combination of calcium and vitamin D have in relation to cancer.

Cancer cells	The effect of vitamin D and calcium
Grow without boundaries	Inhibits cell proliferation
Switch off the 'self-destruct' mechanism	Activates self-destruct (apoptosis)
Form their own blood supply (angiogenesis)	Inhibits angiogenesis in tumours
Invade tissues and other organs (metastasis)	Decreases metastic potential
Puts immunity under stresses	Activates and strengthens immunity

2: CLEAN UP YOUR CARCINOGEN ACT

If you want to increase your risk of developing cancer, just stand in the main street of a polluted city on a hot sunny day; let your skin burn, breathe in the exhaust fumes, eat some French fries, drink a beer and smoke a cigarette. Not many people do all these things at once, but many people's lifestyles do involve significant exposure to oxidants.

One of the reasons for the rapid development of cancer in the 20th century is our increased exposure to cancer-causing factors, especially those that directly damage our genes. These include:

- Tobacco smoke
- Exhaust fumes
- Industrial pollution

- Food and agricultural chemicals
- Burnt, browned or fried food
- Excessive sun exposure
- Radiation
- Alcohol

Although the overall incidence of lung cancer is falling in countries where cigarette smoking is on the decline, lung cancer among non-smokers is actually rising.[157] The late Professor Simon Wolff, who was a toxicologist at University College London, believed that this was almost certainly because of increasing levels of air pollution, particularly from diesel fuel. He pointed out that 'in rural China, where people tend to smoke very heavily and where air pollution is much less, the difference in lung cancer rates between smokers and non-smokers is very small, and lung cancer rates are about one-tenth of the lung cancer rates in industrialised countries.'[158]

The traditional diet in rural China is also higher in antioxidants than the typical diet in industrialised countries. So, there are several factors at work here. Avoiding cigarette smoke is easier now than it used to be, and it's also important to ensure that you include more antioxidants in your diet. Avoiding pollution, pesticides and other industrial chemicals is harder today, but you can watch out for some chemical compounds found in food, such as one called acrylamide, which is produced by frying, barbecuing, baking, and even microwaving, food.

The safe limit is 10 parts per billion (ppb), but some foods have been found to contain more than 100 times this amount! Fast-food-chain chips, crisps, taco shells and breakfast cereals are the worst. Crisps average 1,250 ppb and Pringles 1,480 ppb. Even home-cooked chips can be high. A recent study from the Netherlands reported that increased dietary intakes of acrylamide could raise the risk of kidney cancer by 59 per cent (although not prostate or bladder cancer).[159]

3: LOAD YOUR DIET WITH ANTIOXIDANTS

Point 2 above is one side of the oxidant equation: trying to limit your exposure to oxidants. The other side is antioxidants, which neutralise the oxidants, and we discussed those in Chapter 5. The evidence for the protective effect of having optimal amounts of these anti-cancer nutrients in your diet is substantial and dates back 30 years.

A survey published in the *Lancet* medical journal in 1981, for example, looked at the relationship between beta-carotene status (the vegetable form of vitamin A) and smoking.[160] They found that heavy smokers with a low beta-carotene status had a 6.5 per cent chance of developing lung cancer. On the other hand, a heavy smoker with a high beta-carotene status only had a 0.8 per cent risk. So too did a non-smoker with a low beta-carotene status. Finally, those who had a high beta-carotene status and didn't smoke had no risk. This study suggests that increasing your intake of certain anti-cancer nutrients in your diet is just as important as limiting your intake of carcinogens.

The beta-carotene debate

There's no doubt that eating foods rich in beta-carotene reduces the risk of cancer. The World Cancer Research Fund (WCRF), which reviewed hundreds of studies, concludes that carotenoids – antioxidants found in fruit and vegetables, of which beta-carotene is one – are highly protective. (Others among many include lycopene, which is found in tomatoes, and lutein and zeathanthin, both found in green veg. Collectively, they are probably more protective than any one in isolation.) For example, for lung cancer the WCRF says: 'Overall, the extensive data show a weak to strong decrease in risk with higher dietary intakes of carotenoids.'[161]

There's also no doubt that having a higher beta-carotene level in your bloodstream is beneficial. A ten-year study of several thousand elderly people in Europe, conducted by the Centre for Nutrition and Health at the National Institute of Public Health and the Environment in the Netherlands, found that the higher the beta-carotene level, the lower the overall risk of death, especially from cancer. Eating probably the equivalent of a carrot a day (raising the blood level by 0.39mcmol/l) meant cutting cancer risk by a third.[162]

That's the good news. Unfortunately, all this evidence has apparently vanished from the collective medical memory as the result of a single report a few years ago that found that beta-carotene 'causes' cancer. At least, that was the headline the papers used, and it's that which now sticks in the memory. Countless articles questioning the benefits of taking supplements now frequently end up with a warning that supplements are not as safe as people think – they can cause cancer.

So let's try to nail this myth. It began with a study by the National Cancer Institute in the US, which reported a 28 per cent increased incidence in lung cancer in those who took beta-carotene but who continued to smoke.[163] Another more accurate way of summarising this study is to say that it showed that one smoker out of 1,000 who takes beta-carotene on its own and takes no other antioxidant supplement, and who keeps on smoking, will have a slightly raised risk of cancer. That's it. That is what the 'supplements can cause cancer' canard is based on.

A closer look at the figures shows what was really going on. Out of the 10,000 people in the placebo group, 50 developed cancer; out of the 10,000 getting beta-carotene, 65 developed cancer. That is a 28 per cent increase, but how alarming does it look now? In fact, it didn't even reach 'statistical significance', meaning it could have occurred by chance. And there's another point that's always forgotten, both groups involved people who had smoked for years and probably had undetected cancer before starting the trial.

As if this distortion was not unscientific enough, there was another set of findings in the research paper that never made it into the summary (the abstract), let alone the newspaper headlines. Hidden in the body of the paper, which almost nobody ever reads because they depend on the summary, was the finding that among those who gave up smoking during the trial and took beta-carotene, there were 20 per cent *fewer* cases of lung cancer.

Again, this was not statistically significant, but if one 'trend' is worth reporting, surely another is. Unless you assume that beta-carotene makes moral distinctions, giving smokers cancer while protecting those who give up, the implication of this finding is that there is something about smoking that makes it harder for beta-carotene given alone to have an effect.

And this points towards yet another shortcoming of the trial. It only used beta-carotene or a placebo. But, unlike drugs, which often combine in a harmful way, nutrients, especially antioxidants, usually *reinforce* each other's effects. In fact, giving an individual nutrient to sick people without changing their diet or lifestyle, probably won't do any good. Claiming such trials show supplements can be dangerous is more polemic than science.

For people not 'at risk', not smoking and not supplementing beta-carotene on its own, the evidence for beta-carotene's protective effect remains highly positive overall. One large study involving 13,000 people between the ages of 35 and 60 to investigate the effects of a pill containing a cocktail of antioxidants (beta-carotene, vitamin C and E) found a highly significant 31 per cent reduction in the risk of all cancers in men, plus an overall 37 per cent lower death rate.[164]

Another study found this combination of antioxidants highly protective against colon cancer, but there was no such effect among those who were heavy drinkers and smokers and only took beta-carotene. In fact, for these people there was a very slight increased risk.[165] The British *Daily Mail* had a field day with this story, running a headline that read 'Vitamin pills could cause early death' with a subheading that read: 'vitamins, taken by millions, could be causing thousands of premature deaths'. But you try finding a heavy drinker and smoker who pops beta-carotene on its own! This is about scoring debating points, not trying to understand how best to improve people's health.

Antioxidant nutrients are team players. Their job is to disarm dangerous oxidants, generated by combustion, which can come from a variety of sources – from a lit cigarette to frying bacon. They do this by passing the oxidant through a chain of reactions involving vitamins E, C, beta-carotene, CoQ_{10}, and others you may be less familiar with, such as glutathione and lipoic acid. On their own, these can do more harm than good, by becoming oxidised. This is probably what's happening to beta-carotene among smokers.

So, our advice would be not to supplement beta-carotene on its own if you are a heavy smoker or drinker – and to stop smoking and excessive drinking! But even among smokers, a high dietary intake of beta-carotene is not associated with increased risk.[166] So, keep eating the carrots and supplementing all-round antioxidant supplements or multivitamins, as many other studies show that this combination results in a clear reduction of cancer risk. In relation to cancer, the true danger is not by increasing your intake through supplements.

Antioxidants work together

The problem is that giving single antioxidants, as many negative controlled trials have done, tells us nothing useful at all, because antioxidants work as a team. In the process of mopping up the dangerous oxidant 'sparks', the antioxidants become oxidised and destabilised themselves, and need a partner antioxidant to be 'reloaded', as shown in the illustration below.

The synergistic action of nutrients in disarming a free radical

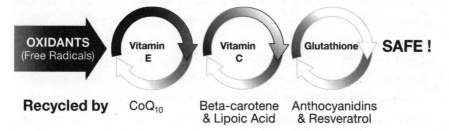

Some examples of this reloading are given below:

- Vitamin E is recycled by vitamin C and CoQ_{10}.
- Vitamin C is recycled by glutathione (one of the most important antioxidants of all), carotenoids (in carrots) and lipoic acid.
- Glutathione is recycled by anthocyanidins (found in berries) and resveratrol (see page 66).

Having a high intake of both vitamins C and E, as well as glutathione and anthocyanidins, is much more protective than just taking one on its own. The synergy of nutrients is also vital, because there are many different kinds of oxidants, each disarmed most effectively by a different kind of antioxidant. So, for all-round protection against all the oxidants that come your way, you need to take in a whole range of antioxidants, including:

vitamin A	glutathione	lipoic acid
vitamin C	anthocyanidins	polyphenols
vitamin E	carotenoids	salvestrols
selenium	CoQ_{10}	resveratrol

These nutrients are found in food and can also be taken in concentrated form as nutritional supplements, but unfortunately this is only part of the story. Even though the subject of antioxidant supplements is contentious (see page 186) there is still good reason to ensure an optimal intake for DNA protection and cancer prevention, since most prevention studies are associated with benefit.[167] From a diet point of view, the simplest way to do this is to eat a multicoloured diet, choosing foods high in ORACs (oxygen radical absorbage capacity).

ORACs: your dietary antioxidants

You can get literally hundreds of antioxidants from foods. The main essential antioxidant vitamins are A, C and E and the precursor of vitamin A, beta-carotene. Beta-carotene is found in red, orange and yellow vegetables and fruit. Vitamin C is also abundant in vegetables and fruit eaten raw, but heat rapidly destroys it. Vitamin E is found in 'seed' foods, including nuts, seeds and their oils, and vegetables like peas, broad beans, corn and whole grains.

There are many other important antioxidant ingredients in food, however, such as flavonoids. Examples are quercetin in onions, catechins in green tea, epicatechin in chocolate, isoflavones in beans, and anthocyanidins, including resveratrol in berries and red grapes. It's far better to eat a varied diet high in antioxidant-rich foods than to simply rely on vitamin C and E. Thanks to research at Tufts University in Boston, there's a way to rate a food's overall antioxidant power. Each food can now be assigned a certain number of ORAC units. Foods that score high in these units are especially helpful in countering free-radical damage in your body.

Our top 20 foods are shown in the table opposite. Each of these food servings gives you 2,000 ORACs. If you can, eat the equivalent of 6,000 ORACs a day. The more ORACs you take in, the more you protect yourself against cancer as well as protecting your memory[168] and your heart.

The chart below shows ORACs of 20 different foods that you can incorporate easily into your daily diet. Each serving contains approximately 2,000 units. Just pick at least three of these daily to hit your anti-ageing score of 6,000.

Top ORAC-scoring foods

1	⅓ tsp cinnamon, ground	11	7 walnut halves
2	½ tsp oregano, dried	12	8 pecan halves
3	½ tsp turmeric, ground	13	¼ cup pistachio nuts
4	1 heaped tsp mustard	14	½ cup cooked lentils
5	⅕ cup blueberries	15	1 cup cooked kidney beans
6	Half a pear, grapefruit or plum	16	⅓ medium avocado
7	½ cup blackcurrants, blackberries, raspberries, strawberries	17	½ cup of red cabbage
8	½ cup cherries or a shot of Cherry Active concentrate	18	2 cups of broccoli
9	An orange or apple	19	1 medium artichoke or 8 spears of asparagus
10	4 pieces of dark chocolate (70% cocoa solids)	20	⅓ medium glass (150ml) red wine

Source: Oxygen Radical Absorbance Capacity of Selected Foods – 2007, US Department of Agriculture

Generally speaking, where you find the most colour and flavour you will also find the highest antioxidant levels. The reds, yellows and oranges of tomatoes and carrots, for example, are due to the presence of beta-carotene. Aim for five to ten servings daily of a wide range of fruits and vegetables to keep your intake high.

Fruits that have the highest levels are those with the deepest colour such as blueberries, raspberries and strawberries. These are particularly rich in powerful antioxidants called anthocyanidins. One cup of blueberries will provide 9,697 units. You would need to eat 11 bananas to get the same benefit as a cupful of blueberries!

One of the simplest and easiest ways to achieve 6,000 ORACs is to have a daily shot of a Montmorency cherry concentrate called Cherry Active, diluted with water. This measures 8,260 on the ORAC scale, which is the equivalent of about 23 portions of regular fruit and vegetables! Other juices claim high ORAC scores, from acai to pomegranate, but this tops the lot.

4: PROTECT YOURSELF WITH VITAMIN C

The antioxidant vitamin C needs special mention because having a high intake has been consistently shown to reduce your risk of cancer, as well as other diseases such as diabetes and heart disease. Furthermore, vitamin C can be taken as a supplement on its own.

Back in 1991, Dr Gladys Block, formerly with the National Cancer Institute, published a review[169] of vitamin C research, which concluded that there was very strong evidence of a protective effect of vitamin C for non-hormone cancers. Of the 46 such studies in which a dietary vitamin C index was calculated, 33 found statistically significant protection. In a further review[170] later that year, of studies linking vitamin C with cancer prevention, Dr Block concludes:

> *Approximately 90 epidemiologic studies have examined the role of vitamin C or vitamin-C-rich foods in cancer prevention, and the vast majority have found statistically significant protective effects. Evidence is strong for cancers of the oesophagus, oral cavity, stomach and pancreas. There is also substantial evidence of a protective effect in cancers of the cervix, rectum and breast. Even in lung cancer there is recent evidence of a role for vitamin C.*

Numerous studies have found a link between high vitamin C intake and low incidence of several different cancers, especially non-hormonal cancers.[171] Also, having a high plasma level of vitamin C cuts your risk of dying from cancer.[172] As we have seen, the evidence for the benefits of vitamin C is strongest for cancers of the mouth, oesophagus, stomach, lung, pancreas and cervix. While one analysis of 12 clinical studies found that 'Vitamin C intake had the most consistent and statistically significant inverse association with breast cancer risk'.

High-dose vitamin C – a possible treatment

Although this chapter is aimed at prevention, it seems worth mentioning a promising but very controversial form of cancer treatment, which involves giving very high doses of vitamin C intravenously or orally. The idea dates back to Linus Pauling, champion of vitamin C, who successfully treated 100 patients over 35 years ago. Those getting vitamin C survived approximately four times longer.[173]

One possible reason why this might work is that in amounts as high as 4g per kilo – which means about 75g given intravenously for an average adult – vitamin C behaves like an oxidant inside the tumour.[174] It causes a build-up of a destructive chemical called hydrogen peroxide only in cancer cells and can reduce tumour size by 40 per cent. A few clinicians use it in the UK and claim that it is effective at shrinking tumours, with virtually no side effects and more cheaply than with chemotherapy. Others recommend oral vitamin C up to bowel-tolerance levels – the most you can take without getting diarrhoea.

A small trial with humans recently found that it produced better results in hard-to-treat pancreatic cancer than chemotherapy alone.[175] Recently, however, the FDA has ordered a small American drug company, McGuff Pharmaceuticals, to stop producing vitamin C for intravenous use on the grounds that when delivered in that way it is an unapproved drug.

5: BALANCE YOUR BLOOD SUGAR

As we saw in Chapter 6, researchers are now exploring the links between high glucose and insulin levels and a raised risk of cancer. One study in Italy found that regularly eating sweet foods, including biscuits, ice cream, honey and chocolate 'may account for 12 per cent of breast cancer cases in this Italian population'.[176]

Eating foods with a *high* glycemic index (GI) and/or glycemic load (GL) has been linked to a higher risk of many cancers, including breast,[177] colorectal,[178] pancreatic,[179] ovarian,[180] thyroid,[181] endometrial (womb),[182] and gastric.[183] Conversely, low-GI and/or low-GL diets are associated with a reduced risk of breast, colorectal, ovarian, and endometrial (womb) cancers.[184] Postmenopausal women with high insulin levels have been shown to have twice the risk of developing breast cancer.[185] Eating a low-GL diet, as we explain in Part Three, Chapter 2, is a fundamental cancer-prevention step.

Although animal studies can't prove that a particular procedure will work for humans, strong evidence for the benefit of a low-carb–high-protein diet emerged from a study reported in June 2011 showing that human tumours implanted into mice grew much more slowly when the animals were fed a diet with very low carbohydrates (15 per cent), high protein (58 per cent) and medium fat (26 per cent) vs a typical Western diet of 55 per cent carbohydrates, 23 per cent protein and 22 per cent fat.[186]

Even more relevant to prevention was the result of research on mice that had been genetically engineered to develop cancer. When they were put on these diets almost half of those on the Western diet developed cancer within a year, whereas none on the low-carb diet succumbed. The low-carb diet even had an anti-ageing effect. Whereas only one of the animals on the Western diet lived a normal life span of two years, more than half of the low-carb group reached two years or more.

Lead researcher, Professor Gerald Krystal, of the British Columbia Cancer Research Centre, believes insulin is responsible for the damaging effect of the Western diet. 'Restricting carbohydrate intake can significantly limit blood glucose,' he said, 'and insulin is a hormone that has been shown in many independent studies to promote tumour growth in both humans and mice.' Even though the link between sugar and cancer has been known since before the Second World War, few oncologists consider something as simple as reducing it in the diet.

It's not just tumours in mice that respond to bringing down insulin, however. When researchers looked at blood samples taken from women in a large study on HRT and postmenopausal women (by the Women's Health Initiative), they found that those with the highest insulin levels were 50 per cent more likely to have developed breast cancer. Among those women who had never taken HRT, insulin had an even larger impact, doubling the risk of breast cancer.[187]

Lead researcher, Professor Marc Gunter, says that when they took into account insulin levels, the link between obesity and cancer became much weaker. 'Women who are obese are more likely to develop breast cancer but now it looks as if it is their insulin levels that are crucial, rather than their weight.' He suggests that screening non-diabetic menopausal women for high insulin could be a useful way of spotting those at high risk for breast cancer.

6: KEEP INFLAMMATION DOWN BY EATING FISH OILS

Omega-3 fats appear on almost every healthy-living list, and cutting your cancer risk is no exception; for example, a six-year follow-up study on 35,000 postmenopausal women in Seattle, Washington found that the use of omega-3 supplements with high levels of EPA and DHA was linked with a 32 per cent reduction in breast cancer, largely of the most common type involving milk ducts.[188]

It is, of course, only an association, but it is not the only one. A group of people who are likely to develop polyps in their colon (known as familial adenomatous polyposis), which makes them much more likely to develop colon cancer, were given either 2g of the type of omega-3 fish oil known as EPA or a placebo. Those getting EPA had fewer (22 per cent) and smaller polyps whereas those on the placebo grew more.[189] The effect was similar to that found with aspirin-type drugs known as COX-2 inhibitors, but they come with a raft of side effects, including gut damage and an increased risk of heart attacks when used regularly.

Omega-3 may also benefit prostate cancer patients, who normally have a high level of inflammation. This essential fat was found to lower the risk of developing an aggressive tumour type. In a group of 465 patients with advanced prostate cancer, those taking the most omega-3 significantly cut the risk of their cancer becoming more aggressive. The ones who benefited most were those who had a particular variation in the COX-2 gene, which affects inflammation. Normally, they would be five times more likely to develop a more aggressive tumour, but that risk was dramatically reversed by taking more omega-3.[190]

7: TAKE SUFFICIENT B VITAMINS

B vitamins are emerging as key players in several of the diseases of ageing. Making sure you have healthy levels, which can be tricky for older people, also appears to be important for reducing your risk of cancer. It's not at all surprising, because, as we've seen elsewhere, they are vital for methylation, which is needed for DNA repair. It's a sensible idea that researchers from the International Agency for Research on Cancer in Lyon, France, set out to test. They used the huge EPIC database referred to earlier. People with higher levels of vitamin B_6 and the amino acid methionine, which is also vital for methylation, had a 50 per cent reduction in their risk of developing lung cancer. The risk reduction was pushed up to over 60 per cent if they had a higher level of the B vitamin folate.[191] For comparison, the widely used cholesterol-lowering statin drugs are usually said to reduce the risk of heart disease by 20–25 per cent.

8: KEEP EXERCISING

It almost goes without saying that exercise can have a beneficial effect on cancer, as it's a key part of healthy ageing. A recent trial suggests that it may also play a valuable role even if your cancer is very advanced. In this case it seems to have outperformed cancer drugs that are priced at $40,000 or $50,000 (£36,000 or £45,000) a year. Patients with advanced recurrent brain cancer who went for a brisk 30-minute walk five days a week were found to live nearly twice as long as those who were sedentary. Survival went up from an average of 13.03 months to 21.84 months.[192] To put this into perspective, drugs are licensed if their benefits are half that result.

FRUIT AND VEGETABLES CAN TARGET CANCER GENES

Many of the newer cancer drugs work by targeting gene variations found in tumour cells but not in healthy ones. Now, that approach is being tried out with plant-based compounds known as salvestrols by Professor Gerry Potter of the Cancer Drug Discovery Group at the University of Leicester. The key discovery was that an enzyme known as CYP1B1, found only in tumours, transforms salvestrols into a compound called piceatannol, known to be highly toxic to cancer cells.[193] What is fascinating is that the salvestrol that does this most effectively is resveratrol, the anti-ageing calorie-restriction mimetic that GlaxoSmithKline paid $700 million for (see Chapter 6). Once again, cutting cancer risk and slowing ageing are closely intertwined.

Potter has found salvestrols in a wide range of plants, so one obvious step would be to incorporate them into our diet. There are a couple of problems, however. Firstly, they taste quite bitter, so many modern varieties have the salvestrols bred out of them. For example, Gala apples have almost none, while Cox's and Pendragon's, if grown organically, are loaded with salvestrols. Secondly, the amount any fruit or vegetable contains varies enormously between the different varieties. It's not helpful suggesting you 'eat an orange', for example, because many types contain little, if any, salvestrol. In fact there's much more in the rind.

You can buy high-dose salvestrol food supplements, which were manufactured following demand from cancer patients once the original 'proof of principle' research was published. If you have cancer and use them in this way, it's recommended that you work with a nutritional therapist to ensure that you are taking the appropriate supplements for your particular type of cancer. Low-dose salvestrols can also be taken for prevention.

We need clinical trials, but there have been a few positive case reports published relating to patients who had various stages of cancers of the lung, melanoma, prostate, breast and bladder.[194]

SUMMARY

To strengthen your body against cancer:

- Don't smoke.
- Eat plenty of antioxidant-rich and anti-inflammatory foods.
- Keep your omega-3 levels up, to reduce inflammation.
- Keep your glucose and insulin levels down with a low-GL diet, such as our Anti-ageing Diet.
- Control your weight.
- Minimise the amount of dairy products you consume.
- Eat plenty of beans and greens (they are rich is phytoestrogens and oestrogen blockers).
- Minimise your intake of deep-fried and crispy foods.
- Eat organic fruit and vegetables as much as you can.
- Do all you can to minimise your exposure to carcinogens and hormone disruptors.

CONTINUED...

In terms of supplements:

- Increase your intake of vitamin D through exposure to sun and taking supplements – whatever you need to achieve a blood level above 100nml/l – normally 2,000iu.
- Supplement at least 2g of vitamin C a day and, ideally, an all-round antioxidant formula.
- Check your vitamin B levels to ensure you have good methylation and DNA repair.
- If you have, or are at risk of cancer, supplement salvestrols and consider upping your vitamin C intake dramatically.

See Part Three, Chapter 7 for your general supplement programme and Recommended Reading for other helpful books on this topic.

KEEP YOUR HEART HEALTHY AND YOUR BLOOD PRESSURE LOW

For most people over 50, having cancer or losing one's memory holds the greatest fear, but in fact more people die prematurely from diseases of the heart and arteries than anything else – 150,000 a year in England alone, roughly half from heart attacks and a quarter from strokes.[195] In the past, many more men than women died from heart disease, but in recent years the numbers have evened out, with more women than men dying from strokes. At least 20,000 deaths occur prematurely every year, in people under the age of 75.

Like other chronic diseases, the causes of heart disease are rooted in how and where we live – a woman living in Scotland, for example, has eight times the risk of a heart attack than her sister living in Spain.[196] People develop heart disease for reasons that are all too familiar: poor diet, smoking, obesity and a lack of exercise, although a serious programme of prevention could cut the numbers dramatically.

If you have a number of risk factors, such as hypertension or excess fats in the blood, or you've had a stroke or a heart attack, your medical professional is unlikely to pay attention to the causes, and you'll probably be prescribed a standard one-size-fits-all cocktail of drugs to lower your cholesterol, bring down your blood pressure and thin your blood.

THE DRAWBACKS WITH DRUGS

There are several serious drawbacks to relying on drugs to protect your heart if you are aiming to live healthily and you haven't already had a heart attack or stroke – and drugs are being prescribed as a preventive rather than as a treatment. The first is simply that if you are now in your fifties you could be taking three or more pills – for cholesterol, blood pressure and blood thinning – for 30 years. Over that period, you would want to ask what the very long-term effects might be, but no one knows.

Several large studies suggest that for healthy people who haven't had a heart attack, a large number of people have to take these medications for just one to benefit, as we first mentioned in Chapter 4, and we'll discuss what this might mean for you later in this chapter. The main problem is not just that you may experience side effects but that many of them are precisely the ones that become more likely as you age anyway, so they are not always recognised as being caused by the drugs. Statins, for example, are linked to an increased risk of muscle weakness, cataracts and poorer blood glucose control.

The combined strategy of changing your diet, improving your lifestyle, and taking the right supplements is a positive step towards reversing cardiovascular disease without the side effects, and surely preferable to taking prescribed drugs. One way to do this is to try reducing your risk factors, following the advice in this chapter, and then asking your doctor for tests to see how you are progressing.

If you are already on medication and the tests show that your risk for heart disease has come right down, then talk to your doctor about coming off medication. Don't make any changes without discussing it, though. Later in the chapter are examples of people who have successfully stopped taking medication following the advice we have here. The point about ageing well is that it takes a bit more planning and research than the more familiar old idea of somehow muddling through with some good genes and a bit of luck.

BEWARE OF STANDARD DIET ADVICE

All health authorities will tell you that you can cut your risk of a heart attack by following a 'healthy balanced diet'. But what exactly does that involve? Unfortunately, for the last 40 years or so, the official advice has been simply wrong. The healthy balanced diet that is supposed to protect your heart is based around the idea that it should be low in fat and low in cholesterol despite clear evidence that these are not the promoters of heart disease. What's more, if you are trying to age well, following a low-fat diet is probably one of the least effective things you could do, because it is likely to push up your insulin, whereas, as you probably remember from earlier chapters, keeping your insulin down is one of the *best* things you can do.

There are a lot of inconsistencies in the data on fat intake and heart disease. Some countries with a high fat intake (for example, Finland) have a high rate of heart disease whereas others (such as Greece) have a very low rate of heart disease. At the end of last year, the American Dietetic Association summarised the findings from decades of research into the benefits of lowering fat and its effect on cholesterol and heart disease.[197] The conclusion was that there was little evidence it made a difference. What difference there was depended on what you replaced the fat with.

'If you replaced saturated fat with polyunsaturated fat there was a reduction in risk [of heart disease],' said Professor Walter Willett, Head of Nutrition at Harvard School of Public Health. 'But if you replaced total fat or saturated fat with carbohydrate, no reduction in risk [was found].' In 2011 the respected Cochrane Collaboration came up with exactly the same conclusion: no clear effect on death rates from cutting down on saturated fat, and no health benefit if the fat was replaced with starchy carbohydrates.[198]

There is a disastrous element in the low-fat diet that has been recommended by dieticians for 40 years, in that it involves eating not just more carbohydrates but more *refined* carbohydrates. The problem starts with manufacturers who have tried to produce low-fat foods but have found that they don't taste as good. In attempting to make those 'healthy' low-fat meals more palatable, many contain added sugar. But, as we have seen, more and more glucose in the blood leads to more insulin, which leads to chronic diseases and poorer ageing.

Fat is needed by the body, so if you want your eyes, blood vessels and skin to age well, low fat is not the way to go.

CHOLESTEROL – IS IT THE KEY?

The story of how fat became unfairly demonised is a long and fascinating one that has been covered by American science writer Gary Taubes in *A Big Fat Lie* as well as by British GP Malcolm Kendrick.[199] You know the official story: cholesterol blocks the arteries; if you stop eating cholesterol-rich foods you will lower blood cholesterol and stop heart attacks. Yet, every single piece of this story is unquestionably wrong. Eating a lower cholesterol diet doesn't make much difference to either your blood cholesterol level or your risk of a heart attack. Study after study has repeatedly failed to find any increased risk of heart disease from eating six eggs a week versus one.[200] One study finds that seven eggs or more a week confers a very slightly increased risk, but this is not confirmed by other studies, whereas two studies find that the risk is slightly higher in diabetics either eating lots of eggs or having a very high cholesterol intake in their diet. So, if you are not diabetic you can assume that it is certainly safe to have six eggs a week. If you are diabetic it may be wise to limit your total cholesterol by having no more than three eggs a week and fewer other cholesterol-rich foods such as prawns; however, it is likely that if your overall diet is healthy even this is unnecessary.

Furthermore, the odds are that if you have a heart attack you won't have high cholesterol. A massive US survey of 136,905 patients found that more than half of those hospitalised for a heart attack had perfectly normal cholesterol levels, and almost half had optimal cholesterol levels (LDL cholesterol less than 1.8mmol/l, below that recommended to GPs by the National Institute of Clinical Excellence).[201] So, what is all this hype about cholesterol?

CHOLESTEROL: THE 'GOOD' AND THE 'BAD'

For years, heart health campaigns have been warning us of the dangers of raised cholesterol and the need to bring it down because of the harm it can do to our arteries. So it's easy to forget how vital this fatty substance is. It forms an important part of the outside wall of every cell in our body and is found

CONTINUED...

---

in the insulation around nerve fibres that allows faster transmission. It's also the raw material that our bodies use to manufacture sex hormones – no cholesterol: no testosterone or oestrogen – and is part of the body's repair system. It is also essential for making vitamin D in the skin from sunlight.

Because it is a fat and doesn't dissolve in the blood, cholesterol like other fats has to be transported to and from the cells by carriers called lipoproteins. The average total cholesterol level in the UK is 5.5mmol/l for men and 5.6mmol/l for women, which is above the level now considered healthy. A European heart charity called R3i claims we need new therapies to prevent heart disease because lowering cholesterol with statins only treats 25 per cent of the risk.

LDL ('bad') cholesterol

The danger from cholesterol comes when too much of the 'bad' sort (LDL) builds up in the blood where it can form plaque, a thick, hard deposit that can narrow the arteries making them less flexible and you more at risk of a heart attack or stroke. But that can't be the whole story because, as some critics point out, cholesterol levels are actually a rather poor marker for heart disease. As we have seen, many of the heart attack patients who are rushed to hospital have fairly normal cholesterol levels. Inflammation is increasingly recognised as playing a role in heart disease and some of the benefit from cholesterol-lowering statins may be because it is also mildly anti-inflammatory. Official advice used to be to avoid fatty cholesterol-rich foods such as eggs but that has been dropped; 80 per cent of our cholesterol is made in the liver.

HDL ('good') cholesterol

The HDL cholesterol is considered 'good' because population studies found that people with higher levels were somehow protected from heart disease. Exactly why isn't clear. One common story is that HDL 'scours the walls of blood vessels, cleaning out excess cholesterol' but there are questions about how exactly it does that. It does take cholesterol back to the liver. Statins don't have much effect on HDL levels and much research has gone into developing a drug that does. The last candidate, Torcetrapib, was found to increase the risk of heart

CONTINUED...

attacks. Non-drug ways to raise it include aerobic exercise, losing weight, stopping smoking and cutting out trans-fatty acids (found in some cakes, biscuits and soft margarines), as well as having a couple of glasses of alcohol. The B vitamin niacin, which lowers cholesterol, is also effective at raising HDL.

The role of cholesterol in your arteries

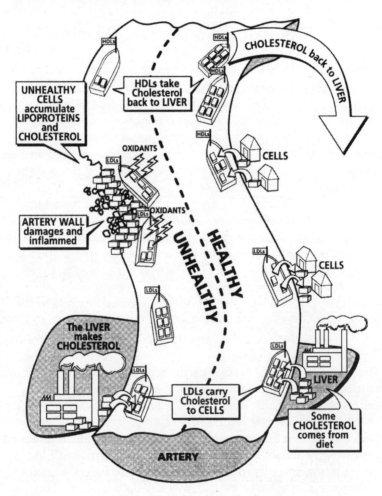

IS YOUR LDL DOWN OR YOUR HDL UP?

Notice in the diagram opposite the role of inflammation in the wall of the coronary arteries. This could be one of the reasons for the benefit that is found with taking statins, which are anti-inflammatory drugs (although there are other ways of dealing with inflammation). But which is more important: to get your LDL down or to keep your HDL up? All of your doctor's attention will be focused on getting your LDL down, and that's what statins do very effectively. Furthermore, your GP's practice receives payments for putting people on statins because the government has put financial pressure on them to reduce heart disease.

This is because, currently, there are no drugs that effectively and safely raise HDL. There is a vitamin, niacin, which does it very effectively, however, but because it can't be patented it is not marketed heavily and GPs are unlikely to be given education seminars promoting its benefits (more on niacin later).

THE TRUTH ABOUT STATINS

For over a decade there has been a worldwide marketing campaign to heavily promote these rather ineffective drugs. At the height of statin fever there was even talk of putting them in the water supply. 'If we can give them a pill in their 30s or 40s, their chances of having a heart attack will be slashed. It could be given to healthy people as a supplement to prevent their arteries becoming clogged,' read one newspaper front page in 2006.[202] In July 2007, the government's heart disease supremo, Professor Roger Boyle, declared that blanket prescribing of statins to all those over 50 would have the biggest effect on saving lives, although he conceded that was unrealistic.

Although the mainstream view is that statins benefit virtually everyone, there is good reason to believe that if you are a man aged over 69, or a woman of any age, they are not going to do you much good, if you haven't already had a heart attack. It's important to make the distinction here between taking statins as *primary prevention* as opposed to taking them if you have already had a heart attack. If you have already had a heart attack and are taking them to cut your chances of having another (called secondary prevention), statins *do* work; however about 75 per cent of people on statins get them for primary prevention: to lower their risk of a heart attack when they haven't had one.

Just how poor the evidence is and how little effort has been made to discover how many people are troubled by side effects was highlighted in a review of statins by the respected Cochrane Collaboration at the beginning of 2010. It analysed trials involving 34,272 people who hadn't had a heart attack and found little evidence that taking a statin would protect people from having a first heart attack unless their risk was classified as high. These are drugs given to about four and a half million healthy people in the UK. And if you are over 65 or female the evidence probably has even less relevance, said the researchers, because most of the trials involved white, middle-aged males, so the results don't necessarily apply to anyone else.

The review also commented on the range of side effects, which include cataracts, acute kidney failure, and moderate or severe liver dysfunction, along with sleep disturbances, memory loss, sexual dysfunction, depression, and (very rarely) interstitial lung disease. Even though the drugs have been prescribed to millions for over a decade, however, the reviewers found that the trials don't give nearly enough information about side effects. Over half the trials didn't report on adverse events at all, and they noted that there had been no attempt to assess the risk of some potentially serious side effects, such as cognitive impairment (brain fog, as some patients call it) or the very real risk of diabetes when cholesterol is lowered too fast.[203]

The myth of a promise of longer life

Even if the evidence that statins cut the risk of having a heart attack is weak, surely they prevent people dying early from a heart attack? Unfortunately not. A study in the *Lancet* in 2007 found that even though the drugs prevented a few heart attacks, none of the patients lived any longer as a result. You will have been told that this pill will cut your risk of a heart attack, so you assume that it will also make you live longer, but that is not the case. Men over 69 didn't benefit from taking statins at all. They didn't live longer and they didn't have fewer heart attacks, and women of any age didn't benefit either.[204]

According to the study's author, Harvard professor John Abramson, you do benefit a little if you have a high risk (officially defined as having a greater than 20 per cent chance of having a cardiovascular event over the next ten years) and you're aged between 30 and 69 years. But the amount is hardly impressive. Fifty people have to be treated for five years to prevent just one event involving the heart. A more recent study on many more people – so the results could be expected to be more accurate – came up with figures for reduction in mortality that were even less impressive.

The study analysed trials involving 65,000 people who didn't have heart disease but just a raised risk. It found that out of 10,000 people who took the drugs for nearly four years, the number of deaths that were prevented (seven) didn't reach statistical significance, meaning the effect could have been due to chance.[205] 'The number of deaths prevented didn't reach statistical significance,' said lead researcher Professor Kausik Ray of St George's Hospital in South London. 'That means it could have happened by chance.' Yet this study and the Cochrane one have made barely a dent in the extent of prescribing. Sadly, this is evidence-based medicine at work.

If you are a woman with a very high risk of heart disease, how much benefit could you expect from taking statins? To answer this question for the GP magazine *Pulse*, Dr Malcolm Kendrick (author of *The Great Cholesterol Con*) analysed a major statin trial called HPS, which is frequently quoted as showing that statins benefit women, and concluded that if you took statins for 30 years, you would gain, on average, just one extra month of life.

Whether or not to take statins has become a complicated topic. The official line is that you should, and experts such as Professor Colin Baigent of Oxford University's Clinical Trials Service Unit are firmly behind it. On the other hand, the chances you will benefit personally are small, and other experts say your chance of adverse side effects have been underestimated; furthermore, some individual GPs writing in the *British Medical Journal* are sceptical about the benefits.[206] One reported an analysis of the benefit in his own practice and found that primary-care patients taking statins had a worse cardiovascular outcome than those without, although he admitted he could have made a mistake with his statistics.

There is certainly plenty of material for you to discuss the issue with your doctor. Either way, drugs are far from a complete answer.

The attraction of the lifestyle approach is that it seems to have the potential to hit so many more targets, and if you do follow our nutritional and exercise advice you'll have a good chance of actually feeling better too – an effect you are unlikely to get from the drugs. Ask your doctor to check after a few months to see if your health markers – blood sugar, cholesterol, blood pressure – are going in the right direction.

The harm caused by statins

All this might not matter too much if there were no downside to being prescribed statins for years. But, as the Cochrane analysis showed, not only are there known to be a range of unpleasant side effects but the companies make little effort to discover just how many people are affected. You might actually be at more risk from serious side effects than from a possible heart attack.

Your doctor will very likely tell you about the risks of muscle pain and weakness (myopathy) and a harmful change in liver function, although he or she will most likely say that these events are very rare. But, again, that may not be the whole story. One study in the *British Medical Journal* found that when 22 professional athletes with very high cholesterol levels were put on statins, 16 of them stopped the treatment because of the side effects.[207] Competitive athletes are known to be more sensitive to muscle pain than other people.

One of the reasons the studies for side effects, which doctors rely upon, report low levels is because people who have any illness or who don't respond well are excluded from the trials. The same *British Medical Journal* article found that in one recent big trial – used to show how safe statins are – almost half the 18,000 people recruited to begin with weren't included. Of course, in the real world those are just the kind of people who would be given the drugs. And this doesn't begin to estimate the effect of adding a statin if you are already taking a number of other drugs.

There is another reason why official adverse drug reaction (ADR) figures for statins are very low: when patients say the drugs are having a bad effect, doctors don't believe them. Although 98 per cent of 650 patients surveyed reported a foggy mental state, only 2 per cent of their doctors accepted it could be linked with taking statins. The figures for nerve pains in hands and feet (96 per cent vs 4 per cent believed) and muscle pain (86 per cent vs 14 per cent) were equally bad.[208]

Even more worrying is the question mark hanging over a possible link between statins and cancer.[209] They certainly give cancer to laboratory animals, and one of the big trials, called Prosper, which involved elderly patients, found taking statins raised your risk. This was dismissed at the time, because no other trials had found it. But because cancer is much more likely to occur in older patients, and because Prosper is the only trial done on older patients, it's quite possible that fewer patients had heart attacks but developed cancer instead.[210]

TAKE COQ$_{10}$, WHETHER YOU'RE ON A STATIN OR NOT

If you have decided to take statins because you have already had a heart attack or because you are at high risk and feel it is worth it anyway, you really ought to take a supplement of the antioxidant CoQ$_{10}$. (Although always check with your doctor if you are taking other medication.) That's because as well as reducing cholesterol production in the liver, statins also interfere with this vital antioxidant. Among other things, CoQ$_{10}$ is vital for proper functioning of the mitochondria (the power plants in every cell that play a major role in ageing – see Chapters 3 and 5). There's plenty of evidence to suggest that this could explain why muscle fatigue and pain are major statin side effects.

Research in the US has shown that a high-dose supplement can reverse muscle pains. Fifty patients who had been on statins for two years were taken off the drug because they were complaining of muscle pains and other side effects. Giving them CoQ$_{10}$ dramatically improved their symptoms.[211] Like others, the scientist in this trial commented that statin-related side effects were much more common than the big studies show. He also found that taking the patients off statins didn't make their blocked-up arteries any worse. A warning on statin packets is now mandatory in Canada, saying that the induced CoQ$_{10}$ deficiency 'could lead to impaired cardiac function in patients with borderline congestive heart failure' (but such a warning is not given on packets sold in the UK or Ireland).

This may be because there are many studies showing that CoQ$_{10}$ has a positive effect on heart and artery health.[212] Controlled trials have shown that it has a remarkable ability to improve heart function and it is now the treatment of choice in Japan for congestive heart failure, angina and high blood pressure, especially among older people. Together with carnitine, CoQ_{10} helps the heart to function more efficiently.

CoQ_{10}, at a daily dose of 90mg, has also been shown to reduce oxidation damage in the arteries, thereby protecting fats in the blood, such as LDL cholesterol, from becoming damaged and contributing to arterial blockages.[213]

So, statins seem a curious choice for heart protection as you get older, when many of the non-drug options covered below – such as omega-3 fatty acids, B vitamins and vitamin D – will not only cut your risk but will also help you to age well.

WHY OMEGA-3 FATS ARE GOOD FOR YOU

The Inuit have a high intake of cholesterol and saturated fat, yet they have the lowest risk of heart disease because of their exceptionally high intake of omega-3 fats, which are now known to be very effective in reducing the risk of cardiovascular disease. They lower cholesterol and triglycerides, raise HDL, prevent blood thinning and lower blood pressure.

Two long-term studies comparing the effects of giving patients with heart failure cholesterol-lowering statin drugs or omega-3 fish oils found that those taking 1g a day of omega-3 fats cut their risk of premature dying by 9 per cent and their risk of admission to hospital by 8 per cent compared to placebo. Those taking statins had no reduction in risk.[214] According to the lead researcher, Dr Philip Poole-Wilson from Imperial College, London, 'The results should humble researchers and remind them that medical decisions should be guided by science, and not strongly held opinion.' There are plenty of other studies that show the benefits from eating fish and supplementing fish oils high in EPA and DHA.[215]

The fat food chain

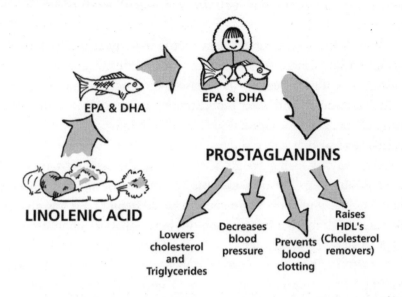

The UK's National Institute of Health and Clinical Excellence recommends all doctors prescribe 1g of fish oil a day to patients who have had a heart attack, for a six-month period – after that the budget runs out! The American Heart Association (AHA) has recommended that all adults eat fish (particularly fatty fish) at least twice a week, as well as vegetables containing omega-3 fats. Walnuts, chia and flax seeds, as we have seen, are the best vegetable sources. The AHA also suggest that patients with documented coronary heart disease consume approximately 1g of EPA and DHA (combined) per day, from oily fish or fish-oil capsules.[216] This means either eating a serving of oily fish, or taking two fish oil capsules. This is especially effective in lowering the high triglycerides, which are one of the risk factors that are becoming increasingly common as obesity levels rise and are often found with lowered HDL. Statins have no effect on them.

EAT A LOW-GL DIET

Given that high levels of blood sugar are linked not only to more fat being put into storage but also to more fatty acids in the blood, it won't surprise you to read that eating a low-GL diet, without any sugar and refined carbs, makes the biggest difference of all to your risk of heart disease.

The well-known Mediterranean diet is low glycemic. It's based on foods that have had little processing, such as fruits, vegetables, pulses and whole grains. These foods release their 'glucose' (that is, energy) much more slowly into your bloodstream. The diet also contains quite a lot of beneficial fats, especially olive oil and omega-3.

This type of diet can reduce your cholesterol levels and is also an effective way of losing weight. Meanwhile, the healthy fats help to protect your heart. A meta-analysis of weight-loss studies concluded that: 'Overweight or obese people lost more weight on a low glycemic diet and had more improvement in lipid [that is, cholesterol and triglycerides] profiles than those receiving conventional [low-fat] diets.'[217] Other benefits were a greater loss in body fat, a reduction in 'bad' LDL cholesterol and an increase in 'good' HDL cholesterol.

You may remember from Secret 3 that recently, I (Patrick) was asked by a group of GPs to put a group of 21 patients who were at a high risk of developing diabetes on my low-GL diet combined with the Zest4Life programme, which provides back up with weekly group sessions to support and encourage people making the necessary diet changes. The doctors were amazed at the improvement that was achieved in just 12 weeks.

Triglycerides, cholesterol and LDL cholesterol all dropped, while 'good' HDL cholesterol increased. Total cholesterol dropped by 13 per cent, from 5.3mmol/l to 4.6mmol, while the cholesterol–HDL ratio dropped by 9 per cent, from 4.1 to 3.7. This scale of improvement is rarely seen on drug regimes. All of this is consistent with a reduced risk of heart disease, as well as diabetes and cancer.

Our low-GL diet is also naturally rich in two other natural cholesterol-lowering compounds: plant sterols (found in beans, nuts and seeds), and soluble fibres (found in oats, barley, aubergines and okra).

Professor David Jenkins, from the University of Toronto, put 34 patients with high cholesterol on several different dietary combinations for a month. Some were on a low-fat diet, another group had a low-fat diet plus statins, and a third group was given lots of plant sterols and soluble fibres.[218] Both statins and the plant sterol-soluble fibre diet significantly lowered LDL cholesterol to the same degree, but nine of the volunteers (26 per cent), achieved their lowest LDL cholesterol while on the plant sterol-soluble fibre diet – not the statins.

If you are interested in trying sterols, this group ate the equivalent of 2.5g per day from the following foods each day:

- 50g of soya (a glass of soya milk, or a small serving of tofu, or a small soya burger)
- 35g of almonds (a small handful of almonds)
- 25g of soluble fibres from oats and vegetables (the equivalent of five oatcakes, plus a bowl of oats and three servings of vegetables)

A LOW-GL DIET LOWERS BLOOD PRESSURE

Eating a low-GL diet is also an excellent way to lower blood pressure (BP), which is one of the top risk factors for heart disease and stroke. Even so, millions of people are given drugs, which are available in four main varieties, and their mechanisms range from relaxing the muscles of the blood vessel walls to making you pee more. You may be prescribed a combination of two different types in one, with the promise of even more effective lowering.

It's easier to decide on a personal treatment plan if you have some idea of how the whole system works. Unlike domestic plumbing, the muscular walls of your blood vessels tense and relax all the time. They narrow to raise the pressure when you're exercising or anxious, but afterwards they should relax. Hypertension happens when they stay tense for too long.

This normally self-regulating system is partly controlled by two pairs of minerals that flow in and out of the cells lining the blood-vessel walls. One of these pairs consists of sodium (salt) and potassium: sodium inside the cell pushes the pressure up; potassium inside brings it down. The other pair consists of calcium and magnesium: calcium raises while magnesium lowers.

This explains why you're advised to keep your salt intake down (more sodium raises BP) and why one of the types of drug is a calcium channel blocker (keeping calcium out lowers BP). But it also highlights the way that half of each pair is largely ignored by the conventional approach. As we'll see below, getting good amounts of potassium and magnesium in your diet or via a supplement is a sensible starting point for any BP-lowering regime.

Understanding the system also highlights the downside to some of the drug treatments, such as the diuretics, which make you pee a lot. The thinking behind this is that there's less liquid in your blood and so the pressure drops. The knock-on effect, however, is that minerals and vitamins are washed out in the process, including potassium and magnesium – precisely the ones you need. There are now potassium-sparing diuretics but, typically, they put you at risk of a potassium overload! And that's not the only drawback to these drugs. According to the recent *Drug Muggers* book,[219] the widely used ACE inhibitors reduce your levels of zinc, magnesium, potassium and calcium, while calcium channel blockers bring down the amount of potassium, vitamin D, calcium and possibly CoQ_{10} – all which are, incidentally, beneficial to the heart.

CASE STUDY: DAVID

David spent ten years trying to sort out his hypertension using drugs, with limited benefits, before he discovered that the low-GL diet could do it in six months. This is his story, which shows how if you are going to age well without drugs you need to be well informed and determined:

In 1996, at the age of 44, David was diagnosed with high blood pressure and told that he would have to take beta-blockers, which stop the heart from being stimulated by adrenalin, for the rest of his life.

'They made it almost impossible for me to exercise. Running felt as if I was carrying a couple of sacks of potatoes.'

So he decided to find another way.

'I had a good diet and I exercised, so I wanted to find out why I was having this problem. I bought a blood pressure meter and I started to do my own research.'

With regular monitoring, he discovered that his blood pressure was very unstable.

'It would be low for a while after I took the drug, but then it would rise out of control. The doctors call it "resistive hypertension".'

He showed his results to a cardiology lecturer who agreed to help, and he ran a lot of tests, which eventually showed David that he had rather high levels of a hormone called aldosterone. The doctor put him on an alpha-blocker instead, which allowed him to start exercising regularly again. But things still weren't right, so David was passed on to a professor at a large hospital in London.

'He was shocked that my blood pressure was so high and he struggled to treat me for a year, but despite more tests and scans we got nowhere. Eventually, we found a high-potassium diet seemed to help. So I went on a diuretic that conserved potassium and two other drugs which brought my blood pressure down, and it stayed down.'

But the idea of staying on those drugs indefinitely didn't appeal. So ten years after he'd started on his quest, David decided to try out Patrick's Low-GL Diet. The results were rapid and impressive.

'Within about three weeks I started feeling giddy and my monitor showed my blood pressure had dropped right down, so I halved my medication. But two weeks later the same thing happened and I had to come off my medication completely!'

Two months later, David took his blood pressure figures to the professor.

'He was astonished and highly delighted. Then I broke the news to him, that those figures had been achieved without any medication at all! The initial look of horror on his face changed to total fascination when I explained it was all the result of the low-GL diet and that a further benefit was that my cholesterol had dropped from 5.7 to 4.6.'

Three years later David is still eating low GL and not taking any tablets. Not everyone achieves a result as good as this, but many are able to come off their pills. It has to be a better way.

THE MAGIC OF MAGNESIUM

David eventually found potassium was important to him. For others, increasing their intake of magnesium may be what's needed. It has been shown to lower blood pressure by about 10 per cent,[220] as well as reducing cholesterol and triglycerides.[221] Unfortunately, a lot of us are deficient in magnesium: the average intake in the UK is 272mg, while an ideal amount is probably 500mg, especially if you have high blood pressure. The richest sources of this mineral are dark green vegetables, nuts and seeds, especially pumpkin seeds. These are all good foods to eat, but if you have high blood pressure or any type of heart disease we recommend supplementing 300mg of magnesium a day. A good multivitamin might give you 150mg, so you'll need at least an extra 150mg. It is cheap, safe and highly effective.

How magnesium lowers blood pressure

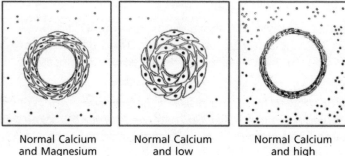

| Normal Calcium and Magnesium | Normal Calcium and low Magnesium | Normal Calcium and high Magnesium |

CUT BACK ON SODIUM

Cutting back on sodium (salt), which tightens up the vessel wall, is part of official advice. We recommend not adding it to foods as a general rule and staying away from salted foods, such as most crisps. Potassium, which is found mainly in fruits and vegetables, also relaxes arteries. Potassium chloride is sold as a salt substitute but doesn't quite taste right.

THE VITAMIN THAT HELPS

Despite the relentless medical focus on reducing levels of LDL cholesterol as a cause of heart disease, 40 per cent of all cardiovascular problems happen in people who have low levels of 'good' HDL cholesterol. But, as yet, there is no safe drug that can raise it. Trials of one mentioned earlier, called Torcetrapib, had to be cut short five years ago because it increased the death rate among those taking it plus a statin. There are several more from the same family under development, however.

Like all the other risk factors for heart disease, though, there are non-drug ways of improving HDL levels. Many of them will be familiar: taking exercise, losing weight, stopping smoking, cutting back on alcohol, having some omega-3 fatty acids. A high-glycemic diet brings HDL levels down; a low-glycemic diet raises them. But according to a major review of what works, in the *New England Journal of Medicine*, 'the most effective way' is with the B vitamin niacin (also called B_3).[222]

A number of studies show that it is effective not only in raising HDL by as much as 35 per cent, but also in reducing LDL by up to 25 per cent. By way of comparison, statins only raise HDL by between 2 per cent and 15 per cent. Niacin also reduces levels of two other markers for heart disease: lipoprotein(a) (a fat that is related to cholesterol) and fibrinogen, which promotes blood clotting.

The most obvious side effect of taking fairly high doses of niacin is a blushing effect, which is diminished by taking it with food, but 'non-blush' or 'extended-release' niacin is now easily available. Other reported side effects include dyspepsia (indigestion), raised plasma glucose and uric acid levels, although these last two have not been confirmed in recent studies.

A recent large review of niacin trials found that because it had a 'markedly beneficial' effect on a particularly dangerous combo of risk factors – a low level of the good cholesterol HDL and high levels of triglyceride fats in the blood – it might be particularly useful in treating people heading towards diabetes;[223] however, the picture has become less clear since a study combining niacin with statins last year was suddenly stopped because of more cases of strokes in the niacin group. It's only one study; no others have linked niacin with strokes, and some critics have described the study as too small and badly designed.[224]

CHECK YOUR 'H' SCORE

As you are now probably well aware, knowing your homocysteine level is a vital statistic in understanding your risk of a number of illnesses.

One of the most exciting discoveries in the prevention of heart disease and strokes over the last decade has been the importance of a raised level of this amino acid in the blood and how it increases your risk of these and other diseases. High levels are a risk factor for heart disease quite independent of cholesterol. In fact, studies have found that homocysteine is a better predictor of cardiovascular problems than either blood pressure or smoking.[225] As you have seen from Secret 1, there's also very good evidence to show that it is linked with the decline in memory that can come before the development of Alzheimer's.

Among elderly people, cholesterol is a very poor predictor of cardiovascular disease death, as was a widely used index of conventional risk factors called the Framingham risk score. According to a study published in the *British Medical Journal*, the best predictor by far is your homocysteine: a level above 13 predicted no fewer than two-thirds of all deaths five years on.[226]

The obvious implication is that lowering these high levels – which you can do with B vitamins – will lower your risk. With over 10,000 studies now published on homocysteine, there's a lot of circumstantial evidence that this is a sensible strategy.

If you suggest this to your doctor, however, he or she may reply that several large trials have found that lowering homocysteine doesn't reduce your risk of heart attacks or a stroke.

It's true that giving homocysteine-lowering B vitamins to people who have heart disease has been disappointing, although it appears that giving them to those without heart disease does reduce risk. Fortification of flour with folic acid (an important homocysteine-lowering B vitamin) in Canada and the US has coincided with a considerable drop in heart attack and stroke rates of between 10 and 15 per cent. Translated into UK terms, that means that increasing folic acid intake could actually save more than 5,000 lives a year.

As far as strokes are concerned, lowering homocysteine by taking folic acid makes a big difference. If taken for three years, it can lower stroke risk by 31 per cent, according to an analysis of trials published in the *Lancet*.[227] (See also page 346 about the link with colon cancer when taking folic acid alone.)

WHY TRIALS OF HOMOCYSTEINE AND THE HEART HAVE PROVED NEGATIVE

We should ask why studies giving homocysteine-lowering B vitamins have failed to reduce the risk of a second heart attack in those with cardiovascular disease, despite clear evidence that high homocysteine is a very good predictor of risk. The explanation is surprisingly simple: lowering homocysteine prevents platelets sticking, which stops blood clots – something aspirin also does, so if people in the trials were already taking aspirin there would be no extra benefit in lowering homocysteine with B vitamins. Aspirin was in fact widely used by participants in the trials because they were mainly conducted in patients who had already had a heart attack or other cardiovascular diseases.

Research led by Dr David Wald at the Wolfson Institute of Preventive Medicine at Barts and The London School of Medicine and Dentistry showed that there was a difference in the reduction in heart disease events between the five trials with the lowest aspirin use (60 per cent of the participants took aspirin) and the five trials with the highest use (91 per cent took aspirin).[228] The observed risk reduction was 6 per cent, but it would have been 15 per cent if no one had been taking aspirin. Research was based on 75 epidemiological studies involving about 50,000 participants and clinical trials involving about 40,000 participants.

'The explanation has important implications,' said Dr David Wald, the lead author of the paper. 'The negative clinical trial evidence should not close the door on folic acid – folic acid may still be of benefit in people who have not had a heart attack because they will generally not be taking aspirin.'

This level of risk reduction suggests that taking the B vitamins instead of aspirin will have a greater protective effect. Unlike aspirin, which damages the gut, the potential side effects of B vitamins are improved memory and mood.

THE OTHER HELPFUL B VITAMINS

As well as folic acid, other B vitamins – B_2, B_6 and B_{12} – also help to lower homocysteine, along with zinc and a nutrient called TMG (tri-methyl-glycine), which helps with chemical reactions in the body.

These nutrients are found in greens, beans, lentils, nuts, seeds and root vegetables.

AVOID RAISING YOUR HOMOCYSTEINE LEVELS

Cut back on alcohol and coffee, reduce stress and stop smoking – all of which raise homocysteine.

VITAMIN C AND THE LIPOPROTEIN(A) FACTOR

At the age of 92, Dr Linus Pauling, a scientific genius with two Nobel Prizes to his name, proposed that the development of cardiovascular disease, the number-one killer in the Western world, may have prevented our extinction. His paper, 'A unified theory of human cardiovascular disease', co-authored by Dr Matthias Rath, attracted considerable interest among leading cardiologists.[229]

According to Pauling and Rath we may have developed the ability to deposit lipids (fats) along the artery walls to protect them from deteriorating and bleeding, in order to increase our chances of surviving during vitamin C-deficient times. Having lost the ability to make vitamin C, we humans are dependent on a high fruit and vegetable diet. As we moved out of Africa, and especially during the Ice Age, we would have been at high risk of dying from scurvy, which is an extreme vitamin C deficiency. In scurvy the arteries start to become 'leaky' because collagen, the intracellular glue, is made from vitamin C. Two proteins that normally accumulate at injury sites to effect repair are fibrinogen and apoprotein. Lipids and apoprotein combine to produce lipoprotein(a) which, in excess, is a very good predictor of impending cardiovascular disease.[230] You want to have a level below 30mg/dl (a level that would be checked by your cardiologist). Above 50mg/dl your risk for cardiovascular disease increases quite substantially.

Pauling and Rath recommended the combination of high-dose vitamin C and lysine to lower lipoprotein(a). Niacin, which raises HDL cholesterol, also works. A study from the University of Arkansas for Medical Sciences, reported a 35 per cent decrease in lipoprotein(a) after

26 weeks on niacin,[231] which proves even more effective in combination with high-dose vitamin C and the amino acid lysine.

Using a nutritional approach to ageing well is not a one-off process. Inevitably, as you get older, your body's self-repair potential is going to decline further, but there are still plenty of options, and nutrition puts you much more firmly in charge. An example of this is what David Holmes did. Writing in the journal *Holistic Health*[232] he describes how he managed to rectify angina with a combination of vitamin C and other supplements.

'At the age of 48 I had a sudden and quite severe heart attack with no prior warning.' After that he devised an excellent nutritional prevention strategy, which kept him healthy for the next 17 years. But then he started having angina pains, even after walking just 20 yards. Blood tests showed healthy cholesterol but a dangerously high level of lipoprotein(a). 'To bring it down I began taking 3g of vitamin C a day plus the same amount of an amino acid called L-lysine which also lowers cholesterol.'

Over three weeks, David gradually doubled the dose and included omega-3 and magnesium. 'On this new regime my angina became less and less frequent and my exercise tolerance increased.' Blood tests showed a dramatic fall in both lipoprotein(a) and a related potentially harmful lipid apolipoprotein A2. After three months David was walking six miles a day.

Vitamin C is one of those all-round health heroes, certainly for heart disease. The higher your intake, the lower your risk.[233] Having a higher intake also lowers your homocysteine level,[234] and reduces inflammation.[235] We take at least 2g a day and recommend you do the same. Also, eat antioxidant and anti-inflammatory foods: lots of fruit, vegetables, herbs and spices, which are all included in our Anti-ageing Diet in Part Three.

VITAMIN D AND THE IMPORTANCE OF SUNLIGHT

Just a few years ago, vitamin D was thought to be only really important for bones, but now, as we've already discussed in earlier chapters, it's emerging as the new supplement superstar that looks like playing a major role in your overall health and reducing the risk of cancer, among other illnesses. A number of studies have also found that people with more exposure to the sun or more vitamin D in their blood are less likely to suffer from heart disease.

Twenty years ago, Dr David Grimes, a gastroenterologist in Blackburn, UK, was intrigued by the failure of a study designed to show that the reason people in the north of Britain were more likely to suffer from a heart attack was because they ate a more fatty diet. In fact, those in the south with the lowest rate ate the most fat. For various reasons, Grimes suspected that lack of sunlight contributed to heart disease. He compared the number of sunny days with the rate of heart disease in three nearby towns – Blackpool, Burnley and Blackburn – and found that the lowest number of heart attacks was in Blackpool, which had the highest level of sunshine.[236]

Although Grimes was a maverick at that time, now he's edging into the mainstream. Vitamin D is increasingly becoming recognised as an important risk factor in heart disease, and many individual clinicians believe it should be tested for and supplements offered, although the gold-standard randomised trials still haven't been carried out. Links between a lack of the vitamin and heart disease are showing up in many different areas of research.

A few years ago, James O'Keefe of the Mid America Heart Institute in Kansas City, commented in a journal article that: 'Vitamin D deficiency is an unrecognised, emerging cardiovascular risk factor, which should be screened for and treated.'[237] Then, in 2011, he reported that testing the vitamin D levels of 239 patients arriving in hospital with a heart attack revealed that 96 per cent had 'abnormally low' levels.[238]

It appears that the problem can start very early in life. Dr Michael Burch, of Great Ormond Street Hospital, London, has estimated that 25 per cent of cases of babies with heart failure are due to vitamin D deficiency. He reports on a few cases where babies scheduled for a transplant recovered rapidly when supplemented with vitamin D.[239]

Exactly how vitamin D protects the heart is not yet clear, but one way is probably by keeping the endothelium (the very fine lining of blood vessels) flexible, making you less likely to suffer with high blood pressure. Researchers checked the vitamin D levels of over 500 healthy staff at Emory University in Georgia and found that those with a deficiency had vascular dysfunction comparable to those with diabetes or hypertension.[240]

You could wait for all the results to come in, or alternatively it might be worthwhile doubling your blood vitamin D level from the average of 54nmol/l with changes to your diet, plus taking supplements and by spending more time outdoors. If this was done all around the world, according to one of the top researchers in the field, it would increase life expectancy by two years overall.[241]

LEARN HOW TO HANDLE STRESS

A major factor that is usually overlooked in conventional approaches to heart problems is stress – both physical and psychological. Of course, stress in the form of exercise or a challenging job can be very good for you, but chronic stress from poor working conditions, a bullying boss or too many deadlines can damage your health and your heart. Studies have shown that those of us who are regularly stressed have a five-fold increased risk of dying from heart-related problems.[242]

Stress affects the heart because you respond to it by producing adrenalin, which pushes up blood sugar levels, raises blood pressure and increases both blood clotting agents and LDL cholesterol. Meanwhile, extra amounts of the stress hormone cortisol encourage the storage of dangerous 'visceral' fat in the abdomen. Visceral fat is strongly connected to metabolic syndrome, which, as you know, is a big risk factor for diabetes and heart disease.

What is noticeable is that the effects of negative stress are similar to the symptoms that show up in men with very low testosterone (see Secret 10) and people who are developing metabolic syndrome, which also leads to heart disease and diabetes. In all cases, they can be significantly helped through diet, exercise and lifestyle changes.

A vital part of any healthy heart regime involves turning off a damaging stress response. There are plenty of ways to do this, such as exercise, watching your football team or organising an enjoyable social evening, and you may remember that in Secret 4 we spoke about the tremendous value of the HeartMath techniques. You can see on page 162 the benefits in reduced blood pressure measured in a workplace study of employees with hypertension after three months of practising HeartMath. The participants also reported improvements in emotional health including reductions in stress symptoms, depression and an increase in peacefulness and positive outlook.[243]

In a hospital study on 75 patients suffering abnormal heart rhythms (atrial fibrillation) who'd been taught the HeartMath techniques and practised it for three months, 71 reported substantial improvements in their physical and emotional health; 56 experienced such improvements in their ability to control their heart rhythms and hypertension that they were able to decrease their medication; and 14 were able to discontinue medication altogether.[244]

You might also want to learn how to meditate: a study run by the Maharishi University of 202 people with hypertension followed up over 19 years found it can drop heart disease deaths by 30 per cent.[245] You can also learn how to shift your outlook from pessimistic to optimistic by using cognitive behavioural therapy (CBT) and how to handle stress; in five-year trials, this produced 50 per cent fewer heart attacks. The exercise system Psychocalisthenics, which includes the breathing exercise Diakath Breathing, is also an excellent way of reducing stress (see Part Three, Chapter 6).

SUMMARY

To protect yourself against heart disease:

- Eat a low-GL diet, such as our Anti-ageing Diet, with plenty of beans, lentils, nuts and seeds, including foods such as oats, chia and flax seeds, which are high in soluble fibre.
- Eat oily fish at least three times a week, and omega-3 rich walnuts and pumpkin seeds. (Chia and flax seeds also contain omega-3.) These are all also high in magnesium.
- Avoid salt. Eat lots of fruits and vegetables, spices and herbs.
- Exercise is also essential. See Part Three, Chapter 4.

In terms of supplements:

CONTINUED...

- Check your homocysteine level and bring it down to below 7 by supplementing a high-dose B vitamin formula designed to lower homocysteine. If your homocysteine is already low, supplement a high-dose multivitamin–mineral.
- If you have cardiovascular disease already, especially high blood pressure, make sure you are supplementing at least 300mg of magnesium a day.
- If you have high cholesterol or a high cholesterol–HDL ratio, take a non-flushing form of niacin, 1,000mg a day until your cholesterol level is normal.
- If you are on statins, supplement at least 90mg of CoQ_{10}. If you have damaged your heart or have heart problems supplement at least 90mg of CoQ_{10} together with carnitine. (Check with your doctor first, if you are taking other medication.)
- Make sure your multivitamin gives you at least 15mcg of vitamin D. You may need more, 25–50mcg in the winter.
- Do all you can to reduce the stress level in your life. Address the causes, practise HeartMath techniques, meditation, yoga, t'ai chi or Psychocalisthenics, all of which help to reduce stress levels.

See Part Three, Chapter 7 for your general supplement programme and Recommended Reading for other helpful books on this topic.

Secret 8

IMPROVE YOUR DIGESTION WITHOUT DRUGS

'**H**aving a strong stomach and good set of bowels is more important to human happiness than brains', so remarked a Harvard School professor of medicine. As we age, we are at a growing risk of digestion and gut problems, such as indigestion, acid reflux and food intolerances. We will also become less effective at absorbing critical nutrients such as vitamin B_{12}. Some of this is just part of growing old, but that doesn't mean that there is nothing to be done about it; however, the situation is often not improved by some of the drugs that are widely prescribed to older people.

The most problematic of these drugs are aspirin – which is linked with stomach ulcers – and the acid-lowering PPIs (proton pump inhibitor drugs, whose commercial names end in '-prazole'). The PPIs are often given to reduce the side effects of aspirin, and the result can be that your absorption becomes even poorer. (See also Chapter 4, where we discuss these in detail.)

That's the bad news. The good news is that by understanding how your digestion works you can avoid these kinds of problems so that you won't need the drugs, and you'll increase the amount of anti-ageing nutrients you absorb from your food.

TUNE UP YOUR DIGESTION

We often hear that 'you are what you eat', but this isn't strictly true, because it is actually what you can *digest and absorb* that is fundamental to good health. In common with other animals, we spend our physical lives processing organic matter and turning it into waste. How effective your digestion is at doing this determines your energy level, your longevity and your physical and mental health.

Over your lifetime no less than 100 tons of food passes along your digestive tract, and you'll produce 300,000 litres (65,990 gallons) of digestive juices – 10 litres (2 gallons) a day – to break it down. The human digestive system is a tube – a 9m (30ft) long tract with a surface area the size of a small football pitch. Amazingly, most of the billions of epithelial cells that line your gut walls make up the barrier between our inside and the world outside. It is only a quarter the thickness of a sheet of paper and is renewed every four days.

The guts are also home to trillions of bacteria that play a vital role in how we break down nutrients and drugs, as well as directly affecting the efficacy of our immune system. It's also here that we make many of the chemical messengers found in the brain that affect our emotional state, as well as the hormones that control whether we feel full or hungry.

If you suffer from indigestion, bloating, abdominal pain or feeling sleepy after meals, or if you often have a stomach upset, diarrhoea or constipation, there are four simple steps that you can take to tune up your digestion.

1: REVERSE ANY FOOD INTOLERANCE

At the root of many digestive problems may be an intolerance to particular foods. This can happen because that fine inner skin lining your guts can be easily damaged; alcohol, antibiotics and painkillers (the average person takes 300 painkillers a year) are the most common culprits. Then there's the fact that we drink too much milk and eat too many dairy products, both of which have a very high allergenic potential. The result is that some of the proteins from your diet that are normally broken down into amino acids are able to pass through the gut walls directly into your bloodstream. There, your immune system identifies them as invaders and attacks them. This is how you develop a food intolerance (but note, this is not the same as a deadly allergy, such as one to peanuts, that flares up in minutes).

You can find out if an intolerance is the reason for any of your digestion problems by using a simple home-test kit that takes a blood test to check if any food types trigger an immune reaction (known as an IgG response) (see Resources for more about tests). This is a milder, less rapid and usually less dramatic reaction than the IgE response you would get to a peanut allergy, for example. An IgE response can be rapidly fatal, as it can cause an asthma attack or the throat to swell. IgG reactions, on the other hand, are more often associated with bloating, IBS (irritable bowel syndrome), headaches, chronic tiredness and aching joints. Once you know the foods your system is reacting to – wheat, milk and yeast being the most common – you can omit these 'allergens' from your diet and give your digestive system a break.

It's an approach that is proven to relieve IBS, the symptoms of which include indigestion, abdominal pain, constipation and diarrhoea. Studies have found that IBS sufferers have significantly raised levels of IgG antibodies to specific foods, so researchers at the University of York devised an ingenious study[246] to discover if cutting out these foods made a difference.

They ran an IgG test on 150 IBS sufferers and then gave their doctors either the real or fake results, along with a diet to follow for three months. Those with the fake results got a random list of foods to avoid. At the end of the period only those following a diet based on their test results reported a significant improvement. What's more, those who stuck to it most strictly had the best results. Level of compliance, on the other hand, didn't make a difference in those on the sham diets.

This is, of course, good news for IBS sufferers, but it has a wider implication for all of us, because we tend to produce an IgG response to more foods as we get older, and it is linked with having a low level of inflammation not just in the guts but elsewhere in the body. This is important because low-grade inflammation is associated with most chronic conditions, such as heart disease and diabetes.

This inflammatory response to IgG has been found in children, but it is also relevant to people as they get older.[247] Research at the Technische Universität München (aptly abbreviated to TUM), has discovered that mini-inflammations in the gut upset the sensitive balance of the bowel.[248] The lead researcher, Professor Schemann, put it this way: 'The irritated mucosa releases increased amounts of neuroactive substances such as serotonin, histamine and protease. This cocktail could be the real cause of the unpleasant symptoms of IBS.' So, if you have IBS-type symptoms, it's worth being tested, as you might find that any feelings of gut discomfort improve and you might also be able to dampen down the harmful effects of inflammation elsewhere in your body.

The good news is that most IgG allergies aren't for life. If you remove the offending item strictly from your diet for four months, this will allow your gut to heal (see below) and you can then lose your sensitivity to that food. (Please note, however, that you can't eliminate the much more severe, but less common, IgE allergy in this way.)

2: SUPPORT YOUR GUT'S BEST FRIENDS

An essential part of your digestive system are the enzymes that break down the different food types. These are: protease, which breaks down proteins; amylase, which handles carbohydrates; and lipase, which allows you to absorb fats. So, another way to lessen the load on your digestive system is to take a supplement of these digestive enzymes with each meal. If you instantly feel better, you will know you've got a problem with some part of your digestion.

If you feel bloated after eating lentils or beans, for example, you might benefit from an enzyme that contains a particular kind of amylase called glucoamylase, which breaks down large carbohydrates. You might not need to take these enzymes forever, and they can be a real boon to take for a month after eliminating your food allergies, or whenever you eat foods that you find hard to digest.

NOURISH YOUR DIGESTION WITH GLUTAMINE

Next, you can help rebuild your digestive tract by feeding it with the amino acid glutamine. Although the rest of your body runs on glucose, the rapidly repairing cells that line your gut walls can run on this amino acid, which is abundant in food but is destroyed by cooking.

It's a clever design that allows your gut – the food delivery system of your body – to get its energy from something other than glucose, thus sparing the glucose, which is needed for the rest of your body's cells to function. Having a heaped teaspoonful (5g) of glutamine, ideally last thing at night in a glass of water, is like a visit to the health farm for your insides. Do this every day for a month, or after any kind of infection, alcoholic excess or course of antibiotics.

LOOK AFTER THE DEFENDERS OF YOUR BORDERS

Inside your body are more bacteria than cells. In fact, if you were to count up the entire DNA in your body, only 10 per cent of it would be human; the rest could come from bacteria. The bacteria flourish in a healthy digestive tract and die off in an unhealthy one. So, once you've improved your digestion, 're-inoculating' your digestive tract with exactly the right strains of bacteria makes a big difference. These are called 'human strain' *Acidophilus* and *Bifidus* bacteria and work much better than the dairy-derived strains found in yoghurt.

Our guts are the wild frontier of our bodies, where all kinds of bacteria and spores arrive by the minute from the outside world. Probiotics are the local militia occupying the space, so the invaders can't set up home. The probiotics produce their own antibiotics and help to maintain the vital integrity of the gut wall by stimulating production of protective mucus as well as repairing the damage that allows allergens through. On top of that, probiotics are increasingly seen as major players in the immune system, both stimulating it in the face of attack and damping it down when it becomes damagingly hyperactive, as happens in IBS.

REVERSE THE DECLINE OF GOOD BACTERIA

As we get older, the efficiency of this whole system gradually starts to decline (along with most other body parts) in a process known as immunoscenescence. The numbers of beneficial bacteria drop and our immune systems become less responsive, making infections more likely and prescriptions for antibiotics more common.

Supplementing with probiotics can help to slow this decline and so help to reduce the time you spend feeling ill or needing drug treatments. They can reduce the severity of diarrhoea caused by antibiotic treatments as well as dealing with the problem of constipation that is widespread in hospitals – and they can cut the risk of infection by the superbug *Clostridium difficile* (see Chapter 4). Older patients can benefit from a strain of the *Lactobacillus* probiotic that boosts the ability of natural killer cells to remove harmful bacteria that are causing chronic inflammation in the guts.[249] Supplements of probiotics contain billions of viable organisms so, even though the stomach acid is a hostile environment, some will still get through to the gut.

Another way of ensuring that you keep getting the benefits of pro-biotics is to eat the food that they like (called *prebiotics*) – especially a type of carbohydrate called inulin that's found in oats, chicory, ba-nanas, garlic and onions. Its importance is shown by the fact that it is also found in breast milk. A product containing inulin, called Bimuno, was found to help IBS patients. It boosted the numbers of a beneficial bacteria called bifidobacteria and reduced the level of several harm-ful bacteria such as *Clostridium*. Symptoms, such as pain and bloating, improved.[250]

Your bacteria also like a type of sugar known as oligosaccharides and a special kind of honey called manuka that comes from New Zealand. (You don't want to eat too much manuka, though, since even this healthy source of sweetener can turn into fat around your middle.) Prebiotics can also help with IBS.[251]

PROBIOTICS: PROTECTION AGAINST FLU

The ability of probiotics to improve the effectiveness of your immune system may turn out to be especially useful in the winter, a time when everyone over 65 is offered a vaccine against the latest flu strain, at a cost of £115 million. Several reports have now raised serious questions about whether the vaccination actually makes any difference to the number of deaths, or even the length of time you'll spend in hospital if you do come down with flu.[252] However, several studies have shown that some of the *Lactobacillus* strains can improve the effectiveness of flu vaccinations.[253]

In the future, probiotics could also be prescribed for more unusual reasons, because they produce chemicals that can have a direct effect on the brain and so can affect our emotions and behaviour.[254] Perhaps they will be used for treating depression.

A RECIPE FOR GUT HEALTH

To promote the good bacteria in your gut, reduce your intake of sugar and refined foods, which encourage harmful bacteria to proliferate. Eat plenty of fibre-rich fruits and vegetables, as well as some live natural yoghurt. If you have been on antibiotics or had some kind of stomach upset, take a good-quality probiotic supplement to help restore levels: having a capsule or powder for up to 30 days is all you'll need to get your inner flora flourishing.

Some supplements contain all three of your 'gut helpers' – digestive enzymes, glutamine and probiotics. Together with cutting out foods you are allergic to, they will relieve the vast majority of digestive problems. If you still feel uncomfortable try identifying any foods or drugs that may be causing a problem.

3: MINIMISE GASTROINTESTINAL IRRITANTS

Alcohol, deep-fried food, burnt meat, coffee, painkillers and wheat damages your digestive tract the most. Wheat contains something called gliadin, which is not found in oats or rice, and which irritates many people's insides. The extreme form of this reaction is called coeliac disease where the lining of your digestive tract eventually degenerates to such an extent that you can't absorb nutrients.

Even if you are not allergic to wheat, it's best not to eat it every day. By 'rotating' a food, which means eating it no more than every four days, you are less likely to develop an intolerance. Fresh fruit, vegetables and soluble fibres (found in oats and vegetables), plus plenty of water, helps digestion, as does chewing well, and avoiding eating when you're particularly stressed.

4: STAY AWAY FROM PPI DRUGS

This relatively new class of drugs is being handed out like Smarties to just about anyone who mentions the words 'indigestion' or 'heartburn'. They are officially licensed for the treatment of ulcers and for gastroesophageal reflux disease (GERD).

GERD is what happens after years of eating the wrong foods. The acid in your stomach begins to leach back into the oesophageal tube that delivers food from the mouth – a process known as acid reflux. One response to this problem would be to find out why the acid was getting out and then to stop it. The pharmaceutical approach is to suppress acid production with PPI drugs, but unfortunately stomach acid (betaine hydrochloride), is absolutely vital for breaking down protein into amino acids, for killing off bacteria in food, and for absorbing vitamin B_{12}.

This class of drugs is generating over \$20 billion worth of sales every year (about the same as antidepressants). But, of course, the PPIs don't do anything about the underlying cause of indigestion or heartburn. Suppressing acid formation does bring temporary relief, but at considerable cost. Your body doesn't produce stomach acid for no reason.

A major cause of GERD is eating a food that you are allergic to. Babies, when given milk too early, regurgitate it. This is the normal response (known as reflux) of the body to get rid of something that doesn't suit it. If you keep eating the wrong foods, this can weaken the circular muscular at the top of the stomach until some stomach acid leaks up into the oesophagus, producing the symptoms of heartburn. Other things that aggravate the digestive tract, including alcohol and NSAID painkillers (such as aspirin and ibuprofen), should be avoided if you have indigestion.

THE LONG-TERM EFFECTS OF SUPPRESSING ACID

PPIs are intended to be for short-term use only, because the long-term effects are not good. These include an increased risk of fractures and infections. Long-term use more than doubles the risk of hip fractures, according to a study in the *Journal of the American Medical Association*.[255] The usual explanation is that stomach acid is required for the absorption of calcium, but there's another possible reason, and one that underlies our greatest concerns about the long-term use of these drugs: that they interfere with the absorption of vitamin B_{12}.

Our body's ability to absorb vitamins declines as we get older, but vitamin B_{12} absorption decreases more rapidly than the others. One in five older people are B_{12} deficient.[256] Why this happens isn't fully understood. Certainly, a lack of stomach acid (known as achlorhydria) is one reason, but indigestion and heartburn can also be caused by not making enough stomach acid rather than having too much. Low production may be linked to a lack of zinc, which the process needs. Many people get acid reflux, which is essentially a mechanical problem, even though they under-produce stomach acid.

Other minerals that are more poorly absorbed as we age include calcium, magnesium and iron.

THE THREAT TO BRAIN AND BONES

As often happens with drugs, the drop in B_{12} as a result of taking PPIs has a knock-on effect on the process of methylation. Vitamin B_{12} is vital for methylation, along with B_6, folic acid, zinc and betaine, which comes from a vitamin-like substance found in grains and other foods – also known as tri-methyl-glycine (TMG).

As we explained in Secret 2, a shortage of these nutrients means that the levels of the amino acid homocysteine will start to rise, causing a reduction in methylation and aggravating two problems that regularly plague older people: a shrinking brain and thinning bones. As we saw in Secret 1, good methylation stops the brain shrinkage that is the hallmark of impending Alzheimer's and, in Secret 2, that methylation is vital for building healthy bones. An estimated two in five people over the age of 60 have insufficient B_{12} in their bloodstream to stop brain shrinkage speeding up, and probably bone shrinkage too. Taking PPIs can be expected to make both of these worse.

If natural alternatives to PPIs really don't work for you, then at least make sure that your doctor checks your homocysteine and ideally your B_{12} level. If they won't, you can do them yourself using a home-test kit (see Resources). Your homocysteine level is also a reliable indicator of your osteoporosis risk, and very probably for Alzheimer's. It obviously makes good sense to take a supplement if your homocysteine is too high and your B_{12} too low.

The real key to any digestive issues, of course, is to improve your diet, drink plenty of water (eight glasses a day) and check for food allergies. If your doctor says indigestion has nothing to do with what you eat, you should probably find a new doctor, or see a nutritional therapist!

SUMMARY

To tune up your digestion:

- Eats lots of vegetables, fruit and fish, and less deep-fried food, alcohol, coffee and wheat. Start each main meal with some salad or something raw.
- Chew your food well and don't eat when you're stressed.
- Drink eight glasses of water every day. Dehydration is the most common cause of constipation.
- If you have IBS, either avoid wheat, milk or yeast for one month (yeast is found in beer but not in spirits, and in bread but not in pasta) or, ideally, test what you're intolerant to with a home-test kit (see Resources).

 For IBS, try these supplements for 30 days:

- Take a heaped teaspoonful of glutamine powder last thing at night to improve the integrity of your digestive tract.
- Take digestive enzymes with each main meal.
- Re-inoculate your gut with beneficial bacteria by taking a capsule or powder of human-strain *Acidophilus and Bifidobacteria*. You can buy combined digestive enzymes and probiotics.

See Part Three, Chapter 7 for your general supplement programme and Recommended Reading for other helpful books on this topic.

Secret 9

STOP YOUR EYESIGHT DETERIORATING

As you get older you're encouraged to have regular eye checks, partly to make any adjustments to your prescription but also to check for the three most common eye conditions that can lead to blindness: AMD (age-related macular degeneration), cataracts and glaucoma. And yet, according to Professor Dan Reinstein of the London Vision Clinic, the way most eye tests are done misses a valuable opportunity. 'The eyes may not be the window of the soul,' he says, 'but they do allow you to have a good peek in at the body and the brain.' This is because the retina – the part of the eye that transforms the patterns of light and shade into electrical information that travels up the optic nerve – is actually an outgrowth of the brain. Recently, researchers have suggested that the health of the retina could be a way of picking up early signs of Alzheimer's disease.

The eyes are also heavily dependent on a healthy cardiovascular system: blocked arteries or high levels of sugar in the blood can play havoc with the incredibly delicate blood vessels in the eye. That's why diabetes is a leading cause of blindness.

'As far as assessing the health of your eyes, the standard NHS test is the equivalent of going into your dentist's surgery, flashing a smile and walking out again,' Reinstein goes on:

> Of course it's vital to check for the obvious disorders but a proper examination can show up so much more …The cornea can show up problems with lung and kidney, the retina can provide clues to cardiovascular problems elsewhere such as high blood pressure. Abnormalities in the tear film, which keeps the eye moist, can tell you about your diet and whether you are deficient in beneficial omega-3 oils such as you get from flax seed or fish.

PROTECT YOUR EYES WITH A HEALTHY HEART

What this means is that, just as with the rest of the body, the gradual deterioration of your eyes that comes with ageing doesn't happen in isolation, it's intimately tied up with your general health. And that means that you have the chance to do something about it. Common features of ageing, such as a decline in hormones, a rise in damaging free radicals or too much inflammation, can all end up threatening your sight.

According to the Royal National Institute for the Blind, there are two million people in UK who are blind or who are suffering with serious sight loss, but half of those cases could have been prevented. The best way to protect yourself is to have regular checks and to make use of the same supplements and nutritional approaches that can slow ageing and the risk of disease elsewhere in the body.

If you're carrying extra weight, you should aim to bring it down, because being obese immediately puts you at a greater risk of cataracts (clouding of the lens), glaucoma (a dangerous rise in the pressure in the eye) and AMD (a loss of the sharp focusing area at the centre of the retina). You need to avoid the high blood sugar that can lead to diabetes and damage to the blood vessels of the eye, so a low glycemic diet would seem a good place to start protecting your eyes.

Typical cardiovascular problems, such as high blood pressure or narrowed arteries, can also have a knock-on effect. Your eyes need a healthy flow of oxygen-rich blood, which also removes waste products. Many of the nutrients that benefit the heart, such as antioxidants, the right omega-3–omega-6 balance, reducing homocysteine with B vitamins, and bio-identical hormones, all have a part to play.

THE EYE DEFENDERS

There are three groups of nutrients that are especially helpful for eye health:

VITAMIN A: THE LIGHT CATCHER

This is perhaps the most important nutrient for the eye, as it is for the skin. It is a key part of the chemical process that turns photons of light into the electrical nerve impulses that travel to the brain. It also maintains the mucus lining of the eye; supports tear production; protects the eye; and prevents night blindness. Vitamin A can only be obtained from the diet and comes in two forms. One is the readily absorbed, fat-soluble vitamin retinol, found in animal tissues; the other is known as beta-carotene and you get it from plants, particularly apricots, cantaloupe melons, carrots, pumpkins, sweet potatoes, spinach, squash and broccoli. Beta-carotene is converted into retinol in the liver.

THE ANTIOXIDANT TEAM

Other major players include the essential antioxidants that help protect against the oxidants created by ultraviolet rays from the sun (see Secret 5) and the likes of cigarette smoke. These include the familiar vitamins C and E, along with CoQ_{10} and some rather more specialised compounds: acetyl-l-carnitine, n-acetyl-cysteine (the precursor for glutathione) and alpha lipoic acid.[257]

These are often provided in antioxidant formulas and are well worth taking to protect your eyes as you get older. CoQ_{10} is particularly interesting, as it has been shown to help prevent both cataracts and AMD (see below) and may soon be available as eye drops. It is naturally present in the eye but the amount declines by about 40 per cent between youth and old age.[258]

THE PROTECTIVE PIGMENTS

Carrots are an especially rich supply of a group of nutrients called carotenoids. Two carotenoids present in the macula of the eye – lutein and zeathanthin – are powerful antioxidant pigments. Rich sources are found in green leafy vegetables and brightly coloured fruits. Lutein and zeathanthin appear to protect the retina and, perhaps, even prevent age-related diseases such as AMD and cataracts. Researchers from the University of Georgia concluded that these carotenoids have a positive effect on the retina, reducing disability and discomfort from glare, enhancing contrast and increasing visual range.[259] A very large study of over 35,000 women[260] found that those whose diets included the most lutein and zeathanthin lowered their risk of developing cataracts by 18 per cent, whereas those in the top fifth for vitamin E – found in fish, nuts and seeds – lowered their risk by 14 per cent. A review of studies found that increased intakes of the carotenoids were associated with a 26 per cent reduction in the risk of late-stage AMD.[261]

Lutein is an oil-soluble nutrient found in vegetables, so if you put a splash of olive oil or a little butter on your vegetables you will actually absorb lutein better than if you eat them without any fat. Egg yolk is another highly bio-available source of both lutein and zeathanthin, whereas foods such as cantaloupe melon, carrots, sweet potato, yams and yellow squash are rich in beta-carotene, another carotenoid, but provide no lutein.

BE CAREFUL OF THE DRUGS YOU TAKE

A number of widely used drugs have been linked with eye problems. A recent analysis of the side effects suffered by people being treated with statins at 368 GP practices in England and Wales found that cataracts were 'significantly associated with statin use'. In fact they were the most common side effect, more so than muscle weakness.[262] Several drugs have been linked to an increased risk of cataracts but the 'most frequently implicated drugs are corticosteroids'.[263]

A few years ago, a review of drugs associated with eye problems found, among other things, a strong link between the bone-building bisphosphonate drugs and various kinds of painful inflammations of the central part of the eye; also, that the epilepsy drug topiramate could cause glaucoma; and that another epilepsy drug, vigabatrin, was linked to the kind of damage to the retina seen in AMD; the erection-boosting drug Viagra may be linked with damage to the optic nerve due to poor blood supply.[264] The authors also warned that drugs derived from vitamin A, known as retinoids, could be linked to raised pressure in the brain and that liquorice could cause temporary vision loss, similar to what can happen with a migraine.

Check your medications for side effects that affect the eyes, and discuss any concerns with your doctor or pharmacist.

What can you do to protect yourself against the three major threats to your eyesight?

TO AVOID MACULAR DEGENERATION: KEEP YOUR RETINA HEALTHY

Imagine that if you looked straight ahead everything seemed swathed in a thick fog; you can't quite make out people's faces; you can't read road signs even with your glasses on. That's what AMD is like, and around half a million people in the UK aged over 65 know how frightening that feels. The number of younger sufferers in their forties and fifties is rising.

So what happens? The cells in a tiny oval patch, no more than 5mm (¼in) in diameter, at the centre of your retina gradually begin to break down. Known as the macular, this is where all your most fine-grained visual processing happens. Without it you can't read fine print, drive a car or watch a movie. This is 'dry' AMD, which affects about 90 per cent of sufferers. Some cases turn into 'wet' AMD as new, abnormal blood vessels begin to grow and leak under the macular, leading to permanent sight loss, although a little vision usually remains around the edges.

Exactly why it happens isn't clear, but besides just getting older, the risk factors are all too familiar: smoking, obesity, high caffeine intake, poor insulin control, low HDL cholesterol and oxidative stress. So, as well as the carotenoids, lutein and zeathanthin, already mentioned above, what else can be done to bring down the risk of AMD?

AN ANTIOXIDANT BREAKTHROUGH

The big breakthrough in treatment came just over a decade ago when a large study of 3,640 people published in the *Lancet* found that a combination of antioxidants (vitamins C, E and beta-carotene), plus zinc, could slow down progression of the disease by 25 per cent and reduce vision loss by 19 per cent.[265] Since then there has been a number of follow-up studies, but not another large randomised trial. (This is in stark contrast to the number of trials there would have been if a drug had come up with the same results.)

There is one study on the way (called AREDS2), but it won't be reporting until 2013, so the official recommendation for the time being is not to take antioxidants for primary prevention but to consider supplementing if AMD has started developing[266] or if you are at high risk.[267] It is a clear example of the difference between the pharmaceutical and nutritional approach. We suggest, though, that you take the supplements, since the risk of harm is negligible and, as we've seen, taking them is very likely to be beneficial in all sorts of other ways.

THE BENEFIT OF B VITAMINS

Antioxidants and B vitamins tend to help with the same conditions, and eye health is no exception. Studies found that patients with advanced AMD had higher levels of the damaging amino acid homocysteine. In this controlled trial of over 5,000 women who had heart disease or a raised risk, it was found that those who took a combination of the B vitamins (which, as we know, bring down homocysteine) had a lower chance of developing AMD – 55 cases vs 82.[268] The participants received high-dose B vitamins for seven years.

EAT FISH OIL, NOT VEGETABLE OIL

Not surprisingly, fish oils show up as being beneficial here as well. Two studies pinpointed the protective effect of eating omega-3 oils, and this makes perfect sense, because the retina naturally contains high levels of one that is important in the brain, known as DHA.[269] Researchers at Harvard Medical School discovered that diets high in omega-6 vegetable fats – found in crisps, French fries, cakes and biscuits – doubled the risk of the disease, whereas two or more servings of oily fish per week, containing omega-3 DHA, lowered it. A further study of over 35,000 women found that those who ate the most DHA had a 38 per cent lower risk compared with those who ate the least.[270]

Combining omega-3 with the antioxidants CoQ_{10} and acetyl-l-carnitine (an amino acid widely used as a supplement) improved the vision and slowed the progression of the disease in a placebo-controlled trial of over 100 AMD patients. Only 1 in 48 (2 per cent) taking the nutrients deteriorated a year on, compared to 9 in 53 on the placebo (17 per cent).[271]

MAKE SURE YOU HAVE ENOUGH VITAMIN D

Another important nutrient to supplement, especially if you live in northern Europe, is vitamin D. High levels of vitamin D in the blood are associated with a decreased risk of developing early AMD before the age of 75. Women who consumed the most vitamin D had a 59 per cent decreased odds of developing early AMD compared with women who consumed the least.[272]

AN UNHEALTHY DIET CAN DAMAGE YOUR EYESIGHT

In a study of more than 4,000 people, researchers from Tufts University in Boston, Massachusetts, discovered that people who regularly eat high-GL foods – white rice, pasta and bread – are also more likely to develop AMD and diabetes. They estimated that 20 per cent of AMD cases could have been prevented had the patients eaten fewer processed foods.[273]

THE POSSIBLE LINK WITH HORMONES

Dr George Rozakis, an American expert in laser eye surgery at the Northeastern Eye Center, Lakewood, Ohio, has a radical new idea about how to treat AMD with a supplement of bio-identical hormones (see Secret 10). The first clues came when it was found that an early sign of the disease – yellow deposits under the retina, called drusen – were largely made up of cholesterol. Most of us think of cholesterol as something that puts you at risk of heart disease, to be brought down with statins, but it is also the raw material for making many of our hormones and the manufacturing process may go awry as we get older.

Rozakis combined this discovery about drusen with two other findings. Firstly, that patients with AMD often have very low levels of the hormone DHEA, which needs cholesterol for its manufacture, and which is then used to make many of the other hormones, such as oestrogen and testosterone.[274] Secondly, hormones play a role in the retina, which can make hormones because it is part of the brain and that's one of the things the brain does.[275]

The idea is that as we get older and hormone levels drop, the retina tries to compensate by setting up a hormone production line starting with cholesterol, except that the process goes wrong. Rozakis is currently running a trial to see if a supplement of bio-identical hormones will stop or slow the development of AMD.

PROTECT YOUR EYES WITH A LOW-GL DIET

The best cure for AMD remains prevention by eating a low-GL diet, rich in fresh fruit and vegetables, together with optimal amounts of lutein and omega-3 fats. If you have to reverse AMD, you will need to follow a supplement programme that covers all the bases, as Daisy did, below.

CASE STUDY: DAISY

Daisy, 82, had been suffering from AMD for six years and could no longer go shopping or enjoy her garden, because she had tripped over several times and hurt herself quite badly. She was taking a number of drugs for high blood pressure, high cholesterol and thinning bones, which could have aggravated her failing sight.

She was keen to try supplements to see if she could at least stop the disease progressing. Daisy took a broad-spectrum antioxidant capsule, a B complex, and an omega-3 essential fat supplement, and then made some changes to her diet. She stopped using margarine and used oat milk instead of cow's milk. After a few months she was able to reduce her prescriptions with her doctor's help, and felt confident to visit her local shops on her own. She has been so pleased with her progress, she's persuaded her younger sister, who has just been diagnosed with AMD, to make similar changes and to take advice on supplementation.

OTHER THINGS TO TRY

As well as eating well, keeping your weight down and exercising, what else can you do to protect yourself? Here are a few more specialised suggestions.

- Lutein supplements in a sublingual form sprayed under the tongue have a much higher take-up compared with those in tablet form.

- Electrical stimulation, which encourages cellular regeneration, applies a micro-current stimulator (MCS) to acupressure points around the eyes. This treatment has produced much interest since Sam Snead, the retired professional golfer, had a series of MCS treatments. The MCS improved his vision, which had been weakened by AMD. Dr John Jarding treated 35 macular degeneration patients with a controlled micro-current and all subjects reported vision improvements.[276] (For more information see Resources.)

- People who have a pale colouring should wear a hat with a brim to shade the strong sunlight and wear sunglasses (see below).

LIFESTYLE TIPS FOR HEALTHY EYES

Here are some ways to protect your eyes from age-related conditions:

- Only wear sunglasses in very strong sunlight, your eyes need certain wavelengths of sunlight for eye health.

- Sleep in total darkness to allow the rods and cones in the retina to replenish. Constant light, even at low levels, disrupts hormone balances in the body leading to disturbed sleep, poor eye health and many other conditions.

- Trayner pinhole glasses can help focusing problems, such as far- and near-sightedness, computer strain, eye strain, headaches and presbyopia (difficulty reading small print). Regular use builds up the eye muscles and reshapes the eyes. Most people are amazed when they put pinhole glasses on for the first time and find that they can instantly read small print and see sharply without their glasses (see Resources).

- If you spend a lot of time on the computer, make sure that you sit squarely facing the computer and aim to position the screen so it's a little below your eye level. Blink very regularly to rest and wet the eyes. Take regular, full breaths to relax all your muscles and also raise oxygen levels in the bloodstream. Take a short break every hour and use the palming technique

CONTINUED...

---

from the Bates Method to increase eye responsiveness (see below). The lighting of your work area should be equal to the computer screen. Avoid shiny, reflective surfaces around you and bright glare from windows or lamps.

Learn the Bates Method

The Bates Method of eye exercises is well worth learning to re-educate the muscles of your eyes safely. It is well known to help common eyesight problems, such as long- and short-sight, astigmatism and old-age sight. One of the simplest Bates exercises to do is palming to fully relax the eyes. Sit at a table to support your elbows. Be quiet and undisturbed; empty your mind. Warm your hands. Shut your eyes and cover them with your palms but do not touch your eyelids. Initially, you are likely to see dull colour until your eyes become totally rested and your vision repairs. You should eventually see total blackness. Alternately visualise seeing something jet black and then picturing a relaxing scene. Take deep, slow breaths and relax all your facial muscles. Ideally, do this about eight times a day for about five minutes each time, but even a few seconds will still be valuable. Build up the eye muscles by looking up, down, far right and far left in turn, then centre whilst palming. Repeat this ten times.

   This is one of a number of eye exercises that many people claim have really helped transform their eyesight. For more information on the Bates Method, read the book *Improve your Eyesight – A Guide to the Bates Method for Better Eyesight without Glasses* by Jonathan Barnes.

CAN YOU PROTECT YOURSELF FROM CATARACTS?

When a cataract forms, a white cloud gradually develops over the normally transparent lens of your eye – initially causing blurred vision and near-sightedness, but eventually leading to loss of detail and ability to see images. There are various forms caused by metabolic disorders such as diabetes, taking medications such as statins,[277] hypertension, alcohol, tobacco, excessive ultraviolet light, radiation, trauma, malnutrition, chemical toxins and heavy metals, as well as the most common associated factor: getting old.

With a good diet and the right prevention steps, however, you can stop this happening to you. Julie Mares from the University of Wisconsin, tracked 1,808 women aged 55–86 to see which factors increase the risk of developing cataracts. Her finding? 'Lifestyle improvements that include healthy diets, smoking cessation, and avoiding obesity may substantively lower the need for and economic burden of cataract surgery in aging American women.'[278]

Cataract surgery is an extremely lucrative business for surgeons but it's not without risk, and it isn't performed until the cataract has become 'ripe', causing poor quality of life for patients while they are waiting. Then, after surgery, some people develop complications or need further surgery after a few years. According to the 'Review of Optometry', up to one in six people who undergo eye laser and Lasik surgery for all types of sight problems will experience complications that affect their eyesight. Predominant complaints are dry eyes, astigmatism, double vision and loss of night vision.

Numerous studies since 1935 have shown that vitamin C has the ability to reverse the damaging effects that high blood sugar, linked with diabetes, can have on the eyes.[279] Last year an Indian study found that those getting higher levels of vitamin C were less likely to develop cataracts and that it was more effective than other antioxidants such as lutein, zeathanthin, beta-carotene and vitamin E.[280] But other studies have had less favourable results.

There are two studies that show that CoQ_{10} stops the destruction of cells in the lens of the eye,[281] which is the cause of cataracts, with some very positive results using CoQ_{10} drops into the eye;[282] however, this research is in the early stages and CoQ_{10} drops are not yet available.

As with AMD, your best bet seems to be a good all-round diet and supplement programme, plus a healthy lifestyle that includes plenty of exercise.

When it comes to diet, aim to eat our low-GL Healthy Ageing Diet, which we will explain in Part Three. It is especially important to avoid all sugars and to limit dairy products, which naturally contain milk sugars, as these destroy vitamin C and glutathione in the lens and stop the lens from keeping itself clear. Dairy products can also cause sinus problems, thus impairing blood flow from around the eyes, so it's best to avoid these if you find you react.

Also, fill your diet with antioxidant-rich foods, such as plenty of yellow and orange vegetables, apples, garlic, onions, spinach, beans, tomatoes and greens, which are high in lutein and zeathanthin. Red onions are particularly high in quercetin, a potent antioxidant and anti-inflammatory, which has been shown to protect against cataract formation.[283] In an animal study, onions have been shown to prevent cataract formation.[284]

The herb eyebright has traditionally been used to treat and prevent cataracts, either taken as a tea or in capsules, and it can also be used as an eyewash.

GLAUCOMA AND THE NEW FINDINGS FOR TREATMENT

The third-leading cause of blindness globally, glaucoma can appear at any age. Most glaucoma sufferers have no symptoms or pain and many have 20/20 vision, but only when looking straight ahead. If not detected and treated, peripheral vision deteriorates until you are looking into a tunnel or, worst still, you go blind.

In a healthy eye, the aqueous humour (the fluid that sits behind your cornea) helps to transmit light rays to the retina. It drains into the bloodstream constantly and the correct amount is replenished. Some people make too much aqueous humour, others have problems draining it; in either case, pressure can build up inside the eyeball, which eventually damages the optic nerve. This is a serious condition requiring medical help to quickly relieve intraocular pressure.

NEWS OF A HERBAL-COMPOUND TREATMENT

There was new hope for glaucoma sufferers in 2010 following a study that found that a combination of French maritime pine bark and bilberry lowered pressure in the eye by 24 per cent. Even more impressive was that when the compound was combined with the standard drug treatment, latanoprost, pressure declined by 40 per cent.[285] The controlled study had 79 participants and a larger one is planned.

The benefits of the drug and the herbal compound were about the same, although the nutrients took much longer to work – 24 weeks instead of four; however, for many people, the big plus of the two plant products is that the side effects of the drug can be fairly unpleasant. They include blurred vision, burning/stinging/itching/redness of the eye, increased sensitivity to light, flu-like symptoms, or muscle/joint pain. Both pine bark and bilberry are powerful antioxidants and have been linked with a beneficial effect on the lining of blood vessels. The compound is called Mirtogenol.

A LACK OF VITAMIN C MIGHT CAUSE GLAUCOMA

A diet rich in vitamin C could be protective against glaucoma. That's the implication of the surprising finding that the retina has to be bathed in relatively high doses of vitamin C, or it doesn't function properly.[286] This was reported in 2011 by researchers at the Oregon Health and Sciences University in America, who said that it implied that vitamin C plays a bigger role in the brain than anyone had suspected (the retina, as we have seen, is part of the brain).

Even more intriguing was that a lack of vitamin C interfered with the working of the GABA receptors, the ones targeted by sleeping pills to boost GABA production and slow down brain activity (see Secret 4). 'This finding could have implications for disorders like glaucoma and epilepsy,' says co-author Dr Henrique von Gersdorff. 'Both are caused by dysfunction of nerve cells in the retina and brain that become overexcited in part because GABA receptors may not be functioning properly.' The research, which was carried out using goldfish retina, is at a very preliminary stage.

OTHER WAYS TO BRING DOWN PRESSURE IN THE EYE

Poor circulation can inhibit eye drainage, and obesity, high blood pressure and arthritis all increase the risk of glaucoma. Damage from the food additive monosodium glutamate (MSG) is also linked to glaucoma. In one study, Japanese researchers fed rats with MSG, resulting in vision loss and thinner retinas.[287]

Medication for glaucoma is usually given as eye drops, often beta-blockers or corticosteroids, but all of them can have dangerous side effects, such as arrhythmias, damage to the central nervous system and even irreversible retinal damage.

Alternative treatments include the herb ginkgo biloba – this may have a protective effect on the optic nerve where glaucoma damage exists. A small study demonstrated that ginkgo biloba treatment improved the ability to see a wider visual field in some individuals.[288] Together with zinc, this may slow vision loss.

It is also good to avoid drinking fluids in large amounts, but rather having little and often throughout the day. Aerobic exercise and regular brisk walking have both been shown to bring down eye pressure.[289]

DRY EYES: A COMMON PROBLEM

With advancing age, the eyes produce about 40 per cent less moisture. As well as feeling dry, symptoms can be that the eyes burn and over-react by producing excessive tears.

Dry eyes can be caused by an under- or over-active thyroid or other autoimmune diseases, where the soft tissues around the eye are attacked by the body's antibodies, creating eyelid retraction and a staring appearance, sometimes leading to double vision.

Hypothyroid patients are almost always vitamin A deficient, as they cannot convert beta-carotene to vitamin A, or vitamin A to the form used in the eyes, a process which depends on zinc.

In women over the age of 40, dry eyes, together with dry mouth and a difficulty in swallowing, can be the result of Sjogren's syndrome, an autoimmune disorder. If you have this, it is best to see a nutritional therapist who can advise you accordingly.

The oil glands in the eye that help prevent eyelids from sticking together depend on balanced hormone levels, particularly androgens and progesterone. The next chapter explains about how to test for, and correct, hormonal deficiencies.

SUMMARY

To keep your eyes healthy as you get older:

- Eat a low-GL diet, such as our Anti-ageing Diet, with plenty of antioxidant rich, brightly coloured vegetables and lots of onions. Eat dark blue berries such as blueberries, bilberries and blackcurrants. These strengthen the eye cells, help your eyes adjust to different light levels and reduce eye fatigue. Eat raw nuts and seeds for essential fats. Stay away from junk food.
- Follow the Lifestyle Tips for Healthy Eyes on page 244.
- Exercise your body and also your eyes with some of the Bates Method techniques on page 245.
- Stay away from smoke and wear good-quality sunglasses in very bright light.
- Don't spend too long staring at a computer screen.
- Make sure you have plenty of light when you are reading, and complete dark when you are sleeping.
- Get your eyes checked regularly and, if you are diagnosed with any of the problems above, act accordingly.

 In terms of supplements:

- Supplement extra antioxidants, including vitamin A, beta-carotene, vitamin C, lutein, zeathanthin, CoQ_{10} and possibly alpha-lipoic acid and acetyl-l-carnitine, which can be found in combination formulas. Also supplement the basics: a multivitamin–mineral with lots of B vitamins, zinc and magnesium; essential omega-3s; and extra vitamin C. If you have eye problems, you'll need a separate supplement of vitamin A.

See Part Three, Chapter 7 for your general supplement programme.

DISCOVER THE NATURAL ANTI-AGEING HORMONES THAT PERK YOU UP

Hormones, with their power to roll back the effects of ageing and boost sexual activity, have always been regarded with a mixture of fascination and alarm. In the first half of the last century, before testosterone or oestrogen were synthesised, there were lurid accounts of wealthy elderly males practising an adventurous and eye-watering form of anti-ageing medicine by grafting the crushed testicles of chimpanzees and other mammals onto their own which, they claimed, was hugely rejuvenating. With the arrival of a synthetic version of testosterone just before the Second World War, the way was open for large-scale hormone therapy.[290]

The response from medical authorities at the time was confused. One report warned of the dangers of turning 'sexual weaklings into wolves, and octogenarians into sexual athletes', while the American Medical Association stated magisterially that 'endocrine preparations invariable fail when they are given to otherwise normal individuals to stimulate sexual desire'. So, hormones were dangerously powerful but also ineffective.

We'll be talking about testosterone later; it's still seen as dangerously potent – it builds muscle and it makes you feel more sexy and self-assertive, but it is also officially not recommended unless you have extremely low levels. Much more concern and confusion now centres on HRT (hormone replacement therapy), which is composed of synthetic versions of the 'female' hormones, oestrogen and progesterone.

THE ADVENT OF HRT

Until 2002, HRT was widely prescribed as the solution to the menopause, when the body's production of those hormones starts to decline. HRT seemed the perfect solution, keeping the skin looking healthier, the hair more glossy, and so on. Not only that, but it reduced menopausal symptoms, such as night sweats and mood swings, as well as protecting the bones and the heart. It seemed a modern panacea.

As everyone knows, the panacea turned out to have a dark side, when HRT was found to actually raise the risk of heart disease and breast cancer following the large Women's Health Initiative study in 2002.[291] This has left millions of women in their forties and fifties in a dilemma. Do you plump for the benefits of HRT and hope to avoid the side effects? Or do you stay off it and hope to find something else? Official medical advice now is that short-term use – two years – is not linked with an added risk. Even so, many have stopped taking it; following the 2002 study, the number of prescriptions in the UK and in the US has halved. In the years after that drop there has also been a significant decline in the number of breast cancers.[292] So what can you do instead?

There is a solution that is widely used in the US but little known in the UK. It involves the same hormones found in regular HRT but they come in a subtly different form known as 'bio-identical', which means that they are exactly the same as the ones your body was making until it reached the menopause. The ones used in HRT are not identical, and this is very probably the reason for the problems they have caused; for example, a type of oestrogen still widely used (over 500,000 prescriptions were issued in England alone in 2010) is known as conjugated oestrogen and comes from the urine of pregnant mares, so it contains types of oestrogen normally only found in horses. The best-known brand is Premarin, which was used in the Women's Health Initiative trial.

The replacement for progesterone that is used in regular HRT is known as progestin (or progestagen), and the best-known brand is Provera. It also has a significantly different chemical structure from progesterone, as you can see from the diagram opposite. This is linked to the very different effects the two have: progesterone is the hormone made in large amounts during pregnancy, it is also a diuretic, it decreases the risk of blood clots, has antidepressant effects and helps to build bone. Progestins, in contrast, can cause miscarriages, fluid retention and blood clots, and it is linked with mood swings and can reduce bone density.

The difference between bio-identical and synthetic hormones

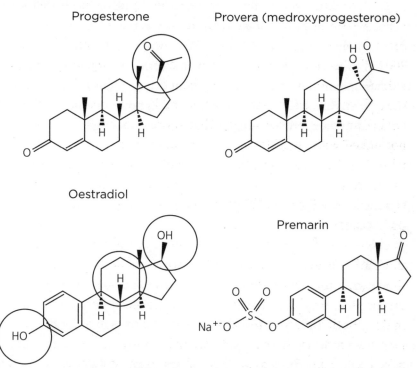

Chemicals in the body have their effect by fitting into a receptor, in the same way that a key fits into a lock. Trying to open an oestradiol 'lock' with a Premarin 'key' will therefore create a few problems.

Bio-identical hormones are manufactured from plants, especially Mexican wild yams and soy, to be chemically the same as the hormones your body makes. The appeal of this is easy to understand. 'Replacing the oestrogen that your body is no longer producing with the versions found in conventional HRT is like replacing parts designed for a Chevvy with those made for a Mercedes,' says Dr Jonathan Wright,

Medical Director of Tahoma Clinic in Washington, DC, who has written extensively on this topic. 'They may be almost the same, but with both engine parts and biology, very precise measurements matter.' He's also reviewed the evidence for the safety and effectiveness of bio-identical hormones.[293]

Progestin was originally made not as a complete replacement for progesterone but to overcome the raised risk of womb cancer caused by the early versions of HRT that only contained oestrogen. Unopposed oestrogen can cause the run-away cell growth that leads to cancer. The original difficulty with replacement progesterone was that it couldn't be taken orally, as it was broken down too fast and it was hard to get enough from a patch or cream. Changing the chemical structure meant that it could be taken in pill form and also allowed it to be patented and far more profitable. Now, however, there is an oral version of progesterone available on the NHS, although few GPs even know about it (see below).

DO WE NEED ADDITIONAL HORMONES AS WE AGE?

There's an obvious parallel between taking nutrients as we get older, because we absorb them less efficiently, and replacing hormones as their levels decline. Should we correct these deficiencies? Both are needed to help your body and brain to adapt to changes around you, and they can overlap. Vitamin D, for example, also functions as a hormone. In fact, ageing could be defined as a loss of adaptive capacity. So, if your aim is to live as long and as healthy a life as possible, the obvious answer is yes.

Attractive as the idea seems, the debate ultimately comes down to whether that actually makes a difference in the real world. There is evidence it does. A review of over 200 studies on bio-identicals in the *Postgraduate Medical Journal* concluded that they were more effective and had greater health benefits than regular HRT.[294] 'Many physicians state there is no evidence they are safer,' says the author, Dr Ken Holtor, who runs a clinic that uses them in America, 'but the medical literature clearly shows they are highly effective and have some distinctly different, often opposite, physiological effects to regular HRT.'

Meanwhile, a follow-up of those in the Women's Health Initiative study found that among postmenopausal women, use of oestrogen plus progestin was associated with more advanced breast cancers and more deaths from them.[295] And the same combination has also been linked with a raised risk of lung cancer.[296]

PROCEED WITH CARE

Hormone 'replacement', however, needs to be approached with considerable caution. Unlike nutrients, such as vitamin C, where the body uses what it needs and then excretes the remainder, hormones directly tell cells what to do, so increasing the level of one hormone automatically affects several others. If you take one you have to make sure that it doesn't unbalance the others. It's worth noting here that when giving conventional HRT, doctors pay no attention to what your actual levels of those two hormones are, nor do they check what effect they might be having on the others. Always get the advice of a doctor who knows about bio-identical hormones and can test you before taking them.

Bio-identical practitioners, like Dr Marion Gluck, a private GP in London, explains that she and other practitioners are trying to return women to the state they enjoyed before the menopause began in the most natural way possible. They don't just replace the two sex hormones found in regular HRT, they also run blood tests to check the levels of these and other related hormones such as testosterone and thyroxine, the thyroid hormone. She will then make up an individualised cream with appropriate doses. 'Hormones work together,' she says. 'Oestrogen, for instance, needs to be balanced by testosterone to avoid inflammation. Low levels of progesterone may affect thyroid function.'

The idea of using hormones to keep people well rather than treating disease is a relatively new one; two American experts reviewed the evidence a few years ago concluding that 'well informed use of hormones in wellness and disease prevention will result in symptomatic improvement.'[297]

THE NATURAL HORMONES THAT BOTH MEN AND WOMEN HAVE

The chart opposite shows the natural fat-based hormones made from cholesterol that we will be talking about, and, as you can see, they get made in a cascade. Progesterone is the 'mother' hormone that gives rise to all the others – DHEA, testosterone and the oestrogens (oestrone, oestradiol and oestriol) – which is why the drop in progesterone at the menopause can have such a knock-on effect. Although only the sex hormones are given in HRT, clinicians giving bio-identical hormones would also consider the stress hormones – cortisol and DHEA – which, as you can see, are closely related.

The stress hormone cortisol is also produced both from DHEA and from the adrenal glands that sit on top of your kidneys. The result is that if you feel stressed all the time it will lower your DHEA level. This in turn means that there is less DHEA available to manufacture testosterone. Chronically low amounts of DHEA is one of the consistent indicators that you are ageing faster than your chronological age, which is why it has become a popular supplement. We'll look at this in more detail later and how to test your levels.

The sex hormones – progesterone, oestrogens and testosterone – are made by both men and women; it's the amounts that make the difference.

The DHEA-lowering effect of stress also has a knock-on effect on the sex hormones because DHEA also makes testosterone. Both sexes are likely to have lower sex drive if their testosterone is too low. Men can also become depressed, put on weight around the middle, develop breasts and possibly be at a raised risk of heart disease – all signs of the male menopause, or andropause. Women need testosterone to cut their risk of osteoporosis and for a healthy sex drive.

The family tree of hormones

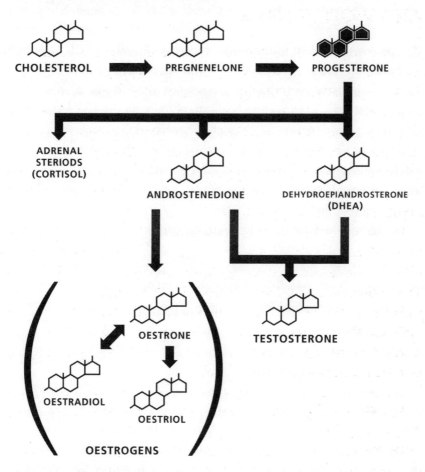

So let's look at the full set of hormones and see how they interact.

THE HORMONES THAT MOSTLY AFFECT WOMEN

Progesterone and oestrogen are the two 'female' hormones.

PROGESTERONE

Many hormone experts think that all post-menopausal women should be on physiological levels of progesterone, because none is produced by the ovaries after the menopause and your body uses it to make all the rest of the hormones. Also, as we saw in Secret 2, it is needed to protect your bones: stimulating the bone-building osteoblasts while oestrogen damps down the demolition team of the osteoclasts. In fact, it could be that progesterone plays a larger role in bone protection than oestrogen. Women who have periods when no progesterone is produced – known as anovulatory – start to lose bone mass;[298] however, the results from trials using progesterone to protect bones have been contradictory; for example, one found that it was four times more effective than oestrogen HRT, with none of the associated risks,[299] whereas two more found no effect, although menopausal symptoms, such as hot flushes and night sweats, were reduced.[300]

Could you be deficient? These are the symptoms to watch out for:

- Anxiety, depression, irritability and mood swings
- Loss of bone mass/increased risk of osteoporosis
- Increased pain and inflammation
- Insomnia
- Decreased HDL cholesterol
- Excessive menstruation

If you have two or more positive answers you could well benefit from seeing an expert. But how can you be certain that you won't be at the same risk of cancer as women taking HRT? You can't be absolutely certain, but there is evidence that combining oestrogen with progesterone is considerably safer than the progestin–oestrogen combination. Inevitably, randomised trials haven't been done, but there is a very interesting natural experiment underway in France where both progestins and progesterone are widely used, because some women prefer one and some the other.

Researchers have followed over 80,000 women to see what happens to those in each group, and the result was a convincing win for progesterone, which caused no increase in cancer. Those getting the progestin combination, however, had their risk raised by 69 per cent. Taking oestrogen alone raised the risk by 29 per cent.[301]

The oral progesterone used in France is now licensed in the UK for treating the menopause – called Utrogestan. Doctors can also prescribe

Pro-juven, a transdermal progesterone cream, as an unlicensed medicine.

CASE STUDY: SHARON

'Starting the menopause was hell,' says Sharon, an advertising executive, who was 46 at the time and had two teenage children and a husband who, she admitted, was losing patience with her wild mood swings.

'They'd always start two weeks before my period. I was like Jekyll and Hyde, so it seemed likely that the problem was connected to my monthly cycle.'

But when she went to her GP he didn't even discuss the possibility.

'I think doctors are wary of using HRT these days, because of the risks, but I'd probably have taken it if he'd suggested it; I was desperate.'

The only treatment she was offered, however, was an antidepressant. There is some evidence that they can temporarily help with hot flushes, but they also come with side effects such as loss of libido, stomach upsets, dry mouth and nausea.

'I refused them because I knew I wasn't depressed, I just wasn't myself any more.'

It was then that Sharon heard about Dr Gluck.

'The first thing she did was to listen to me. I felt that everyone else was trying to offer me a ready-made solution. She then did something else that, oddly, no one else had done, which was to measure what my hormone levels actually were.

'It turned out that my oestrogen level wasn't too bad but that I had almost no progesterone, so my oestrogen wasn't being balanced.

'She explained that progesterone affects a brain chemical called GABA, which is targeted by tranquillisers, and this is why it has a calming effect.'

Sharon was given a progesterone cream to rub in, and within six weeks the mood swings had gone and she was functioning normally again.

OESTROGENS

During middle age, a woman's level of the three oestrogen hormones begins to decline, because these hormones are no longer needed to prepare the womb lining for pregnancy. One effect of this is that menstrual flow becomes lighter and often irregular, until eventually it stops altogether. Other signs of a declining level of oestrogen include:

- Thinner, older skin with more wrinkles
- Vaginal dryness
- Increased risk of urinary tract infections
- Decreased sex drive
- Loss of bone mass

Once again, if these seem familiar, you could benefit from being checked out. Even if your oestrogen level is low, you could still be suffering from a condition called 'oestrogen dominance', symptoms of which include water retention, breast tenderness, mood swings, weight gain around the hips and thighs, depression, loss of libido and cravings for sweets. This seems counterintuitive, but it's because oestrogen and progesterone need to be kept in balance. So if you are in your forties and having anovulatory periods, you could be in a state of oestrogen dominance, even though your oestrogen is low, because your progesterone levels are even lower.

The result can be too many growth signals to the cells of the breast and womb, raising the risk of cancer. This is why you need a good practitioner. Just replacing low oestrogen without checking what else is going on might not make you feel better and could lead to cancer. To complicate matters further, you don't just replace 'oestrogen'. It comes in three varieties – oestradiol, oestrone and oestriol. And, furthermore, they are present in very different proportions. Oestriol is the weakest, and premenopausal women normally have lots of it; it makes up about 90 per cent of the total amount. The next most abundant is oestradiol, the most potent one, at around 7 per cent, followed by oestrone at 3 per cent.

In regular HRT, the quantities of oestrogens aren't present in similar proportions. One of the most common brands, Premarin (made, as you may remember, from mare's urine), is what is known as 'conjugated oestrogen'. Not only are the proportions very different, but it also contains extra horse oestrogens. Oestrone shoots up from being the least to the most abundant at 75 per cent; next comes oestradiol which, together with two other horse oestrogens, makes up between 6 and 15 per cent. And finally you get 5–19 per cent of another horse hormone called equilin. Premarin, plus one of the progestins, is the HRT that was given to the women in the Women's Health Initiative trial and is still widely prescribed in the UK.

Bio-identical practitioners will test to find the proportions of your oestrogens and then prescribe accordingly. 'I often find that oestrone levels are elevated in postmenopausal women,' says Dr Gluck 'while oestradiol and oestriol are too low.' More than half her patients are prescribed progesterone along with a combination of bio-identical oestradiol and oestriol.

Hormonal problems, especially an imbalance between oestrogen and progesterone, often go hand-in-hand with poor eating habits, stress and anxiety. For that, the basic low-GL Anti-ageing Diet will help – see Part Three – as well as one of the ways to handle stress, such as HeartMath (page 159), relaxation or exercise. More specifically, you can help your liver remove the extra oestrogen by eating broccoli, because it contains chemicals called indoles that help to detoxify excess oestrogens and oestrogen-like chemicals.

You can also supplement these as I3C (indole-3-carbonol) or DIM (di-indolyl methane). Supplements that contain I3C should also contain betaine hydrochloride, which helps to activate this compound to mop up excess oestrogens. These supplements can also help to stop a common hormonal problem that affects middle-aged males – the conversion of testosterone into oestrogens (see below under Testosterone).

If regular visits to a private doctor are not a financial option, then bio-identical oestrogen is available on the NHS, so ask your doctor about it. There are patches or creams containing bio-identical oestradiol, which is then absorbed directly through the skin; brands include Estrogel and Estraderm. One called Hormonin will give you the three oestrogens in a bio-identical form.

WHAT THE EXPERTS DO: DR MARION GLUCK GP

'I went into menopause at the age of 49, and since then I have been taking low doses of bio-identical oestradiol and oestriol, progesterone, DHEA and pregnenolone.

'It's important for me to keep a balance between work and the rest of my life, so I always make time for dinner with family or friends. I eat pretty well. I have lots of fruit and vegetables, as much organic meat as I can, although I avoid red meat, and plenty of fish. I only have carbs and white flour or sugar rarely.

'Ideally, I exercise for half an hour a day but that can be hard to fit in, so a personal trainer visits twice a week.

'The supplements I take are the obvious ones: antioxidants, CoQ_{10}, magnesium, B vitamins, vitamin D and fish oils.

'But the most important thing about all of this is not to beat yourself up if you don't do it all. I have an 80/20 rule: if you do 80 per cent of what you'd ideally like, then you're doing OK.'

DHEA – DO YOU NEED IT?

DHEA is the most abundant hormone in the body, but production for both men and women peaks at age 20 and it is reduced to half that rate by age 40, and by the time you are 65 you will only be producing 10–20 per cent of your youthful level. It's part of the pathway that produces the sex hormones, so it is likely to have an impact there and it is also the hormone that balances cortisol, the stress hormone. This means that low levels can reduce the effectiveness of the immune system, which becomes less responsive when you're stressed. So there is certainly a logical case for restoring your levels. DHEA supplements benefit mice, but there is not yet any hard proof that they slow down ageing in humans.

Symptoms of a deficiency include:

- Feeling burnt out
- Unable to cope with stress
- Insomnia
- Lack of drive or motivation

Your body naturally produces 35–60mg of DHEA a day, which can be accurately measured in both saliva and blood. Practitioners are likely to prescribe between 15mg and 50mg. If you are taking DHEA, you should then re-check your level after about 90 days.

The other way to increase your DHEA level is to reduce your stress and so bring down your cortisol level. Some very simple exercises that can do this have been developed by the HeartMath Institute, and we discuss these in Part Three. They are designed to eliminate negative thought loops and to promote sustained positive emotional states. In one study with 45 volunteers, the 15 who did the exercises for a month saw their cortisol drop by 23 per cent, and their DHEA level increase by 100 per cent.[302] They also reported feeling much less stressed and more positive. There was no change in the others.

THE HORMONES THAT PARTICULARLY AFFECT MEN

Although testosterone is also present in women, it is men who experience most of the problems when levels are low. In women this is strongly linked to lack of sex drive.

TESTOSTERONE

Just as the decline of oestrogen and progesterone lead to many of the key signs of female ageing, falling testosterone does the same for men. In both cases there is a decline in sex drive, along with thinning bones, thickening waists, fading memory, emotional swings, aching joints and night sweats.

Although keeping women looking and feeling younger with replacement hormones is the norm, and bio-identicals offer the promise of doing it in a safer and more sophisticated way, men don't get shortages in sex hormones taken nearly so seriously. In fact, medical attitudes don't seem to have moved on much since the 1950s' experts veered between worrying about creating ancient sexual athletes and declaring their treatment useless.

PROTECT YOUR HEART

According to Dr Malcolm Carruthers, who has conducted a number of surveys, around a fifth of men over the age of 50 complain about a loss of potency, sex drive and morning erections, along with mild to moderate depression, irritability and an earlier-than-usual decline in memory and concentration. And yet the idea that this forms some kind of syndrome comparable to the menopause – otherwise known as the andropause – is too frequently dismissed out of hand by most doctors.

CASE HISTORY REG

Reg was in his mid-forties and very busy running a successful electronics business when he first started feeling irritable much of the time. Over the next few years things got worse – he began having night sweats, his memory became poorer, he had outbursts of irrational anger and his libido plummeted.

'I no longer felt like myself,' he said. 'I went right off sex, I had no energy whatsoever and my memory was so bad I had to write simple instructions on my hand, such as "lock office door".' His long-term partner, Anita, a computer programmer, thought he was having an affair.

At first, Reg put it down to the stress of his job but then he began to worry that he was becoming really ill, so he went to see his GP. However, after doing a battery of tests, the doctor told him he was simply getting old and nothing could be done about it. Help finally came one morning when he was lying in bed. 'I just couldn't be bothered to get up and I was listening to *Woman's Hour* when I heard a doctor being interviewed who was describing my symptoms exactly.'

The speaker was Dr Malcolm Carruthers and Reg immediately arranged to see him at the Centre for Men's Health clinic in Harley Street. This time blood tests revealed that Reg's testosterone level was less than 10 pg/ml of 'free', or available, testosterone – the normal range for men is 14–40 pg/ml.

'I had half the normal level for a 70-year-old man – and I was still in my 40s,' Reg said. Dr Carruthers prescribed testosterone capsules, and the results were extraordinary. 'Within two days my memory returned, my depression had lifted and my libido had returned. I felt sharp, bright and full of energy.' His other symptoms took several months longer to respond, but eventually they all disappeared.

We'll come to what you can do to boost your flagging libido shortly, but recently a few doctors have been pointing out that the testosterone drop is also linked to the bigger picture of ageing in general. The symptoms are also very much like what happens when you are at raised risk of chronic illnesses like diabetes and heart disease and that boosting testosterone can reverse that.

'Until very recently doctors have largely ignored just how remarkably similar the symptoms of erectile dysfunction and diabetes are,' says Dr David Edwards, a Gloucestershire GP with an interest in sexual medicine. 'They are both linked with being overweight, having raised blood sugar levels, high levels of fat in the blood and becoming very fatigued. It's what's called metabolic syndrome and there is evidence that having a testosterone boost can improve it.'

EXCESS OESTROGEN IS NOT GOOD FOR MEN

Whereas women lose oestrogen as they arrive at middle age, men are at risk of getting too much of it. They start making less testosterone and produce rather more oestrogen. 'First you produce less because of general ageing but to make things worse, more of what you do make is turned into oestrogen,' explains Professor Ashley Grossman, an endocrinologist at Bart's Hospital, London. 'This rise in oestrogen leads to more fat being laid down round your middle and that then pumps out more of the enzyme that turns testosterone into fat.'

And there's another threat emerging to older men's precious testosterone supplies. It's more likely to be inactivated by something called 'sex-hormone-binding globulin' (SHBG). So, if your testosterone level is normal, but your SHBG level is high, you are still effectively testosterone deficient. This is a bit like insulin resistance, discussed in Secret 3, where you become increasingly insensitive to insulin. Even the testosterone you do make doesn't work so well because it has to run the gauntlet of SHBG. And there is worse. Men are being shifted in a feminine, oestrogen-driven direction by our pesticide and chemical-drenched modern world, filled with compounds that mimic oestrogen and increase the amount in our bodies.

'Too much oestrogen does not agree with men at all,' says Professor Maryann Lumsden, a gynaecologist from Glasgow University. 'A study a few years ago, which involved giving men large doses of oestrogen to try and reduce their risk of heart disease, had to be stopped because some men developed blood clots.'

Professor Hugh Jones, an endocrinologist at Barnsley Hospital, recently reported research showing that around 40 per cent of people with type-2 diabetes (developed later in life) have low testosterone. There is also some research showing that having a healthy testosterone level is linked with living longer and suffering fewer of the classic risk factors associated with diabetes and heart disease.[303] Another study found that among 800 men aged over 50 living in care homes (who had been studied for 20 years), those who had a testosterone level in the lowest quarter were 40 per cent more likely to die in the period than those with levels in the top quarter.

Patients treated for low testosterone very often report the additional benefits of improved libido and sexual functioning.

WHAT TO DO

So, if your get-up-and-go has got up and gone, and sex isn't what it used to be, or you have some of the signs of an early risk of heart disease, it would be worth having your testosterone levels checked by an expert. There is an increasing range of testosterone treatments available, including pellets, injections, pills and, more recently, transdermal creams. Try one that suits you for at least three months.

Of course, it's important to also make the lifestyle changes that reduce risk as well. But if a man has lost his enthusiasm for life and love, you can often kick-start these by correcting testosterone deficiency and then he may have more enthusiasm to reduce stress, cut back on alcohol, lose weight and make changes to his diet. Eating more protein tends to push up testosterone and bring down SHBG, unlike a strict vegetarian or vegan diet with a lot of fibre, which tends to increase SHBG. So the low-GL Anti-ageing Diet, explained in Part Three, is good for your sex drive.

ARE THERE ANY DOWNSIDES TO TAKING TESTOSTERONE?

After the cancer links that have shown up with HRT, clinicians have been concerned that testosterone could either raise the risk of prostate cancer or make it worse if it had already started. Some trials recently suggest that this isn't a problem. One discusses testosterone replacement and declares that, 'no evidence to support this risk exists'.[304]

In a small study reported in 2011, 13 men, with an average age of over 58, who had testosterone deficiency and untreated prostate cancer, were given a testosterone supplement for two and half years. Their testosterone levels went up nearly three times but there was no increase in the size of their tumours or prostate-specific antigen (PSA) score. Half found their cancer had disappeared.[305]

According to testosterone expert Dr Malcolm Carruthers, 'Although I see no evidence that testosterone therapy could initiate prostate cancer it could conceivably aggravate it. For this reason I always measure a man's PSA, which is a potential marker for prostate cancer. If it is raised, then a diagnosis is made on the basis of ultrasound study and/or biopsy. Screening for older men is a good idea anyway. By pre-screening over 2,000 men I've identified early stage prostate cancer in 12 patients to date, which can then be treated.'

If you would like to read more on this subject, we recommend Dr Malcolm Carruthers's book *The Testosterone Revolution* (see Recommended Reading).

CHECKING OUT YOUR THYROID GLAND

The thyroid hormone is produced from a tiny gland that curves across the windpipe just below the Adam's apple; called thyroxine, this hormone's job is to keep the body's various functions working at the right pace. Too much and everything goes too fast – you lose weight, you can't sleep and your heart races; too little and your systems slow down – and you suffer from fatigue, dry skin and constipation.

Too little (hypothyroidism) is much the more common, four million people are tested for it every year and three million are put on a thyroxine supplement. It's the most common hormonal deficiency, affecting many more women than men. Some cases are caused by your body mounting an autoimmune response to the thyroid gland, which can also be damaged by stress and certain drugs. Patient groups like Thyroid-UK – set up in 1999 to fight for better treatment for this condition – controversially claim that pollutants, and even a lack of fruit and vegetables, can also reduce your thyroid gland's output.

THE SYMPTOMS OF THYROID PROBLEMS

The effects of hypothyroidism can be devastating. 'You put on weight; your muscles are so weak that you can only hold a book for a few minutes,' says Sarah, a 58-year-old one-time administrator in local government. 'Your concentration is so poor that you have to re-read what you've written four of five times. Your joints are throbbing and painful, you're so tired you fall asleep several times a day. Your flat turns into a slum because you have no energy to do anything.' Other effects include poor digestion, because thyroxine is needed to make stomach acid and digestive enzymes, and constipation, because the hormone also affects the muscles that push food through the guts.

Many of these are the same as the symptoms found in other conditions we've been looking at. They are similar to the metabolic syndrome that can come with low testosterone or simply be part of the decline that can come with ageing. 'Patients often say that when they go to their doctor complaining of tiredness and depression, they are offered antidepressants and told to eat less and exercise more,' says Dr Gluck. 'Others might be told that it's just part of the ageing process and they need to accept that they are slowing down.'

MEASURING YOUR TSH

The business of diagnosing hypothyroidism can be hugely controversial. When your levels of thyroxine (also known as T4) start dropping, the amount of another hormone produced by the brain – thyroid stimulating hormone (TSH) – starts rising, telling the thyroid gland that there's not enough, so make more! It's TSH that doctors normally measure so, slightly confusingly, the higher your level of TSH, the lower your T4. T4 is then converted into T3, the active hormone.

The big debate comes around the issue of how high your TSH has to go for you to be diagnosed as hypothyroid. In the US, the Association of Clinical Endocrinologists recommends treating anyone with a level above 3. In Belgium and Germany it's above 2.5. In the UK, however, not only is anything above 5 and even below 10, considered OK, but practitioners have been hauled in front of the GMC (General Medical Council) for treating patients below 5, even though they had all the classic symptoms. There are harrowing stories of people like Sarah above who were unable to get proper treatment for years because their TSH levels were considered 'fine'.

If you have some of these symptoms:

- Poor concentration
- Confusion, memory problems
- Cold hands and feet
- Weight gain
- Menstrual problems
- Sleep disorders
- Dry skin
- Thinning hair and low energy levels
- Lethargy and depression
- Indigestion and constipation

go to see a hormone specialist with an interest in bio-identical hormones, who will usually measure all three markers: TSH, T3 and T4. They shouldn't rely only on blood tests; symptoms are extremely important too. If you've seen a regular doctor, always ask for a copy of your test results so that you can see what the actual levels are. Most specialists will also test for food allergies.

You can run into problems if you react badly to the regular T4 supplement. There is an older form of treatment that was used regularly on the NHS until 30 years ago known as Armour Thyroid, which is a dried extract of pig thyroid containing T3. Mainstream doctors will say that T4 is more consistent in quality and lacks the risks associated with treating with animal extract. But its supporters claim that Armour Thyroid is more like the natural human hormone T3 and that some patients do very well on it. It is no longer licensed in the UK, but it can be obtained from the US and doctors can issue a private prescription for it.

As with all hormonal problems, it is vital to find a sympathetic and knowledgeable doctor. In addition to more or less extensive blood tests for an under-active thyroid some may also recommend using the Barnes temperature test, which involves taking your temperature first thing before rising on five consecutive mornings (for women, in the first half of your cycle if you are still menstruating). If it falls below 36.6 °C (97.8 °F), it can indicate the need for further checks.

NUTRITIONAL SUPPORT FOR YOUR THYROID

The thyroxine pathway

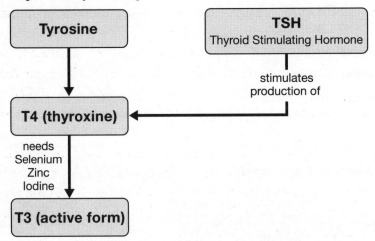

As the illustration shows, thyroid hormones are made from the amino acid tyrosine, which is converted into thyroxine (T4), then into T3. This process is carried out by enzymes that depend on zinc, selenium and iodine. B vitamins are also important. So, make sure you are taking a high-strength multivitamin–mineral that contains iodine, zinc (at least 10mg) and selenium (at least 35mcg). You might want to try adding extra zinc (up to 20mg a day in total) or extra selenium (up to a maximum of 200mcg in total). Kelp is also a good source of iodine, as is seafood.

You need about 1,000mg of tyrosine (some people need twice this), taken on an empty stomach, or with a carbohydrate snack, such as a piece of fruit or an oatcake. This improves absorption. Some supplements provide tyrosine together with adaptogenic herbs such as the ginsengs.

Most of all, put yourself on a strict low-GL diet (see our Anti-ageing Diet in Part Three), eating lots of fresh fruit, vegetables and whole foods, and minimise stress and stimulants (caffeine and nicotine). You may also want to supplement 200mcg of chromium, since this often helps to lift low energy and low mood, improving insulin sensitivity, which helps to stabilise both your blood sugar levels and stress hormones, which compete with thyroxine.

HUMAN GROWTH HORMONE

The human growth hormone (hGh) is the most controversial candidate for replacement. Made in the pituitary gland in the brain, it's vital for proper growth in children, and synthetic hGh is licensed to treat children who don't produce enough. In adults, very low levels are linked with less muscle, more fat, fatigue, lack of memory, sleep difficulties, thinning skin, mental disturbances and personality changes in later years.

The hormone is used in high doses by body builders to bulk up their muscles, despite a fearsome roster of possible side effects, which include causing cancer and diabetes, as well as muscle and joint pain, high blood pressure and carpal tunnel syndrome (a painful condition involving trapped nerves in the wrist).

An editorial in the *British Medical Journal* some years ago stated flatly: 'little or no evidence exists of an important positive functional effect [of hGh] on the process of ageing'. Consequently, using it as an anti-ageing treatment, 'amounts to exploiting people and exposing them to unnecessary risk'.

In the US, however, daily hGh shots to stave off the effects of ageing are seriously big business. Claims that it will turn back the clock, like some kind of hormonal plastic surgery, form the basis of a $100 million industry, and its use has been vigorously defended by the American Association of Anti-Aging Medicine.

Dismissing the concerns as a 'disinformation campaign' based on 'self-serving studies', the Association has claimed that, far from causing cancer, treatment with hGh can reduce the risk and that the unpleasant side effects show up only with high doses.

'If you take hGh with the right levels of the other hormones,' says Dr Cecelia Tregear, a hormone specialist in London's Harley Street, 'you get a reduction in osteoporosis, a drop in levels of cholesterol and other lipids in the blood reducing your cardiovascular risk, and an improvement in memory and concentration, youthful looks and levels of energy, good libido and a better quality of life. All very real health benefits.'

Other anti-ageing experts are not convinced. In his book *Transcend: Nine Steps for Living Well for Ever*, Dr Ray Kurzweil comes down against hGh on the grounds of cost (at least $10,000 a year), the inconvenience of daily injections and the risk of side effects. Our main concern is that hGh may abnormally increase insulin-like growth factor (IGF-1), which is strongly associated with increasing cancer risk, particularly of the breast, prostate and colon.

If you are adopting a more healthy lifestyle, a number of the changes it will embrace will have the effect of raising hGh levels naturally anyway. Lifestyle changes include deep sleep, exercise – especially resistance or strength training – eating a good amount of protein and staying on a low-glycemic diet. Supplementing with the amino acids arginine, glutamine, glycine and ornithine can make the pituitary gland produce more hGh and so can the hormone DHEA.

IN CONCLUSION

Depending on your symptoms and test results, there may be real benefit in correcting the hormones you are deficient in by using bio-identical hormones given in the dose equivalent to that which your body would normally make. In Part Three we give you some more details on testing for deficiencies. See Resources for ways to find a hormone-friendly doctor or natural practitioner. We recommend that you are reassessed after three and six months, because some hormone imbalances will be corrected so that you won't need to keep taking as much. There is one other hormone, melatonin, that is worth considering supplementing, but this has been discussed in Secret 4, with more details in Part Three, Chapter 5.

Will natural hormones extend your healthy lifespan? The odds are good, but there's no definitive proof yet.

SUMMARY

Hormones affect almost every part of your system so, not surprisingly, when your levels drop too low you can suffer a confusingly wide range of symptoms – and most of these could also be caused by something else! If you've been suffering from any of the following for a while, it's worth having your hormones checked to see if they could be contributing:

- Anxiety, depression, irritability and mood swings
- Increased pain, inflammation and aching joints. Insomnia, night sweats and weight gain
- Thinner, older skin with more wrinkles
- Decreased libido and lack of energy and drive
- Confusion and memory problems

See Recommended Reading for other helpful books on this subject.

Part Three

YOUR ANTI-AGEING ACTION PLAN

What can you practically do, right now, to surf the Silver Tsunami and reduce you need to rely on drugs? The good news, as you will have realised in Part Two, is that all the different Secrets are remarkably consistent when it comes to the actions you can take that are also likely to turn back the clock. They involve changes to what you eat, taking exercise on a regular basis, getting enough sleep, spending some time just chilling out, having a positive attitude, keeping prescription drugs to a minimum and taking the appropriate nutritional supplements. You may also supplement any hormones you are deficient in along with getting enough, but not too much, sun exposure. In this Part we show you what to do and how to do it.

Chapter 1

YOUR STRATEGY FOR HEALTHY AGEING

You are unique. How you are right now is the sum of your genes, what you have exposed them to – largely through what you eat, drink and breathe – plus all your life experiences and stresses, your mental attitude and health habits, both good and bad. All these factors make you who you are right now, and all of these are changeable, including your genes, or rather the way some are expressed.

What no study can tell you yet is what happens when you combine all the things we've been discussing into your own personal healthy-ageing strategy. What evidence *does* exist, though, suggests that the combination of even a few positive actions can have a dramatic effect. For example, not smoking, having a low alcohol consumption, eating five servings of fruit and veg a day and keeping physically active, can add up to 14 years to your life. (This is according to a 13-year study of 20,000 people by Professor Kay-Tee Khaw at the University of Cambridge.[1])

The keys to healthy ageing

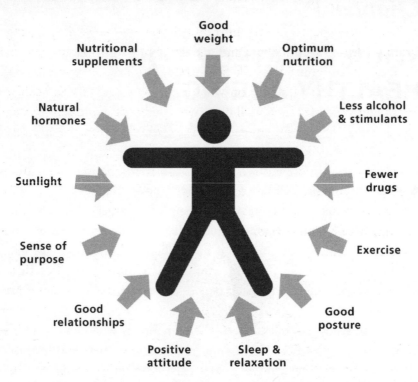

Just imagine what might happen if you also add in all the easily doable anti-ageing actions we've set out in the book that relate to your personal health profile. The truth is, we don't yet know but, like us, you will become part of an intelligent ongoing experiment into healthy ageing and, provided you've completed your free online 100% Health Check, which gives you a measure of your biological age, we'll be inviting you to stay in touch by tracking your progress year on year. That way, we'll be able to research what works, and feed that learning back to you. Also, you'll have the opportunity to join our 100% Health Club and become part of a community of like-minded people around the world, sharing and learning from each other's health-promoting experiences. If you like, you can attend our regular seminars and courses covering aspects of nutrition, exercise and psychological health.

THE HEALTHY BASELINE

In Part One, Chapter 1, we introduced you to the healthy-ageing pyramid (shown again below) and explained how it works for you. In this Part we are going to work from the bottom of the pyramid up, by giving you clear guidance on what and how to eat to stay healthy throughout your life. Then we'll move on to exercise – and how to stay fit and strong as you age. In each area we will focus on the simplest changes that are likely to have the maximum effect. Some you may already have incorporated into the way you live, whereas others may mean you have more work to do.

The healthy-ageing pyramid

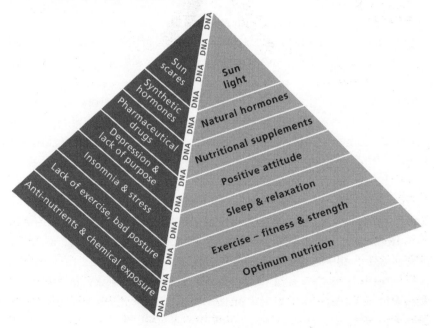

Your goal is make sure you are taking positive actions for all the bands of the pyramid.

If you have completed your 100% Health Check it will help you to see which areas need the most attention and which you've already got covered. If you take part in the 100% Health Programme, you can opt to have daily prompts on your key goals, as well as a monthly reassessment and access, by phone, to a nutritional therapist to keep you on the right track.

The important point is to make the changes become habits so you effortlessly continue them on a regular basis. Steady steps forward like this are more important than short-lived bursts or New Year resolutions that soon fade.

THE 3-6-36 RULE

It takes 3 weeks to break a habit, 6 weeks to make a habit and 36 weeks (9 months) to hardwire a habit. So, your first commitment must be to create a regime for yourself that you will stick to for 6 weeks. We will show you how to do this.

Most people start to feel different within five to ten days, the first signs often being increased energy, mental clarity and a more balanced mood. Then, after a few weeks, you will start to look better: you will have clearer skin; lose inches off your waist, if you need to; and your body will begin toning up. If you are already suffering from some of the common age-related health problems, from arthritis to weight gain, it is probably going to take you up to three months to really see a significant benefit. The body is constantly rebuilding, but it takes much longer to rebuild cartilage, for example, than it does skin.

You may remember Ruth from Secret 2, who changed her whole diet and lifestyle to relieve her painful rheumatoid arthritis. Ruth is one of hundreds of people diagnosed with 'degenerative' diseases, who are often told they are 'incurable', but who have made a full recovery to a level of health they had never dreamt was possible, by applying the kinds of principles contained in this book. Now, 25 years on, Ruth is super-healthy and looks really good for her age.

If you do have a medical condition, you might benefit greatly from some one-to-one professional advice. We have a growing team of qualified and registered nutritional therapists, not only in the UK and Ireland, but all over the world. You can find one near you in our nutritionist directory in the 'advice' section on the website (see Resources).

We also have our highly successful local groups, called Zest4Life, run by nutritional therapists, which you join and attend once a week for 12 weeks, to get you started on the right road. During this time we work to get you 'hardwired' for health. This is highly recommended if you are someone who knows what to do but just doesn't do it. Our Zest4Life practitioners are masters in helping you break through the barriers stopping you developing a super-healthy, feel-great lifestyle. Also, we have exercise groups that you can attend, for example, three times a week, to upgrade your level of fitness and hardwire exercise into your weekly routine. They work with you at whatever your level to start with, often outdoors in local parks, but they also give you simple exercises that you can do at home without any expensive equipment or having to join a gym.

The bottom line is that we want you to successfully transform the way you live so you can maximise your chances of staying well, and avoiding pain and disability, throughout your life. The next chapter starts with your anti-ageing diet.

Chapter 2

YOUR ANTI-AGEING DIET

The first thing we'd like you to know is that you can follow anti-ageing diet principles and cook meals that, by any standard, are absolutely delicious. Over the years we've collected recipes that adhere to our healthy-ageing principles from top chefs and our own kitchen wizard, Fiona McDonald Joyce. We'll be recommending several recipe books to introduce you to low-GL eating, but you can also use the principles in this chapter to create your own recipes using healthy ingredients.

Secondly, you don't have to follow these principles rigidly every day. In fact, we recommend eating in this way for six days out of seven. The important point is to develop food habits that stick and become instinctively 'just what you eat'.

The core principles are:

A low-glycemic load, Mediterranean-style diet that keeps your blood sugar level even, thus reversing metabolic syndrome and reducing hunger. As a result, you'll naturally eat fewer calories, which is a key to living longer and healthier.

A high intake of anti-ageing antioxidants by choosing naturally bright-coloured fruits and vegetables, and using plenty of flavourful herbs and spices.

Ensuring essential fats from oily fish and seeds with an emphasis on increasing omega-3 fats, which have the most positive anti-ageing properties because they reduce inflammation.

Maximising your intake of vitamins and minerals from the most nutrient-rich foods that will become part of your staple shopping list.

You'll lose weight this way if you need to and any markers of unhealthy ageing will improve. As we showed in Secret 3 on page 143, by following this way of eating for 12 weeks, a group of people who had metabolic syndrome, on the edge of diabetes, were able to not only lose an average of 6.3kg (1 stone/14lb) but also significantly lower high damaging levels of glucose in their blood, bring down their cholesterol and reduce other signs of 'internal global warming'.

This way of eating is consistent with, but even more effective than, a Mediterranean diet, which is associated with increased survival among older people.

If you really want to push out the anti-ageing boat, we'll also show you how to apply the Alternate Day Diet principles, once you've got the hang of low-GL eating.

HOW TO MASTER YOUR BLOOD SUGAR BY EATING LOW GL

The reason we want you to focus on the carbohydrate content of foods is because the other two main food types – fat and protein – don't have any appreciable effect on blood sugar. In fact, I recommend you eat some fat and protein with your carbohydrate, because this will further lessen the effect the carbohydrate has on your blood sugar, thereby lowering the glycemic load of the meal.

So, for balancing your blood sugar, there are only four rules, as you'll remember from Secret 3:

THE THREE RULES TO LOSE WEIGHT

Rule 1 Eat 40GLs a day (plus 5GLs for a dessert, drink or additional snack).
Rule 2 Always eat protein with carbohydrate.
Rule 3 Graze don't gorge – have three 10GL meals a day, and two 5GL snacks.

THE THREE RULES TO MAINTAIN A HEALTHY WEIGHT

Rule 1 For most people this would be eat no more than 50GLs a day (plus 10GLs for a dessert, drink or additional snack).
Rule 2 Always eat protein with carbohydrate.
Rule 3 Graze don't gorge – have three 10GL meals a day, and two 10GL snacks.

Also, whether you want to lose weight or maintain it, it's important to cut back on stimulants (Rule 4).

GL is a precise measure of what effect a food has on your blood sugar balance (see the box opposite). The examples given in this chapter are based on 40GLs a day (plus 5GLs for a drink or dessert): the amount needed to lose weight. If you don't need to lose weight, then you don't need to be so strict on the carbohydrate portions and can eat a maximum of 65GLs a day.

All animal produce, plus any type of seed, nut or bean, is protein. Combining, for example, nuts with fruit, or an egg on toast, fulfils the second rule of eating carbohydrate with protein, and it helps to keep your blood sugar level stable for even longer.

The third rule means eating little and often. So always eat breakfast, lunch and supper – and introduce a healthy snack mid morning and mid afternoon. This way you'll provide your body with a constant and even supply of fuel, which means you'll experience fewer food cravings.

The fourth rule is especially important if you are in the habit of drinking coffee with a carbohydrate snack, such as a croissant. According to research at Canada's University of Guelph, this is a deadly duo as far as your blood sugar is concerned. Participants were given a carbohydrate snack, such as a croissant, muffin or toast, together with either a decaf or caffeinated coffee. Those having the coffee–carb combo had triple the increase in blood sugar levels, while insulin sensitivity was almost halved.[2]

We'd like to take you through a typical day, starting with breakfast, so that you get a good idea of how to apply these rules in your daily life.

But first, it's worth understanding what glycemic load means and which kind of foods are high or low GL.

UNDERSTANDING THE GLYCEMIC LOAD

The glycemic load combines the glycemic index with the concept of measuring carbohydrate intake to provide a scientifically superior way of controlling blood sugar. Put simply, the glycemic index (GI) of a food tells you whether the carbohydrates in the food are fast or slow releasing. Fast-releasing foods (such as those made with refined flours and sugar) are bad for blood sugar, causing highs and sudden dips; as a result they also create excess weight, if eaten to excess. The GI, therefore, is a 'quality' measure. It doesn't tell you, though, how much of the food is carbohydrate. On the other hand, carbohydrate points, or grams of carbohydrate, tell you how much of the food is carbohydrate, but they don't tell you what that particular carbohydrate does to your blood sugar. It's a 'quantity' measure. The glycemic load (GL) of a food is the quantity × the quality. It's the best way of telling you that you'll gain weight if you choose a particular food.

Here are some examples of high- and low-GL carbohydrates so that you can understand which kinds of foods to choose. Ideally, you want to eat 5GLs for a snack as part of a weight-losing diet (and you'll have two a day) and 7–10GLs for the carbohydrate portion of a main meal (if you don't need to lose weight, your snacks will be 10GLs each). The low-GL foods are shown in **bold** and the high-GL foods are shown in *italics*.

Food	Serving looks like	GL
FRUIT		
Blueberries	**1 large punnet (600g)**	5
Apple	**1 small (100g)**	5
Grapefruit	**1 small**	5
Apricot	**4 apricots**	5
Grapes	**10 grapes**	5
Pineapple	**1 thin slice**	5
Banana	*1 small banana*	*10*
Raisins	*20 raisins*	*10*
Dates	*2 dates*	*10*

CONTINUED...

STARCHY VEGETABLES

Pumpkin/squash	**large serving**	**7**
Carrot	**1 large**	**7**
Beetroot	**2 small**	**5**
Boiled potato	*3 small potatoes (60g/2¹⁄₈oz)*	*5*
Sweet potato	*1 sweet potato (120g/4¹⁄₄oz)*	*10*
Baked potato	*1 baked potato (120g/4¹⁄₄oz)*	*10*
French fries	*10 fries*	*10*

GRAINS, BREADS, CEREALS

Quinoa	**65g/2¹⁄₄oz (cooked)**	**5**
Pearl barley	**75g/2³⁄₄oz (cooked)**	**5**
Brown basmati rice	**small serving 70g/2¹⁄₂oz)**	**5**
White rice	*¹⁄₂ serving (65g/2¹⁄₄oz)*	*10*
Couscous	*¹⁄₂ serving (65g/2¹⁄₄oz)*	*10*
Rough oatcakes	**2–3 oatcakes**	**5**
Pumpernickel-style rye bread	**1 thin slice**	**5**
Wholemeal bread	**1 thin slice**	**5**
Bagel	**¹⁄₄ bagel**	**5**
Puffed rice cakes	**1 rice cake**	**5**
White pasta	*small serving (75g/2³⁄₄oz)*	*10*

BEANS AND LENTILS

Soya beans	**3¹⁄₂ cans**	**5**
Pinto beans	**1 can**	**5**
Lentils	**large serving**	**7**
Kidney beans	**large serving (150g/5¹⁄₂oz)**	**7**
Chickpeas	**large serving (150g/5¹⁄₂oz)**	**7**
Baked beans	**large serving (150g/5¹⁄₂oz)**	**7**

For a complete list of foods and their GL scores, log on to www. holforddiet.com.

WHAT TO EAT FOR BREAKFAST

First of all, don't skip breakfast. It's your most important meal of the day. Many people, when they wake up with a low blood sugar level but a firm resolve to lose weight, make the fatal mistake of trying not to eat anything for as long as possible. Unless propped up with liquid stimulants (coffee or tea), nicotine, or instant sugar in the form of a piece of toast or a croissant, that resolve becomes weaker and weaker as their blood sugar level dips lower and lower, until the chances of making the right food choices becomes slimmer and slimmer. So they buckle under the strain and end up bingeing on high-GL foods. Does that sound familiar?

That's why you must eat breakfast. The only questions are what and how much? There are three fundamental breakfasts that give you the right balance of both carbohydrate and protein. These are:

Balanced breakfasts

Carbohydrates		Protein
Cereal/fruit	+	seeds/yoghurt/milk
Bread/toast	+	egg
Bread/toast	+	fish (such as kippers or smoked salmon)

The questions are which and how much cereal, fruit, toast and so on? Let's kick off with the cereal-based breakfast, sweetened with fruit rather than sugar.

THE BEST CEREAL-BASED BREAKFASTS

A good cereal-based breakfast needs to include a low-GL cereal, a low-GL fruit as a sweetener, and a source of protein and essential fats, with the goal being no more than 10 GL points.

In the chart below you'll see how much of the following seven cereals equals 5 GL points. As you can see, the best 'value' in terms of your appetite are oat flakes, either cooked as porridge or eaten raw, just like you would cornflakes. Basically, you could eat as many as you like, given that two servings will fill anybody up.

The GLs for cereal servings

Cereal	5 GL points
Oat flakes	2 servings or cups
All-Bran	1 serving (½ bowl or 1 cup)
Unsweetened muesli	1 small serving (less than ½ bowl or ¾ cup)

Alpen	Half a serving (¼ bowl or ½ cup)
Raisin Bran	Half a serving (¼ bowl or ½ cup)
Weetabix	1 biscuit
Cornflakes	Half a serving

On the right-hand side of the chart below you can see how much of each of these seven fruits you could eat to equal 5 GL points.

The GLs for fruit servings (breakfast)

Fruit	5 GL points
Strawberries	1 large punnet
Pear	1
Grapefruit	1
Apple	1 small (can fit into the palm of your hand)
Peach	1 small
Banana	less than half
Raisins	10

So, your all-time best bet would be to have unsweetened oat flakes with as many strawberries as you could eat. Alternatively, you could have a bowl of All-Bran and a grapefruit, or a bowl of unsweetened muesli without raisins in it, with a small grated apple.

As far as protein is concerned, there's some in cow's milk (or in soya milk). Rice milk is quite high in GLs and is best kept to a minimum. Oat milk is lower GL than rice milk but higher than soya milk. But yoghurt (unsweetened) is high in protein, so it is a reasonably low GL. So having a spoonful of yoghurt on your cereal helps to stabilise your blood sugar.

Another source of protein – as well as countless vitamins, minerals, essential fats and fibre – are seeds. I recommend you have a tablespoonful of ground seeds on your cereal as well. This really adds flavour and, by giving yourself the healthy essential fats you need, you won't crave less desirable food sources of fat.

EGG-BASED BREAKFASTS

Although it is true that more than half the calories in an egg come from fat, the kind of fat depends on what you feed the chicken. Most eggs come from battery chickens. If you knew how unhealthy they were, you probably wouldn't want to eat their eggs, which are high in saturated fat; however, there are some types of eggs, which are laid by free-range chickens fed omega-3-rich feed; for example, flax seeds (Goldenlay Omega-3 Free Range eggs is one example – it's sold in most large supermarkets). Either these or organic eggs are much better for you. If your intention is weight loss, I recommend you have up to seven eggs a week (they don't raise your cholesterol), but only these kinds of eggs. Have either two small eggs, or one large egg. Poach them, boil them or scramble them, but don't fry them, as the high heat damages the essential fats.

As eggs are pure protein and fat, what carbohydrate can you have with them? If this is your breakfast choice, you can use up your entire 10 GL quota by having any of the following bread servings.

The GLs for bread and bread-substitute servings for breakfast

Bread	10 GL points
Oatcakes	5 biscuits
Pumpernickel-style rye bread	2 thin slices
Sourdough rye bread	2 thin slices
Rye wholemeal bread (yeasted)	1 slice
Wheat wholemeal bread (yeasted)	1 slice
White, high fibre bread (yeasted)	less than 1 slice

As you can see, your best 'value' breads are either oatcakes, a favourite from Scotland, or Scandinavian-style pumpernickel breads or sourdough rye bread, made without yeast. These are real breads; unlike the light, white, fluffy 'fake' breads we've been conditioned to eat by adding flavour enhancers, sugar and numerous chemicals. So, even if it's a shock at first, do try these breads, as they are more sustaining for your appetite, they are naturally high in fibre and cooked slowly (in the case of pumpernickel) or risen without adding yeast (in the case of sourdough), thus keeping the GL score lower.

WHAT TO EAT FOR SNACKS

Many diets cut out snacks completely, as they can be the downfall of many individuals. Those with sugar sensitivity are likely to reach for snack foods to compensate for changes in blood sugar levels and hormonal responses. Most commercial snacks are incredibly high in sugar or fat. A Mars Bar, for example, is almost two-thirds sugar with the rest being mainly fat, while even some so-called 'muesli' bars are deceptively unhealthy, made with refined sugar, dates, raisins and large quantities of hydrogenated fat.

Research clearly shows, however, that 'grazing' (eating little and often) is healthier for you than 'gorging' – having one or two big meals in the day.[3] One advantage is that it keeps your blood sugar level even. For this reason, we recommend you have a mid-morning and a mid-afternoon snack. The ideal snack is one that provides no more than 5 GL points (if you're on the weight-losing diet) as well as some protein. The simplest snack food is fruit. Let's see what you'd need to eat to stay within 5 GL points for your snack.

The GLs for fruit servings (snacks)

Fruit	5 GL points
Strawberries	1 large punnet
Plums	4
Cherries	1 small punnet
Pear	1
Grapefruit	1
Orange	1
Apple	1 small (can fit into the palm of your hand)
Peach	1 small
Melon/watermelon	1 slice

Berries, plums and cherries are your best 'value' fruit snacks. Berries include raspberries, blueberries, blackberries and any others that you can get your hands on in season. They are low GL because the principal type of sugar they contain is called xylose. This has about half the GL of fructose, the principal sugar in apples and pears. This, again, is about half the GL of glucose or dextrose, the principal sugar in grapes, dates and bananas. You can further lower the glycemic load of these fruits by eating them with five almonds or a dessertspoonful of pumpkin seeds, which are both high in protein.

Another snack option would be some kind of bread with a protein-based spread. Cottage cheese, hummus or nut butters such as peanut, almond or cashew, are good examples. Hummus is very low in GL and tastes great with oatcakes or rye bread, or with a raw carrot (a large carrot is still less than 5GLs). If you choose hummus or nut butter without added sugar, plus a slice of one of the bread servings described above, this will give you the right mix of low-GL carbohydrate with protein to keep your blood sugar level even.

So, here is a selection of 5 GL snacks to choose from:

- A piece of fruit, plus five almonds or a dessertspoonful of pumpkin seeds.
- A piece of bread or two oatcakes and half a small tub of cottage cheese (150g/5½oz).
- A piece of bread/two oatcakes and half a small tub of hummus (150g/5½oz).
- A piece of bread/two oatcakes and peanut butter.
- Crudités (a carrot, pepper, cucumber or celery) and hummus.
- Crudités or berries and cottage cheese.
- A small, plain soya or dairy yoghurt (150g/5½oz), no sugar, plus berries.

WHAT TO EAT FOR LUNCH AND DINNER

The easiest way to get the balance right for your main meals is to imagine your dinner on a plate. Half the plate will consist of very low-GL vegetables. These vegetables, listed on page 295, will not account for any more than 4 GL points.

The perfect diet plate

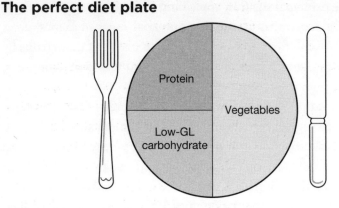

The other half of your plate is divided into two, one for protein-based food, such as meat, fish (or tofu, for example, if you are vegetarian) and the other for more 'starchy' vegetables, accounting for 6–7 GL points. So, a quarter of what's on your plate is protein-rich, a quarter is carbohydrate-rich and half is made up of very low-GL vegetables. You'll soon get the hang of it. It's very straightforward.

STARCHY VEGETABLES

As a rough guide, the serving size of the carbohydrate-rich 'starchy vegetable' food should be more or less the same weight, or size, as the serving of the protein-rich food. If you are eating chicken, which is quite dense and heavy, with rice, which is quite light, the serving size of rice is somewhat larger than the piece of chicken for each to be roughly the same weight.

But let's take a look at what quantity of different starchy vegetables you can eat to keep within the 10 GL points per meal rule, leaving 3 GL points for the 'unlimited vegetables' which make up half your plate.

The GLs for starchy vegetables

Starchy vegetables	7 GL points
Pumpkin/squash	big serving, 185g (6¾oz)
Carrot	1 large, 160g (5¾oz)
Swede	big serving, 150g (5½oz)
Quinoa	big serving, 130g (4½oz)

Beetroot	big serving, 110g (3¾oz)
Cornmeal	serving, 115g (4oz)
Pearl barley	small serving, 95g (3¼oz)
Wholemeal pasta	½ serving, 85g (3oz) cooked weight
White pasta	⅓ serving, 65g (2¼oz) cooked weight
Brown rice	small serving, 70g (2½oz) cooked weight
White rice	⅓ serving, 45g (1½oz) cooked weight
Couscous	⅓ serving, 45g (1½oz) soaked weight
Broad beans	serving, 30g (1oz)
Corn on the cob	½ cob, 60g (2⅛oz)
Boiled potato	3 small potatoes, 75g (2¾oz)
Baked potato	½ potato, 60g (2⅛oz)
French fries	tiny portion, 45g (1½oz)
Sweet potato	½ potato, 60g (2⅛oz)

As you can see, there are some obvious winners. Wholemeal pasta, for example spaghetti, and brown basmati rice are much better than white pasta and white rice (there are some specialist low-GL pastas, called Dreamfield, and also specific strains of low-GL rice, called Maharani rice, available from Totally Nourish – see Resources), which allow you to increase the portion size. Both taste delicious. Another pasta option is Del Ugo's chickpea pasta (available in some supermarkets). Swede, carrot and squash are much better than potato. Boiled potato is better than baked potato, which is better than French fries.

BEANS AND LENTILS

The best foods for balancing your blood sugar and giving the correct mix of protein and carbohydrate are beans and lentils. In fact, it's the combination of protein and carbohydrate in beans and lentils that keep their GL scores low. These are also traditional foods that are no longer eaten in many of the world's fattest nations. So, any meal containing beans and lentils as both the protein and the carbohydrate source can be quite generous with the portion size because you are getting both protein and carbohydrate from the same food.

When you are eating these foods as your source of protein, however, only combine with half the serving size of a carbohydrate-rich food, instead of an equal serving. So, for example, if you were making a bean and rice dish, you'd have a cup of uncooked lentils and half a cup of uncooked brown rice. This is because beans and lentils also contain a significant amount of carbohydrate. This is how much you can eat, assuming you are not eating another starchy vegetable, to stay within 7 GL points.

The GLs for beans, chickpeas and lentils

Beans and lentils	7 GL points
Soya beans	2 cans
Pinto beans	¾ can
Green/brown lentils	¾ can
Baked beans	½ can
Butter beans	½ can
Split peas	½ can
Kidney beans	½ can
Chickpeas	⅓ can

NOTE A 400g (14oz) can is roughly equivalent to 75g (3oz) dried beans.

A soup made with canned butter beans and vegetables or red lentils, for example, takes minutes and makes a perfect snack or meal with a salad and oatcakes.

NON-STARCHY VEGETABLES

Now it's time to move on to the other half of your plate. This is made up of what I call the 'unlimited vegetables', although there are, of course, some limits even to vegetable choices, but these particular vegetables are those for which a serving is less than 2 GL points. A serving, in this context is quite small – a cupful of peas for example. I want you to eat two servings of unlimited vegetables, one serving of 'starchy' vegetables and one serving of protein-based food – and feel full at the end of every meal.

Non-starchy vegetables

Asparagus	Cucumber	Peas
Aubergine	Endive	Peppers
Beansprouts	Fennel	Radish
Broccoli	Garlic	Rocket
Brussels sprouts	Kale	Runner beans
Cabbage	Lettuce	Spinach
Cauliflower	Mangetouts	Spring onions
Celery	Mushrooms	Tomato
Courgette	Onions	Watercress

ANTI-INFLAMMATORY FOODS

There are certain vegetables that are quite potent anti-inflammatories, reducing pain naturally, but also calming down your whole system. These include red onions, peppers and anything from the pepper family, plus the spices cinnamon, ginger and turmeric, which we use in many recipes. Also, on page 191 there's a list of the top antioxidants, including oregano, mustard, berries and other brightly coloured foods. These are also anti-inflammatory so make sure you eat plenty of them too.

DESSERTS

Provided the basic foods you choose are low GL you can have your cake and eat it without gaining weight or losing energy. It just needs to be the right kind of cake!

In *The Low-GL Diet Bible* and *The Low-GL Diet Cookbook* we allow an additional 5GLs for drinks or snacks for those wishing to lose weight (if you don't have a weight issue, you don't have to be quite so strict). This means you could have a dessert on Monday, a glass of wine on Tuesday, a drink and a dessert on Wednesday, but neither on Thursday. That's as hard as it gets. In these books Fiona McDonald Joyce has created all kinds of low-GL desserts. For those into gourmet food for entertaining you'll also find more delicious dessert recipes in *Food GLorious Food* and *The 10 Secrets of 100% Health Cookbook*. Some of our favourites are listed overleaf.

ANTI-AGEING RECIPES

As well as choosing low-GL foods and meals, you need to eat nutrient-rich foods that provide plenty of methylation-friendly B vitamins, antioxidants and omega-3 fats, both from oily fish and seeds, and nuts and seeds, such as chia, flax, walnut and pumpkin.

On page 191 we showed you some groups of antioxidant-rich foods. The foods with strong colours – mustard and turmeric; blueberries and blackcurrants; kale and spinach; butternut squash and carrots; cinnamon and chocolate – come out top for antioxidants.

B vitamins are generally to be found in whole and fresh foods. Fish is a particularly good source of both B_{12} and other methylation nutrients.

Although you can obviously make your own meals and recipes, choosing anti-ageing foods, here are a few of our favourite combinations:

Hot smoked trout with scrambled eggs and watercress
Salmon and asparagus omelette
Kippers with spinach
Porridge with almonds and goji berries or strawberries
Chicken broth with oriental spices
Peppers stuffed with olives and feta cheese
Poached haddock with cannellini bean mash
Salmon with butter beans and leeks
Chicken with cherry tomatoes and crème fraîche
Stir-fried chicken with soba noodles
Chicken satay skewers
Braised lamb with flageolet beans
Quinoa-flour pancakes with blueberries
Pears with oat and nut crumble

MORE MOUTHWATERING LOW-GL MENUS FOR LOSING WEIGHT

If you need to lose weight, the recipes with the lowest GLs come from *The Low-GL Diet Bible* and *The Low-GL Diet Cookbook*. Here are a few of our favourite recipes to tempt you:

Snacks, light lunches and starters:

Walnut and Three Bean Salad	*The Low-GL Diet Cookbook*
Quinoa Tabbouleh	*The Low-GL Diet Bible*
Chestnut and Butterbean Soup	*The Low-GL Diet Bible*

Lunches and dinners:

Tuna Steak with Black-eyed Bean Salsa	*The Low-GL Diet Bible*
Sticky Mustard Salmon Fillets	*The Low-GL Diet Bible*
Trout with Puy Lentils, Roasted Vine Tomatoes	*The Low-GL Diet Cookbook*
Spicy Mackerel with Couscous	*The Low-GL Diet Bible*
Thai Fish Cakes	*Food GLorious Food*
Mushroom and Pot Barley Risotto	*Food GLorious Food*
Wild Rice and Puy Lentils with Lemon and Asparagus	*Food GLorious Food*

Desserts:

Apple Flapjack Crumble	*The Low-GL Diet Bible*
Carrot and Walnut Cake	*The Low-GL Diet Cookbook*
Apple and Almond Cake	*The Low-GL Diet Cookbook*

If you decide to look at these books you will not be short of recipes and menu options – we think you'll be surprised at how sustaining and flavourful they are.

ALTERNATE DAY DIETING

Once you've got the hang of anti-ageing eating, you can, if you wish, push the boat out further by applying the anti-ageing principles of Alternate Day Dieting. You will remember that in Part One we explained how eating every other day controlled the amount of calories you consumed without causing you to put on weight the day that you ate normally. We saw that some people, the ultra-anti-agers, were using this system (combined with supplements) to keep young. Although there is no really hard evidence that this works in humans yet, the results with animals are quite extraordinary, and many people who have applied these principles, which are designed to switch on the anti-ageing gene (called Sweet Sixteen – see page 82) and to switch off the Grim Reaper gene (that switch on the genes for conditions such as diabetes), are very encouraging.

CASE STUDY: MARGARET

Margaret is a 60-year-old property developer.

'I'd been putting on a pound every year for 20 years and I finally decided they had to come off.'

The problem was that Margaret had tried 'every diet known to woman'. So when she heard about the eat-every-other-day diet she was immediately interested.

'It was something new and the theory behind it was intriguing and plausible.'

She found the 'down' days extraordinarily easy.

'I was limiting myself to 500–800 calories – about as much as you'd get on a strict low-calorie diet, but it was easy, because you knew you could have more tomorrow. But I never wanted to gorge the next day. It was like being offered jam tomorrow, but when tomorrow came you didn't actually want it. In fact, I found myself seeking out more nutritious food for the "down" days to get the most benefit from the calories I was allowed, and that carried over to the "up" days.'

The most immediate effect was that Margaret lost 4.5kg (10lb) in two weeks.

'What was really noticeable was where it went from. I got my waist back! I can't see any reason not to eat like this all the time. Unlike many diets, it is really easy to fit in round the family and social occasions. You can't do that with a raw-food diet for example. I'm now doing a relaxed version, maybe two days on, one off. But if the pounds start creeping back I'll just get a bit more strict.'

In order to trigger this change in genetic expression using Alternate Day Dieting you need four weeks of eating every other day. After the first four weeks you can switch to two days eating normally, and one day off, eating no more than 500–800 calories on the 'down' day. By eating normally, we mean eating a low-GL, highly nutritious diet, as shown above.

Since a total fast for a day is quite challenging for many, the best way to follow a modified fast of 800 calories is to have one of the following options:

- A Get Up & Go shake, made with low-fat milk, soya or oat milk and a handful of berries and a 30g (1oz) scoop of Get Up & Go (see Resources). With milk and a handful of berries it's under 300 calories so you can have this twice a day and still be well under 800 calories. You can even add a teaspoonful of chia seeds to increase the protein, fibre and omega-3 content. Add a heaped teaspoonful of a super fibre such as glucomannan (from konjac fibre) or PGX, and it will really fill you up.

Get Up & Go is a powder that you blend with a piece of fruit, choosing from any of the 5 GL servings of fruit shown earlier, plus 350ml (12fl oz) skimmed milk (or sugar-free soya milk, if you are allergic to dairy).

Get Up & Go is made from a special blend of quinoa, brown rice and soya flour, giving an excellent quality of protein. This is balanced with carbohydrate, mainly from whole apple powder, together with oat bran, rice bran and psyllium husks for added soluble fibre, plus sesame, sunflower and pumpkin seeds, and some almond meal, cinnamon and natural vanilla for flavour. In addition, it has added vitamins and minerals, including 50mcg of chromium and 1,000mg of vitamin C, plus all the B vitamins.

This is our top recommendation, because it also gives you a very good all-round intake of protein, low-GL carbs, and vitamins and minerals, and it fills you up the most, being high in soluble fibres.

- A small bowl of porridge, made with half water and half low-fat milk or sugar-free soya milk, plus seeds and berries. You can eat this twice a day. To stay within 800 calories, have no more than two heaped teaspoonfuls of seeds in total for the day.
- An egg for breakfast with two oatcakes and a small bowl of soup in the afternoon.

- Fruit (ideally berries, plums, cherries, a peach or half an apple) with a small amount of seeds or nuts (a tablespoonful) four times a day. The daily allowance for seeds or nuts is a small cup.

- A thin slice of lean meat or fish (such as smoked salmon), with a thin slice of Scandinavian-style bread or two oatcakes. To stay within 800 calories you need no more than 100g of meat or fish – chicken breast or smoked salmon being good choices – with two oatcakes or a slice of wholegrain bread, three times a day.

When you are hungry or thirsty, drink water. Keep yourself well hydrated. Do not do strenuous exercise on your 'fasting' days although stretching and yoga-type exercises are good.

A word of caution: Alternate Day Dieting is not for the faint hearted. If you have diabetes or heart disease, or any other condition that might be adversely affected by big drops in blood sugar levels please check with your doctor first before embarking on this kind of approach.

It is worth getting well established on low-GL diet principles first. When you are Alternate Day Dieting you don't need to be so strict on the 40GLs a day (or 45GLs with drinks/dessert), which is for maximum weight loss. Eat 60GLs a day on your 'up' day, which is for maintenance. The low-GL diet books and recipes mentioned above give you recipe options for 60GLs a day.

An important point, whether you do Alternate Day Dieting or not, is not to get to the point where you are so hungry that you go off the deep end and eat anything and everything, since that defeats the purpose. It appears that you need four weeks of one day on, one day off, to switch on the anti-ageing genes. This way of eating is also excellent for shifting unwanted weight, as we've seen with Margaret above.

Once you have done this, and your weight is under control, a 20 per cent difference in calorie intake may be enough to maintain the effect. This would be the equivalent of 45GLs one day (following the diet really strictly) and then 65GLs the next, eating at maintenance level. This is not so difficult to do.

Chapter 3

WHAT TO DRINK

What you drink makes a big difference to the ageing process for three reasons. Firstly, one of the consistent measures of increasing age is dehydration. In simple terms, you can predict a person's biological age by the percentage of water in the bones and brain. Keeping yourself well hydrated is a simple and effective anti-ageing step.

Secondly, most of the increase in sugar in our diets has crept in through drinks. So, choosing the right low-GL drinks makes all the difference.

Thirdly, there are mixed messages out there about whether or not it is good or bad to drink a little alcohol or even quite a lot. To date, the oldest person ever recorded is Madame Jeanne Calmant from Arles in France who died at the age of 122 in 1997. Madame Calmant was not a health fanatic; she gave up smoking at the age of 117 and drank two glasses of port every day until her last decade. She had a penchant for dark chocolate and olive oil, kept reasonably fit and had a good mental attitude. The longest living man, Shigechiyo Izumi, is claimed to have lived until 120; he was a lover of wine, women and song. In his case his alcoholic drink of choice was a daily shot of sake. Both kept fit and had a positive mental attitude – could that be their secret, or did they just throw the right genetic die? Or perhaps we should all be drinking port or sake? Read on to find out more.

HOW MUCH WATER DO YOU NEED TO STAY YOUNG?

We tend to take water for granted but, as Professor Jamie Bartram of the World Health Organization, says, 'Water is a basic nutrient for the human body and is critical to human life. It supports the digestion of food, absorption, transportation and use of nutrients and the elimination of toxins and wastes from the body.' Not only is water our most important nutrient but it is also by far the most abundant in our bodies – so drinking plenty is essential. Approximately two-thirds of your body is water. Your brain is about 85 per cent water, whereas muscles are 75 per cent, and even bone is 22 per cent.

You need about eight glasses of water a day, and more if you live in a hot climate. If you only drink when you're thirsty, your body is already in a state of relative dehydration. Not drinking enough makes you tired and dries out your skin and your joints. It's also a major cause of constipation. The long-term effects of not drinking enough can be more serious – including kidney stones.

The trouble is that hunger is often confused with thirst, so when you're hungry, drink a glass of water. There is some evidence that either drinking water with a meal,[4] or eating water-rich foods,[5] such as fruit and veg, makes you likely to eat less, so this would be important if you need to lose weight. Water may also speed up your metabolism in such a way that could encourage weight loss.[6]

Dehydration also causes a loss of concentration. Drinking water needs to become a habit if you want to age healthily. In our 100% Health Survey of over 55,000 people we found that:

- 81 per cent of respondents had less than one bowel movement a day.
- 56 per cent of people had dry skin.
- 48 per cent of people frequently had headaches or migraine.
- Those who drank the equivalent of eight glasses of water a day were nearly twice as likely to be in optimal health compared to those who drank less than a glass of water a day.

YOUR BODY'S NEEDS FOR WATER

Apart from feeling thirsty, there are many ways your body tells you that you need to take in more fluid. These are some of the more obvious and short-term signs of dehydration:

- Headache

- Dizziness
- Increased body temperature (inability to sweat)
- Loss of concentration/mental ability
- Decreased physical performance
- Hunger
- Lack of energy/fatigue
- Dry membrane surfaces (mouth, eyes, skin)
- Dark, strong-smelling urine
- Constipation/poor digestive function

The more long-term consequences of not drinking enough include the increased risk of kidney stones, premature ageing, high blood pressure, digestive problems, certain cancers, depression and cognitive decline, asthma and allergies, and possibly weight gain. Apart from kidney stones, these conditions are not only caused by a lack of water, but not drinking enough makes them worse. In fact, just about every biochemical reaction in your body depends on water. Most digestive juices, for example, are principally water, and your body releases 10 litres (17½ pints) of the stuff into your digestive tract on a daily basis, much of which then becomes reabsorbed into the body. If you don't eat enough fibre in your diet, your stools become dehydrated, leading to constipation. Constipation, in turn, is a major driver of digestive health problems.

HOW MUCH DO YOU REALLY NEED?

Nowadays, with the bottled-water industry worth over $60 billion globally, water is big business, so there are certainly vested interests in telling us to drink more. Nevertheless, as explained above, drinking sufficient water is essential. The average man needs between 1.2 litres (2 pints) and 3 litres (5¼ pints) per day, whereas a woman needs between 1.2 litres (2 pints) and 2.2 litres (3¾ pints) – that averages out at about eight glasses or more of water-based liquid a day. We get about 19 per cent of our requirement from the food we eat, with fresh fruit and vegetables containing the most. So the more fruit and veg you eat the more water you take in. Conversely, concentrated foods with a high sugar or protein content increase your need for water to dilute the excess sugars or break down the products of amino acids in the bloodstream.

Dehydration is defined as a 1 per cent, or greater, loss of body weight as a result of fluid loss; however, we feel thirsty when dehydration reaches 0.8 to 2 per cent. In other words, you can be dehydrated (and have lost over 1 per cent of your body weight) but not yet feel thirsty.

DOES IT MATTER HOW WE DRINK IT?

What you drink your water with also makes a big difference. Your body retains much more if you drink little and often, rather than having it all in one go.[7] Also, if water is drunk with sugar, which is so often the case in sugary drinks, the water is less well retained by the body.[8] This will also be the case if drunk in tea or coffee. One of the popular myths is that caffeinated drinks are so dehydrating that you actually lose more water than you gain. This is not true. For many reasons, though, it is best to get your water from non-caffeinated and non-sweetened drinks. In fact, there's nothing better than drinking water itself as a first port of call, or a herb tea.

HOW ESSENTIAL FATS HELP YOU BENEFIT FROM WATER

For cells in the body to retain the correct fluid levels inside and out you need the cellular membrane to be waterproof, allowing water in and out as needed. That waterproofing is produced by essential fats woven into the matrix of your cells' membranes. A lack of essential fats can therefore lead to too much water in the wrong places, causing water retention and weight gain, and not enough in the right places, leading to dry skin.

HOW PURE IS YOUR WATER?

There's a lot more to water than pure H_2O (hydrogen and oxygen). Water can also provide many minerals, especially if you're drinking mineral water, which means the water is effectively filtered as it's pushed up to the surface through cracks in underground rocks. You can get a tenth of your calcium needs for the day from some mineral waters. Tap water in a soft-water area, on the other hand, provides as little as 30mg of calcium a day.

In addition, tap water can contain traces of nitrates, trihalomethanes, lead and aluminium, all of which are anti-nutrients in their own right. In most areas of Britain the levels of these pollutants don't exceed maximum safety limits. In rural parts of Scotland, however, about 5 per cent of water tested exceeds the permissible levels of trihalomethanes, a potential carcinogen and a by-product of treating organic-rich water with chlorine or bromine. Lead is not generally present in the mains water supplied, but it can be picked up through contact with lead plumbing in some homes and buildings. You can check whether your home has lead plumbing – it's unlikely to if it was built after 1970. Your water company can help check this for you.

Concerns over pollutants in water have led many people to switch to bottled, distilled or filtered water. Overall, it is much more important to drink tap water than to avoid water altogether if you live in the UK and that is your only option, as it does contain small levels of nutrients. But if you are a purist and want your water super-clean, it is best to fit a water filter onto a tap you use for drinking water. This is what we do, using a high-quality carbon water filter unit plumbed in under the sink. This also improves the taste of the water, which makes you more likely to drink it. Plumbed-in water filters are the most cost effective, with new cartridges costing as little as £25, once or twice a year depending on your household use of drinking water. That's certainly a lot cheaper than drinking mineral water. Some filtering processes remove not only impurities but also many of the naturally occurring minerals, and the same applies to distilling water. This once again pushes up the need for minerals from food, which is not a problem if you eat a wholefood diet: nuts, seeds, beans and root vegetables are all good sources of minerals.

SIMPLE WAYS TO INCREASE YOUR WATER INTAKE

Here are some simple steps you can take to increase your intake of water and hydrate your body optimally.

- On a normal day, drink around 2 litres (3½ pints) – eight glasses – of water.

- Start by drinking a glass of fresh water when you get up in the morning.
- If you are not used to drinking water regularly, replace one of your other drinks each day with fresh water, increasing your consumption as the weeks go by.
- Ask for a glass of water to go with your coffee and tea in cafés – if you're still having them!
- Drink a glass of water with each meal.
- Have a herb tea or hot water with fresh mint, lemon balm, ginger or lemon.
- Carry a bottle filled with filtered water with you whenever you leave the house.
- During exercise, drink at 10–15 minute intervals.
- Keep a check on your urine. It should be plentiful, pale in colour and odourless.
- Ask for water with your meal when in restaurants, and always drink water with an alcoholic drink.

LOW-GL DRINKING

To keep your blood sugar under control, you need to be really careful about what you drink. Estimates suggest that two-thirds of the increase in sugar in our modern-day diets come from drinks – including natural fruit juices. It's a lot easier to drink a glass of grape juice, for example, than to eat a whole bunch of grapes. It is better to eat fruit rather than to drink it. At the other end of the scale, a 2 litre (3½ pint) bottle of cola has roughly 45 teaspoons of sugar in it! The chart opposite shows you what you can drink for 5GLs.

Drinks for 5GLs

Drink	5GLs
Tomato juice	600ml (20fl oz/1 pint)
Carrot juice	small glass
Grapefruit juice, unsweetened	small glass
Cherry Active concentrate	small glass, diluted 50:50 with water
Apple juice, unsweetened	small glass, diluted 50:50 with water
Orange juice, unsweetened	small glass, diluted 50:50 with water; or juice of one orange
Pineapple juice	½ small glass, diluted 50:50 with water
Cranberry juice drink	½ small glass, diluted 50:50 with water
Grape juice	2.5cm (1in)-worth of liquid!

A good rule of thumb is to have no more than one glass of juice a day, diluting it as you need to in order to have no more than 5GLs a day. So have, say, either a glass of carrot juice, or a diluted apple juice or cherry concentrate. Cherry juice is especially good because the predominant sugar is xylose, making it very low-GL. Cherry Active, a pure concentrate of the Montmorency cherry, is an absolute winner as far as antioxidants is concerned, so this is probably the best all-round choice (see Resources for details).

Remember, bananas and grapes are fast-releasing, apple and pears medium-releasing (predominantly fructose) whereas cherries, berries and plums are slow-releasing (predominantly xylose). So, if you pick a smoothie, don't go for one where the top two ingredients are bananas and grape juice. Most of all, stay away from all fizzy, sweetened, caffeinated drinks and sugar-sweetened cordials.

WHAT ABOUT ALCOHOL?

Whole books have been written extolling alcohol's merits and dangers. There is no doubt that alcohol is bad news for the liver – it's strongly associated with an increased cancer risk and it damages the gut. But small amounts may not be so much of a problem and may even be a benefit. One obvious attraction that is rarely factored into the alcohol equation is that it relaxes you, and that your stress hormones, as we saw in Secret 10, rapidly age you, promoting metabolic syndrome and accelerated brain shrinkage. Benefits of light drinking have also been reported in relation to cardiovascular disease risk and Alzheimer's.

In our 100% Health Survey, drinking a small amount of alcohol, up to a glass a day of wine for example, had no negative effect in relation to mood or energy. In fact, there was a hint of a benefit in relation to mood and memory. The benefits of light drinking – for example a glass of wine in the evening – have also been reported in relation to a reduced risk of cardiovascular disease and Alzheimer's. From a GL or blood sugar point of view, small amounts of 'dry' drinks such as dry wine, champagne, or spirits such as whisky, are not a big issue. The mixers, such as tonic and cola are more of a problem. Beer has a higher GL value so, again, it is better to go for dry lagers. On page 310 we'll show you the best low-GL alcoholic drinks.

GOOD FOR THE HEART?

One plus for alcohol in moderation is the well-established finding that it increases HDL ('good') cholesterol. This is true for both beer and wine, and seems to relate more to the quantity drunk than the type of drink. Red wine, in particular, may confer additional cardiovascular benefits by virtue of being high in proanthocyanidins and resveratrol, the antioxidants found in grapes and berries. Alcohol itself, however, is an oxidant.

Another potential benefit of alcohol is a mild reduction in platelet aggregation – in other words, it makes your blood thinner. This occurs because alcohol blocks the formation of prostaglandins from essential fats. For the body to make use of essential fats, however, these fats must be converted into their active compounds – a process which is blocked by alcohol. So the combination of being essential-fat deficient and drinking alcohol is especially bad.

The bone of contention is the dose: does a glass of wine a day confer benefit? Most reviews conclude that there is a clear risk reduction from light or moderate drinking; the positive benefit being primarily for red wine, which is high in resveratrol. Some studies, however, show a link between moderate to heavy alcohol consumption and increased blood pressure and the incidence of strokes. Diabetes risk also appears to be lower with light or moderate drinking, but not with heavy drinking.[9]

ALCOHOL AND WEIGHT GAIN

You have to be careful with alcohol in relation to weight gain. It acts very much like a sugar and can turn into fat. A recent survey that tracked over 120,000 people in the US over four years found that, on average, a person gains 185g (6½oz) a year for every daily drink.[10] So, if you have two drinks a day, that's close to 450g (1lb) a year; however, a study of women finds that those who drink a light to moderate amount of alcohol appear to gain less weight and have a lower risk of becoming overweight and obese than non-drinkers, according to a report in the Archives of Internal Medicine. This survey of over 19,000 non-obese women followed up over 13 years finds that those who drink 15g of alcohol a day, which is equivalent to a glass of wine, a shot of a spirit or 600ml (20fl oz/1 pint) beer, compared to those who drank none, were almost 30 per cent less likely to become overweight or obese. The most positive association was found with red wine, followed by white. A beneficial effect was also apparent at 30g a day, but no longer apparent at 40g a day.

From a glycemic-load point of view we'd be cautious about the pint of beer, because this represents 20GLs – a large proportion of the ideal daily limit for maximum weight loss, which is 45GLs, or the 60GLs for maintenance. On our low-GL diet we allow 5GLs a day for drinks or desserts, which is the equivalent of half a pint of beer every other day or a low-carb lager every day (or a glass of wine). This amount of alcohol is also consistent with maintaining a good homocysteine level, whereas larger intakes raise it. A low homocysteine level also predicts less risk for heart disease and Alzheimer's disease.

Here are the options:

GL and units for alcohol and your daily maximum

	GL	Units	Daily max
Beer/lager 300ml (10fl oz/½ pint)	10	1	150ml (5fl oz/¼ pint)
Red wine 115ml (3¾fl oz) small glass	2	1	1 glass
White wine/champagne 115ml (3¾fl oz)	1	1	1 glass
Spirits 30ml (1fl oz)	0	1	1 shot
Spirits + 125ml (4fl oz) orange juice	6	1	1 small glass

(Assumes that alcohol carbs = 100 GI)

Our advice is to have an occasional drink, perhaps four times a week, not every day. If you do drink every day, limit it to one glass of a good-quality wine or spirit. There is certainly good logic to having a good-quality red wine, high in resveratrol. The chances are that an organic red is more likely to be a good source.

If you find you have to drink every day, or are gradually drinking more, or that you drink to numb negative feelings, it's time to give it a break for a couple of weeks and to face whatever it is that's making you feel bad.

The truth is, we are all different and, for some people, alcohol is especially bad news. For most of us having a drink a day is no big deal, and may even confer benefits. For all of us too much alcohol is a major promoter of disease and premature death.

Chapter 4

EXERCISE FOR LONGEVITY

All the lifestyle changes we've been recommending throughout the book have multiple benefits, and none more so than exercise. And yet 95 per cent of the populations of the UK and the US don't even get the official recommended amount of 30 minutes 'moderate to vigorous' physical exercise a day. Life in the West conspires massively against it. Cars, remote controls, food processors, home-delivery restaurants, 'home entertainment centres', escalators, lifts … every year, there are more gadgets and mod cons that do away with the need to expend energy.

In fact, if governments wanted to do just one thing that would have a major impact not just on levels of obesity but on diabetes, heart disease, stress, high blood pressure and dementia, getting everyone on an effective regular exercise programme would probably be the fastest and most cost-effective way to do it. Recently, Dr Richard Weiler, an expert in sport and exercise medicine at Imperial College in London, set out the case for this in the *British Medical Journal*.[11] According to sports medicine professor Wayne Derman, from the University of Cape Town, 'Exercise is the closest thing to an anti-ageing pill.' There's even evidence that it increases telomere length, thus enhancing cell rejuvenation (see Part One, Chapter 3). For 21 years researchers at Stanford University in California have been studying the effects of consistent exercise on runners aged 50 and over, compared with a control group. So far, after 21 years, 65 of the runners have died from cancers and disorders of the heart and brain compared with 98 of the non-runners.[12]

One of the obstacles to achieving this is that for years exercise has largely been promoted as a way of losing weight, and you don't need to be a maths wizard to work out that if you are doing it to lose calories it looks like a fearsomely laborious task. Twenty minutes of jogging equals one chocolate chip cookie; running a mile equals 300 calories. How motivating is that? But, as we shall see, cumulative exercise does reap big rewards.

The weight-loss approach reflects a very outdated 'calories in = calories out' view of how our metabolism works; however, there is so much more going on when you exercise than the calorie equation. Exercising – not only regularly but also in the most effective way – has to be at the heart of any healthy ageing programme. As we'll be discussing, there are two kinds of exercise that you need to do to reap all the benefits: aerobic and resistance exercise. Aerobic is exercise that makes your heart beat faster, such as walking fast, running, dance fitness or cycling. This exercise strengthens the heart and burns calories, and it is also the best way to lose the dangerous belly fat stored around the middle that increases inflammation, according to a study in the *American Journal of Physiology* in August 2011. Resistance exercise, which involves pushing up weights or pulling against stretchy exercise bands, builds and maintains muscle which you will otherwise lose as you get older (see Part One, Chapter 1). You also need to maintain suppleness and flexibility by stretching – yoga and Pilates are both excellent ways of doing this.

THE BENEFITS OF EXERCISE

Here are some of the virtuous spiral effects of exercise that the calorie equation misses out:

1. The effects of exercise are cumulative. Burning up 300 calories a day, three days a week for a year equals 22,000 calories, or a loss of 5kg (11lb)! And the exercise-multiplier effect kicks in right away – the fatter and less fit you are, the more benefit you'll derive from small bouts of exercise.

2. Moderate exercise decreases your appetite. Exercise can actually make you less hungry. Without exercise, your body stops listening to the chemical messenger that tells it to turn off your appetite. Once you start exercising, you'll often find that, after a burst of activity, you don't actually feel like eating. This is important if you are overweight and inclined to eat out of boredom.

3. Exercise boosts your metabolic rate. What's really important about the food you take in is not its calorie count but how fast your body burns it up – what's known as your metabolic rate. According to Professor William McArdle, exercise physiologist at City University, New York, 'Most people can generate metabolic rates that are eight to 10 times above their resting value during sustained cycling, running or swimming.'[13] What's more, that effect doesn't just happen while you are doing it but also for up to 15 hours afterwards. So, you could be using up much more than a biscuit during a hard run. This speeded-up metabolism is one of the best ways to get your blood sugar down to a healthy level and to restore insulin sensitivity which, as we've seen throughout the book, is vital for healthy ageing. As a bonus, amounts of the ageing glycosylated haemoglobin – the protein and sugar gunky combo – that is behind wrinkled skin and cataracts also comes down.

4. Resistance exercise benefits hormone production. Along with the benefit of maintaining muscle mass, resistance training in particular also boosts your production of several hormones that start falling off as you get older (see Part Two, Secret 10). These include human growth hormone (hGh), testosterone and DHEA. Growth hormone has a number of anti-ageing benefits – but it possibly also has dangerous side effects when given as an injection. Increased testosterone can be very beneficial to older men who are putting on weight, and adequate levels of DHEA are linked with a better immune response. Although these hormones go up naturally through exercise, the stress hormone cortisol, which is a major promoter of insulin resistance, goes down.

5. Exercise is a great way to reduce stress. As we learnt in Secret 4, stress and excess weight gain go hand in hand. Exercise will bring down your stress levels and promote a much more positive and creative mental state. It also helps you to sleep well, and increases the amount of slow-wave sleep, which helps to rejuvenate the body.[14] (But it's best not to exercise too close to bedtime – so the morning or afternoon are better.)

As we have seen, exercise has real benefits as you get older because, even if you are fairly healthy, your blood sugar can begin to creep up, bringing with it all the damaging side effects. One of the many benefits of physical activity in middle and old age, especially the sort known as aerobic, which raises your heart rate and gets you breathing faster, is that it improves insulin sensitivity, thereby helping to stabilise blood sugar levels and weight.[15] Athletes have vastly improved blood sugar control, enhanced insulin sensitivity and faster metabolic rates.[16] This kind of exercise will also improve your production of good prostaglandins (the body's anti-inflammatory agents) and boost circulation (and thus the supply of oxygen and nutrients to cells). But you don't have to be training at top-athlete level to get the benefits. Most exercise research has been carried out on adults who are already taking regular exercise; more is needed to pinpoint the specific ways you can benefit if you are older and just starting to exercise or taking it up again after a break.

EXERCISE AND FAT BURNING

Another of the benefits of aerobic exercise is that it will increase your ability to burn fat. Resistance exercise, the sort that involves lifting weights, or pulling against stretchy exercise bands, doesn't burn fat in the same way, but it helps you to build more muscle which, in turn, burns more fat.

The best kind of exercises to help to burn fat efficiently are brisk walking, jogging, cycling, swimming, aerobic dance, stepping, cross-country skiing, circuit training or any aerobic exercise that is steady, continuous and of a certain intensity. Check out if there are any local classes aimed at the over-fifties that do aerobics or dance fitness such as Zumba for a fun way to work out. Exercising in water – aquarobics – is also a good option if you want to start gently and is appropriate even for people in their eighties and nineties.

MUSCLE IS HEAVIER THAN FAT

A word of warning for the scale-watchers, though: when you start a committed exercise programme and begin to lose fat and gain lean muscle, you will lose inches faster than pounds. In the first month you'll look trimmer and feel fitter, but you may lose less weight than you might have wished. This is because muscle is denser and hence heavier than fat. In other words, 450g (1lb) of muscle takes up less space than 450g (1lb) of fat.

Remember, the enemy is not so much your weight, but having too high a body-fat percentage (high ratios of body fat to lean tissue have been linked to heart disease, diabetes and some cancers). So, if you have access to a body-fat monitor, check this rather than only jumping on the scales. The more lean muscle you gain, the more ability you'll have to burn fat – and that's what counts in the long run.

THE BENEFITS DON'T STOP THERE

Such exercises also tone the body and reduce the risk of osteoporosis. They will strengthen your heart and lungs, reduce your risk of heart disease, help control stress and improve circulation. (See the benefits of muscle building in Secrets 2 and 3.)

In short, exercise offers a huge array of benefits. If you haven't really got into it before, it opens up an undiscovered world of vitality, health – and sheer enjoyment. As your energy returns on the Anti-ageing Diet you'll soon find you really do gain health and vitality through regular exercise. If you have never been active before, it may seem rather daunting, and perhaps you may feel it is hardly worthwhile to start on an exercise regime in your sixties or seventies, but the benefits of exercise are so good that it really is worth getting started at any age. You can begin gently and build up your exercise as you progress – and you should feel the benefit almost immediately. A gentle walk is an ideal way to start or you can join a class and start to move your body; it's a fun way to meet other people – and you don't have to take it terribly seriously, just enjoy yourself.

FINDING RESISTANCE EXERCISES THAT HELP

According to some sources, only 12 per cent of people over 65 do any kind of resistance training to build muscle, even though they are the age group that could benefit the most. Without it you are likely to lose

40 per cent of your muscle mass between the ages of 20 and 80.[17] You could work out on the sort of barbell weights and machines found in gyms or you may prefer the much cheaper and simpler pieces of equipment you can use at home, such as resistance bands or resistance tubes, which come in various thicknesses. They are readily available on the internet or at most sports stores.

With weights or bands, work up the repetitions gradually, as explained in the accompanying leaflets when you buy your equipment; you should be aiming for 8 to 12 repetitions, with the last few being a bit of a challenge. Your movements should be slow and controlled, keeping up the tension until each exercise is finished. Make sure you warm up before you start by walking on the spot, going up and down the stairs or anything that involves continuous movement. On Patrick's website you'll find some simple resistance exercises that you can do at home.

You may need to get some advice from a fitness instructor to create your own perfect resistance-training routine. The Zest4Life groups also offer fitness training, designed by former gladiator Kate Staples and Olympic athlete Daley Thompson (see Resources). Rather than using gyms, they get you outdoors and show you how to use your natural environment to create the perfect mix of both aerobic and resistance training. It will also get you out in the sun – which is good for pushing up your vitamin D levels (see below). Don't be worried that they are top athletes, their aim is to get everyone, whatever their fitness level, working to the best of their ability. And if there isn't a group within easy reach, make use of leisure centres or fitness classes in your area.

BUILDING DAILY EXERCISE INTO YOUR LIFE

If you are over 40 and haven't been exercising on a regular basis, don't forget to check with your doctor before starting on an exercise programme, especially if you have a history of heart disease or have had any symptoms such chest pain, dizziness or back pain. Ask your doctor if you should have an exercise stress test. It's also a good idea to go to a local gym or leisure centre at first so that you have some supervision when you are starting out. And don't overdo it. Make sure you start off gently and build up as you get fitter. 'No pain, no gain' is not a good motto until you've got up to a good level of fitness.

If you join an exercise class of any kind, the trainer will advise you how to begin. The advantage of an exercise class is that, contrary to what you might believe, most people who are taking part are not super-fit but just ordinary people of all fitness levels working hard to improve their fitness, and the classes are often very friendly. There are lots of classes for the over-fifties and many classes for the under-fifties are also suitable for older people if you are reasonably fit.

HOW MUCH EXERCISE WILL YOU NEED TO DO?

If you are doing the right kind of exercise (that is, a mixture of aerobic and resistance), all you need to do is 20–30 minutes a day. If you want to confine your exercising to five days a week, you can do 30 minutes a day with two days off. If you are doing less strenuous exercise, you may need to increase your daily time of exercising to 30–45 minutes a day, but it is important to build up the intensity. Our advice is to make an appointment in your diary to exercise, just like you would to attend a meeting or see a friend. Then, don't break it.

AEROBIC EXERCISE

Depending on your current level of fitness, aerobic exercise can be anything from brisk walking to playing golf, going for a swim or a bike ride or joining an exercise class, but the key is that you get your heart rate into your 'training heart-rate zone'. This is a measure of your pulse in relation to your age.

To find your training heart-rate zone, you need to subtract your age from 220, then calculate 65 per cent of this amount for the lower end of your training zone and 80 per cent for the upper limit:

220 – [age] × .65 = lower limit
220 – [age] × .80 = upper limit

For example, for a 50-year-old:

$220 - 50 = 170 \times .65$ = lower limit = 110 beats per minute

$220 - 50 = 170 \times .80$ = upper limit = 136 beats per minute

You want to be exercising for at least 15 minutes with your pulse in this training heart-rate zone. If you measure your pulse for 10 seconds, then multiply it by 6, you'll find out if you are exercising hard enough, or too hard.

An overweight, out-of-condition person may reach their training heart-rate zone by walking just a few hundred yards. A fitter, leaner person may have to walk briskly for at least five minutes to push their pulse up to their training zone. This is why you need to monitor your pulse while exercising to make sure you do not over- or under-exercise, and to achieve the best benefits for burning fat. As you get fitter and leaner, you'll find that you will have to push harder – perhaps by walking faster or adding more hill walking to your programme – to reach your training zone. You can buy a heart-rate monitor quite inexpensively or, for a rough rule of thumb, you are probably in the zone if you are walking or jogging at a speed where it is hard to keep up a conversation.

THE MUSCLES USED IN RESISTANCE EXERCISE

Resistance exercise is all about building muscle, but you don't need to be lifting a whole ton of weight to do this! It can involve weights or bands – see above – but it can also involve a more intensive sort of workout that uses different muscles to those exercised by aerobics. Whereas aerobics mainly develops one sort of muscle fibre known as 'slow twitch' – used if you are running much more than a few hundred metres – resistance training is needed to work another sort of muscle known as 'fast twitch', which gives you the explosive power of sprinting or jumping. The slow twitch is powered by oxygen, which is why you end up panting. A fast-twitch sprint needs more oxygen than you can supply – and this is why this kind of exercise is known as 'anaerobic' – so your system switches to burning glucose.

Try 30-second bursts

The interesting thing is that if you do the right kind of high-intensity resistance exercise – using and developing both types of muscle – you don't need to do it for long. It can literally be a 30-second burst of intense exercise, five to eight times. That's it. Do this three times a week and you'll get a great result. It makes your heart muscle work hard, so you'll be really panting at the end of your 30 seconds, and this can increase your growth hormone level by up to five times, which then both re-sensitises you to insulin and builds muscle.

One of the original proponents of this type of exercising is Phil Campbell, author of *Ready Set Go!* (see Recommended Reading), which is a great book to read if you want to go into this in more detail. He's a trainer of top athletes and sportsmen, but don't be put off by that – the principles are really simple and can be used by people who are in their fifties, sixties and beyond. You can see for yourself by watching the YouTube video, made by Dr Joseph Mercola, who describes a version of these principles as the *Peak 8 System* (see Resources). This is based on eight sprints, in this case done on an exercise bike, but you can do it with any kind of exercise – swimming or cycling, for example.

The basic guidelines are as follows:

1. You warm up for three minutes.

2. Now exercise as hard and fast as you can for 30 seconds. You should feel like you couldn't possibly go on for another few seconds.

3. Recover for 90 seconds.

4. Then do it again.

5. Repeat this cycle a total of eight times.

That's the goal, but Rome wasn't built in a day, and it is really important to build up to this if you are currently not in good shape. That might mean doing the sequence only two or three times first time, then adding a repetition as you become more able.

At the first level, for example, you might be walking for three minutes, then have a 30-second burst of walking or jogging as fast as you can, then you stop. You want to get your heart rate up into the top end of your training heart-rate zone.

You know you've reached it when it's hard to breathe and talk due to the temporary oxygen debt; you start to sweat; you feel hot; and you get some muscle ache. But simply doing this three times a week will make a big difference to your health. This whole sequence takes 20 minutes.

YOUR WEEKLY ROUTINE

Choose the kind of training that appeals to you, making sure the aerobic exercise will raise your heart rate into the training zone. Don't try to do too much to start with. If you are very unfit or overweight it is good to get some professional guidance and support at the beginning. You need a mix of aerobic activities like running or cycling, some resistance training of the sort you can do at home with bands or a gym work out, and for best results some of the short bursts of explosive activities.

Warm up before aerobic exercise by starting off slowly, and before resistance exercises warm up by walking or stretching. Cool down from aerobics by walking more slowly for three to five minutes to allow your heart rate to return to normal, and after resistance exercise do some stretches. Stretching exercise, such as yoga, also has a resistance element to it.

Now plan your week ahead. A typical weekly routine might look like this, but you will need to build up to it if you are very unfit:

Monday – resistance training (20 minutes)
Tuesday – aerobic exercise (30-plus minutes)
Wednesday – resistance training (20 minutes)
Thursday – aerobic exercise (30-plus minutes)
Friday – resistance training (20 minutes)
Saturday – aerobic exercise (30 minutes)
Sunday – day off

WHEN TO EXERCISE

The best time to exercise is two hours after eating. No self-respecting animal would eat before exercising. From an evolutionary perspective the purpose of exercise is to get food to eat. If you exercise first thing in the morning, make sure you have breakfast straight after. When you eat after exercising, your muscles and liver are geared up to deal with the carbohydrates in your food so that you don't get such big spikes in your blood sugar.

Having said that, going for a stroll after a main meal – for example after Sunday lunch – then having your dessert after the walk, also helps to stabilise blood sugar levels.

Don't exercise late at night. Also, if possible, exercise in natural daylight, because you'll make vitamin D, which strengthens bones and muscles.

INCREASE YOUR BASE-LINE ACTIVITY

One great way to increase your general level of exercise is simply to get more active generally. Use the stairs instead of the lift. Walk or cycle instead of driving everywhere. Run around with your grandchildren, or take up a sport. There are many ways in a day to develop fitness, and soon this way of living will become a habit.

Get fit by taking the alternative way

The fat way	The fit way
Take a lift	Use the stairs
Drive to work	Walk or cycle some of the way
Drive to the shops	Walk to the shops
Spend the night watching TV	Take up an active hobby
Get other people to bring you one too!	Get up and do it yourself!
Use power tools for gardening and DIY	Use manual tools when it's just as quick
Go upstairs as little as possible at home	Run upstairs as often as possible
Use automatic car washes	Wash the car yourself
Stick your grandchildren in front of the TV	Actively play with them
Have business meetings inside	Go for a walk where possible

A small effort to keep fit, supple and strong as you age will reap big rewards – and you'll feel them as soon as you start.

KEEP YOUR MUSCLES IN SHAPE WITH VITAMIN D

You probably don't need any more encouragement to ensure that you have a healthy level of vitamin D in your blood – something over 100nmol/l. But it's worth mentioning here that the vitamin probably plays a role in maintaining healthy muscles. Dr John Cannell from the US, a psychiatrist and leading researcher into vitamin D, has written up research dating back 60 years showing a link between levels of the vitamin and athletic performance. He has noted that sports people perform better in the summer, when their vitamin D levels are likely to be higher, than in the winter. The vitamin may also protect against muscle strain and injury, especially in older people.[18]

'The Ancient Greek athletes had the right ideas, they used to train in the nude,' says Professor Tim Oliver, Professor Emeritus at the Institute of Cancer, Barts Hospital in London, who has had a long-standing interest in combining the benefits of sunshine and exercise. 'Athletes today aren't likely to follow suit, but I am involved in a project to encourage school children to get as much of their exercise outdoors as possible.'

One of his research team is gathering data on vitamin levels in members of the British Olympic team and is hoping to show that bringing them up to optimum levels, which many don't reach at present, will improve their performance.

There are three ways to increase your blood level of vitamin D – eat it, supplement it or expose yourself to sunlight, thus making it in the skin. If you make a point of eating three servings of oily fish a week (a serving of salmon or mackerel provides around 350iu) and six free-range eggs a week (an egg provides 20iu), you'll be getting about 200iu a day from your diet. Better-quality high-potency multivitamins should give you an additional 15mcg (600iu) (although most have a third of this, providing the completely outdated RDA of 5mcg (200iu)). That brings you closer to 25mcg.

During the winter months in Northern Europe (November to April in the UK), the above quantity of vitamin D is certainly not enough, so it's probably worth supplementing an additional 25mcg (1,000iu) and possibly more, especially if you are older and live further north. You can take vitamin D drops, each giving 25mcg (there is no harm in doubling this). That will get you up to 50mcg a day from diet and supplements in total.

Chapter 5

IMPROVE YOUR SLEEP AND REDUCE STRESS

An often-heard complaint, as people get older, is a lack of sleep. A third of people over the age of 65 report difficulties in either falling asleep or staying asleep.[19] Although it is often said that perhaps you don't need so much sleep when you are older, almost all the research suggests that sleep is as vital a nutrient as any you can obtain from food – and we all need at least six hours of it. In fact, you can survive longer without food than you can without sleep.

People who sleep well have a better quality and quantity of life, so a German study of people with insomnia has found.[20] Whereas 3 per cent of those without insomnia rated their quality of life as bad, a much greater number of those who did suffer with insomnia – 22 per cent – gave their quality of life a thumbs down. In terms of overall health, you live longer and feel better if you can get at least six, but no more than eight hours, of undisturbed sleep.

Before explaining how to achieve this anti-ageing goal, it helps to understand why we need to sleep. During sleep you progress through different stages, which are classified according to the changes that occur in the pattern of your brain waves:

- For the first 90 minutes our sleep gradually gets deeper and deeper, while our brain wave patterns change, our temperature drops and heart rate slows. After about an hour we are most deeply asleep in a stage known as delta, when most of the repair and regeneration goes on.

- After about half an hour there we move up into a much more busy stage known as REM (rapid eye movement), when we do most of our dreaming and the brain and other body systems become more active. REM sleep is critical for consolidating memories and discharging unexpressed emotions. Sleeping pills can cut the amount of time we spend in REM.

- After maybe 20 minutes in REM we then start drifting back down towards delta again. We normally cycle through these stages four or five times a night spending more time in REM as the night goes on.

From the point of view of slowing ageing, you want to have more slow wave sleep and, from the point of view of feeling good and discharging the stresses of the previous day, you need enough REM sleep. About 70 per cent of all the growth hormones your body produces to stimulate new cell growth are made while you sleep.[21]

HOW CAN YOU ENSURE A GOOD NIGHT'S SLEEP?

There are two main 'chemical' reasons why people find it hard to fall asleep or to stay asleep (see Secret 4). These are, firstly, a lack of tryptophan that you get from food, the brain chemical serotonin or the hormone melatonin, each being made from the other. The other is an inability to turn off adrenalin, which is controlled by an amino acid and neurotransmitter called GABA. If you are in the habit of not sleeping too well, it is well worth taking a combination of these nutrients for a month to bring your brain's chemistry into balance. Magnesium also helps you to relax. Here's what to take:

	Supplement	When to take
5-hydroxytryptophan	100–200mg	1 hour before bed
or melatonin	3–6mg	1 hour before bed
Magnesium	200mg	in the evening
GABA*	500–1,500mg	1 hour before bed

* GABA is not available over the counter in the UK, although it is in Ireland, South Africa and the US. If you can't get it, either try a sleep formula that contains glutamine and taurine (the chemicals it's made from) or try the herb valerian, 150–300mg an hour before bedtime.

Caffeine suppresses melatonin production for up to ten hours, so have none after noon. Eat a low-GL dinner so that your blood sugar level is even at around the time you want to go to sleep.

Exercise reduces the time it takes to fall asleep, increases sleep duration and increases the duration of slow-wave sleep. But don't do it too close to bedtime.[22] Feeling stressed and anxious is the most common reason for not being able to get to sleep. Practising something like yoga or t'ai chi, however, can be very helpful for promoting a good night's sleep, because it has the effect of calming and centring the mind and body. A walk in the evening can also have the same effect.

Any technique that switches off the stress reaction is good news. In the next chapter we'll talk more about how to do this using simple psychological exercises designed to reduce your stress response, including the HeartMath techniques and a simple meditation using a breathing exercise.

One highly effective way is to listen to 'alpha' music, as we explained in Secret 4. Our favourite CD is called *Silence of Peace* (see Resources). Play it quietly, in the background, as you go to bed and you'll find it rapidly switches off an active mind. If you do wake up, you can always put it on again. We have received many testimonials from people who have found almost immediate relief from insomnia by listening to this CD. Some people with more active minds prefer another CD called *Orange Grove Siesta* (see Resources). They are both worth trying.

HOW TO STAY ASLEEP

Many people have no difficulty falling asleep but frequently wake up in the night and then can't get back to sleep. A lack of serotonin or melatonin can make you sleep very lightly, but practical steps to reduce disturbance can make a big difference.

According to research carried out by Dr Max Hirshkowitz, associate professor at Baylor College of Medicine, Department of Psychiatry and Medicine, the major causes of awakenings are: the need to pee; outside noise or light; a noisy or restless partner; temperature; and thirst. Some of these, obviously, you can minimise; for example, wearing an eye mask can cut out light. If you do wake up in the night to pee, and have difficulty getting back to sleep, play the alpha music quietly. That will help you.

Bear in mind, however, that you may not need as much sleep as you think. Several people have reported that, on following optimum nutrition principles, they feel fully refreshed after between six and seven hours' sleep. Six undisturbed hours of sleep is very healthy. If you wake up early, perhaps at dawn, this is completely consistent with our evolution. Why not seize the day and get up and do something you enjoy? You can always have a siesta in the afternoon.

BE MORE COMFORTABLE BY REDUCING PAIN

Another common cause of not being able to sleep well is physical pain, especially affecting the neck and hips. To a certain extent you can mitigate this by choosing a good mattress such as those containing memory foam, which adjust their shape to even out the pressure across your body. Losing weight, if you need to, makes a difference, too, and our tips in Secret 8 for digestion problems may also give you some pain relief. Try taking the natural anti-inflammatories before bed (see Secret 2 and Chapter 7 in this Part).

Of course, there are other symptoms that can interfere with sleep. Night sweats during the menopausal years, for example, are a problem for many women. We hope that by following the advice for balancing hormones naturally (see Secret 10 and Chapter 8 in this Part) this will not be an issue.

SWITCH OFF THE STRESS

In the next chapter we'll give you some simple exercises for switching off the stress reaction, which can be excellent to do as you go to bed. Please remember, though, that it is also important to deal with issues that arise in the day, or at different times of your life. The predominant feelings that you experience in dreams can give you a clear clue. If you are having nightmares or fearful dreams, what is it, in real life, that you are fearful about?

Negative feelings and unresolved conflicts are common sleep robbers. Having someone to talk to who really understands you is a big blessing. So, if you are worrying about something, speak to a friend in the evening, or, even better, go to see them face to face. Having a good psychotherapist can also be helpful, especially if you are going through a major transition in your life, such as retiring, or the death of a close friend or relative, or any other significant loss. Most of all, make sure you have support. We all need a little help from our friends.

Sometimes, as you lie in bed, you remember things you'd forgotten, or torment yourself about unresolved issues. Have a notebook by your bed and write down anything you want to deal with tomorrow. You'll finds this helps you to let go.

If you really find it hard to sleep, read a good book, or practise a simple meditation (there's more on this in the next chapter) before you turn in. Find a routine for you that works. As you sleep, your body is hard at work rejuvenating itself. That's a comforting thought.

Remember to practise the Sleep Hygiene on page 163 and make your night-time ritual one that is as stress-free and relaxing as possible.

Chapter 6

DEVELOP A HEALTHY MINDSTYLE

Your state of mind has a remarkable effect on how you feel as you age, and also on ageing itself. The worst attitude you can have is that of cynicism, while the best is a positive engagement in life. An extraordinary illustration of the power of the mind was a study by Professor Ellen Langer who took a group of men aged 75–80 years old on a country retreat. Half were asked to think about the past. The other half were invited to stay in a house that had all the artefacts from the year 1959. They listened to music, watched films and ate food from that era. Within five days, several of their signs of ageing had improved, including more joint flexibility, better vision, better breathing and better cognitive function.[23] This shows how your state of mind has a direct effect on your body and the physiological markers that we associate with ageing.

DON'T WORRY, BE HAPPY

Happiness comes from knowing you are on track in life. Being positively engaged, and successful, in activities that you believe in makes all the difference. An example of this is the fact that Academy Award winners live 3.9 years longer, and Nobel Prize winners live two years longer, than other nominees.[24]

There have also been other studies looking at whether an optimistic outlook has any affect on life span; in one, those with a high level of optimism had a 55 per cent lower risk of premature death from all causes and a 23 per cent lower risk of cardiovascular death,[25] and another found that the risk of dying in the next two years was halved in those with a positive attitude.[26] Yet another study on Catholic nuns found that the happiest nuns lived an extra 9.5 years.[27]

Being conscientious, purposeful and working hard might also extend your life. The most extensive study of the effects of one's psychological profile on ageing is that of the Longevity Project, begun by Dr Lewis Terman in the 1920s, and now written up in the book called *The Longevity Project* by Howard Friedman and Leslie Martin. Terman selected 1,500 bright boys and girls, all born around 1920, and his researchers studied their lives in meticulous detail at ten-year intervals right up to the children's deaths. The main findings were that conscientious, purposeful and hard-working people lived longer. They found that the quality of being conscientious was fairly hardwired – it didn't change from youth to old age – and that conscientious people were generally prudent, persistent, responsible, not overly impulsive, and honest. They lived longer.

Contrary to the view that stress is always a bad thing, they found that the longest-living people often worked hard, often not retiring. They were purposeful and generally liked their jobs even if they were hard work and stressful. They also possessed the quality of resilience and found meaning even in the face of difficult circumstances.

Doing something you love was also a key attribute of those living the longest. Another attribute was having a high level of social connectedness, with stable relationships, frequent contact, and interactions that care for others.

The emotions associated with a longer, healthier life are positivity, optimism, resilience, self-esteem, happiness, life satisfaction, love, friendship and hope. (Interestingly, though, in the Longevity Project they found that those individuals who were too optimistic, perhaps not truly experiencing and learning from the difficult times in life, didn't live longer.)

If you don't currently enjoy the positive feelings listed above, there are a number of ways that you can make yourself more open to them.

BE MORE FLEXIBLE

There is a tendency in life to become less flexible, both physically in the body and in the mind as the years go by. As people age they tend to become set in their ways and less able to deal with new circumstances. For this very reason it is important to learn new things, to travel, and to be open to new experiences. Catch yourself whenever you hear the words 'I can't' or 'I don't know how to' coming out of your mouth – remember that it is never too late to learn or to change.

CYNICISM IS BAD FOR YOU

As we said at the beginning of this chapter, the worst emotion for longevity is not depression or stress – it's cynicism. A cynic is more likely not to engage emotionally in activities, and, through questioning everything, closes down opportunities to have new experiences and to try things out.

Cynicism raises 'inflammatory markers' in the body, and the more cynical a person is the more those markers are raised. A study showed that being stressed was worse than being depressed, but the worst of all was being cynical.[28]

Cynicism is a state of insecurity masquerading as sophistication. Everyone and everything else is fraudulent and fake. It comes in many forms, from jeering at big-hearted emotions and displays of affection to rejecting anything new until it has been proven by science. A scientific demand for evidence is admirable but anyone practising preventative non-drug therapies is all too familiar with how that demand can become a cynical witch-hunt when applied in ways that don't increase knowledge or benefit patients.

The trouble with this kind of thinking is that it shuts off the possibility of new experiences and creative expression, blocking you from trying something different and taking risks. It is a negative outlook that springs from a lack of trust in life, making it hard to find meaning or joy anywhere. Even gloomy predictions are often self-fulfilling. And that, according to the science, is bad for you.

TRANSFORMING STRESS INTO RESILIENCE

A large part of stress is self-induced by perceiving a change of circumstances in a negative way – by resisting the opportunities that life presents us with, rather than embracing them. In Secret 4 we explored simple techniques developed by the HeartMath Institute for turning off stress reactions. Scientists there have developed a measure of how people handle stress, known as 'heart rate variability'. A monitor called an Emwave (see Secret 4) has a small screen that allows you to see if your response is effective and coherent or erratic and unfocused. The trick is to bring your breathing into sync with your heart rate. Because you can see your response changing on the screen, you can quickly learn to produce the coherent state that fits very well with the psychological attributes of long-lived people. It is the same state that meditators achieve after years of practice, where you are able to fully participate in life, be present and be open to new experiences.

The researchers found that activities, feelings or exercises that were more heart-centred were the most effective at turning off harmful stress hormones.

The HeartMath Institute runs workshops around the world to help people learn how to transform stressful reactions into resilience (see Resources). In the UK we sponsor one every year (see Resources). These teach people simple techniques to switch off stressful, negative reactions and to settle into a positive mind-frame. You can also consult a practitioner on a one-to-one basis. Here are three simple 'quick coherence' techniques from HeartMath that you can learn and can then apply whenever you are feeling stressed:

EXERCISE: heart focus, breathing and feeling

1: heart focus

Focus your attention on your heart area – the space behind your breastbone in the centre of your chest between your nipples (your heart is more in the centre than on the left).

2: heart breathing

Now imagine your breath flowing in and out of your heart area. This helps your respiration and heart rhythm to synchronise. So focus in this area and aim to breathe evenly; for example, inhale for five or six seconds and exhale for five or six seconds (choose a timescale that feels comfortable and flows easily).

CONTINUED...

Take a few minutes to get the hang of the heart focus and heart breathing stages, then introduce step three:

3: heart feeling

As you breathe in and out of your heart area, recall a positive emotion and try to re-experience it. This could be remembering a time spent with someone you love, walking in your favourite spot, stroking a pet, picturing a tree or scenic location you admire or even just feeling appreciation that you ate today or have shoes on your feet. If your mind wanders, just bring it gently back to the positive experience.

These three steps, when practised daily for five minutes, can help you to de-stress, feel calmer and more content. Your heart rhythms will become coherent and your heart-brain communication will optimise to help you think more clearly. For your daily HeartMath practice, it's a good idea to find a regular time when you can sit down quietly and undisturbed (such as first thing in the morning, during your lunch break or when you get home from work). This way it's more likely to become a habit and you can give the exercise your full attention.

Once you've got the hang of HeartMath, you can then use it any time you encounter a stressful event; for example, if you start to feel tense in heavy traffic, or you become overloaded at work or sense you are about to face a difficult emotional situation. Just a few HeartMath breaths can help you to stay calm and coherent instead of becoming stressed. And you can do it with your eyes open, as you walk or talk – so you have a tool to control stress at the direct point you encounter a situation likely to trigger a negative reaction.

MONITOR YOUR STATE WITH AN EMWAVE

The HeartMath exercises sound very simple, or basic, but they can have a deep effect, especially if you can use the EmWave Personal Stress Reliever (PSR), which gives you instant feedback to enable you to learn how to go into a state of coherence.

The EmWave PSR has an ear clip that attaches to your ear lobe to pick up what is known as your heart rate variability (HRV), through the pulse registered in your ear lobes, and then feeds this data through to a hand-held device that tells you how coherent you are. The device easily fits into your pocket.

There are three zones – the 'red' or incoherent (the state most of us are in), 'blue' for more coherent and 'green' for fully coherent. There is also a 'breath pacer' to help you regulate your breathing, and different levels and modes so that you can adapt your practice as you get the hang of it.

Using the EmWave PSR gives you an objective measure of what works and, even the very act of knowing, through this 'biofeedback', can help you calm down. You can also plug it into the USB port of your computer and track your state. In this way you can try out different techniques for changing your state. One woman found that stroking her cat immediately brought her into a state of coherence. (Perhaps James Bond's Blofeld was on to something!) If you happen to have a cat around, this might be a useful way of bringing yourself back into a positive state. If not, try one of the exercises above.

We are all different, and the trick is to find what really gets you into the zone. It might be exercising, listening to specific music, gardening and growing your own vegetables, learning pottery, painting, playing a musical instrument, helping others or studying a particular subject. One thing that is neat about the EmWave is that you can literally find out what does it for you. We recommend it as an anti-ageing device. It is also excellent to use as you go to sleep, as it trains you to let go of your stresses.

PRACTISE MEDITATION

Another way to find a more coherent, less stressful state is meditation. In meditation, you become aware of your thoughts, emotions and physical sensations and, in the process, become detached. There are many ways to approach meditation, although many people find it difficult to stop the 'chattering' in the mind. In some meditative techniques you focus on the breath, in some the heart, and in others on the vital-energy centre of the body, known as the tantien in t'ai chi and also called the Kath point by the philosopher Oscar Ichazo. (Ichazo has thoroughly researched methods of generating vital energy, known as 'chi' and of attaining higher states of consciousness.) Some people also use a word or a mantra to repeat silently.

DIAKATH BREATHING

An example of a technique to induce a more coherent and meditative state is Diakath breathing based on the Kath point. Although not an anatomical point as such, the Kath point is the body's centre of gravity, and by placing one's awareness at this point, rather than in the head as we most often do, it is possible to become aware of the whole body. All the martial arts, in their pure form, are practised with this awareness, which gives a more complete and grounded experience of oneself. You can experience this for yourself by practising the simple breathing exercise shown below.

EXERCISE: Diakath Breathing

This breathing exercise (reproduced with the kind permission of Oscar Ichazo) connects the Kath point – the body's centre of equilibrium – with the diaphragm muscle, so that deep breathing becomes natural and effortless. You can practise this exercise at any time, while sitting, standing or lying down, and for as long as you like. You can also practise it unobtrusively during moments of stress. It is an excellent, natural relaxant and energy booster, helping you to feel more connected and in tune.

The diaphragm is a dome-shaped muscle attached to the bottom of the rib cage. The Kath point is located three finger-widths below the belly and 2.5cm (1in) in. If you place your index finger in your belly button your little finger will be in the Kath point. When you put your awareness in this point, it becomes easy to be aware of your entire body.

Ideally, find somewhere quiet first thing in the morning. When breathing, inhale and exhale through your nose. As you inhale, you will expand your lower belly from the Kath point and your diaphragm muscle. This allows the lungs to fill with air from the bottom to the top. As you exhale, the belly and the diaphragm muscle relax, allowing the lungs to empty from top to bottom.

CONTINUED...

Diakath Breathing

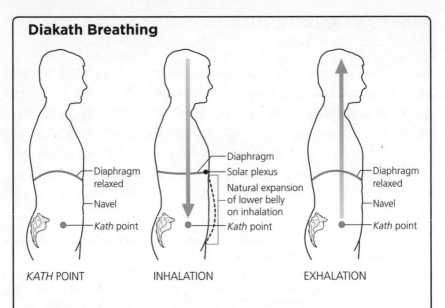

KATH POINT | INHALATION | EXHALATION

1. Sit comfortably, in a quiet place with your spine straight.

2. Focus your attention on your Kath point.

3. Let your belly expand from the Kath point as you inhale slowly, deeply and effortlessly. Feel your diaphragm being pulled down towards the Kath point as your lungs fill with air from the bottom to the top. On the exhale, relax both your belly and your diaphragm, emptying your lungs from top to bottom.

4. Repeat at your own pace.

- Every morning, sit down in a quiet place before breakfast and practise Diakath Breathing for a few minutes.
- Whenever you are stressed throughout the day check your breathing. Practise Diakath Breathing for nine breaths. This is great to do before an important meeting or when something has upset you.

(© 2002 Oscar Ichazo. Diakath Breathing is the service mark and Kath the trademark of Oscar Ichazo. Used by permission.)

The purpose of such practices is to centre yourself, to take yourself out of small-minded stressful and fearful thoughts, and thus become of more use to yourself and others. There are, of course, many different ways of doing this, some of which we list in the Resources. Exercises such as yoga and t'ai chi are great ways to increase your sense of connection and also to reduce stress. So too is walking the dog, gardening and being in beautiful natural environments.

CASE STUDY: ROBERT

Robert, aged 66, took up t'ai chi when he retired. Here's how he describes the benefits:

'I've never been an athletic person or good at anything physical. T'ai chi, however, I enjoy immensely. I like the feeling of being "in control" of my body. It gives me an aesthetic pleasure. I do it almost every day for 20 minutes. It increases my energy and clears my mind. It gives me a kind of equilibrium that has many benefits, such as helping me to play my violin better and helping me to stay detached when things are bad. I find it very calming when I'm stressed or feeling fraught.'

In Patrick's book *The 10 Secrets of 100% Healthy People* the eighth secret is 'generate vital energy' with practices such as yoga and t'ai chi; the tenth is 'finding your purpose' and connecting with spirit; and the ninth is 'get your past out of your present'. You might want to read this book to find out more about how to achieve these secrets, which are reported by the healthiest people as part of the reason for their good health.

Getting the past out of the present refers to the inevitable accumulation of negative emotions – fear, anger and sadness – that we feel and 'store', becoming more and more bound in our ability to react spontaneously and positively to new things and inevitable challenges. In the book Patrick talks about ways to release the emotional charge of past memories and how to free yourself up in the present.

GETTING CONNECTED

Of course, there are many other techniques, systems and approaches for getting into a heightened and positive state of awareness. This is the basis of all spiritual traditions. One can think of 'spiritual' as the greatest sense of connection, be it the love of another, your family, nature, the planet, humanity and life itself as a mysterious adventure.

Psychologist and former nurse Elizabeth Register, who is associate professor at the College of Nursing at the University of South Carolina, is somewhat of an expert in the subject of what really gives a person a high quality of life as they age. Her views are not new and are shared by others who study what conditions make people contented. Her conclusion is that quality of life is largely about connectedness,[29] and she has compiled a Scale of Connectedness that is now being used to measure how people feel and whether the care systems provided are helping or hindering them to age healthily.

There are six aspects to being connected.[30] These are:

1. Being metaphysically connected Having an awareness of oneself within a larger universe.

2. Feeling spiritually connected Being aware of a higher power and/or searching for meaning and a purpose in life.

3. Being biologically connected Optimising your functional capacity and participating in activities that relate to promoting and maintaining your health.

4. Feeling connected to others Enjoying human interpersonal relationships that are free of spatial or temporal constraints.

5. Being environmentally connected Working to connect yourself with your personal living and natural environment.

6. Feeling connected to society Having a relationship with a personal social system, your extended family, community and the global community of society.

'Connectedness is pivotal to successful aging as it can influence both physical and emotional health.'[31]

GIVING AND LOVING

The process of prayer is all about making a connection with others and sending love. Of course, some people don't do this as an internal meditative practice, but through acts of kindness and charitable giving to those who are having a difficult time. Whether one has a spiritual belief or not the act of reaching out to others is a natural instinct that is associated with living a longer and healthier life. As one man said, 'When I do good I feel good, when I do bad I feel bad. That is my religion.'

We also need to give to ourselves. Everyone has the desire to be happy and free of pain. The Dalai Lama says that his daily practice is to remember that his desire to be happy and free of pain is of no greater or lesser importance than that of the people he interacts with. So, there is a balance between taking care of yourself and helping others. Too much either way isn't good for you.

Chapter 7

NUTRITIONAL SUPPLEMENTS

As you get older, the case for taking nutritional supplements on a regular basis gets stronger and stronger. This is not only because several nutrients are less well absorbed later in life but also because the body systems become less efficient and need more support to function fully. If we decrease our exercise, we eat less, and with less food we take in fewer nutrients. In the early Victorian age, the average intake of nutrients for people in the 'mid-working class', regardless of age, was much higher than today, because people were more physically active – there were no cars to fetch large amounts of food from the supermarket, and no freezers for storage – so people took more exercise buying their food daily.[32] Also, the quality of the soil used for growing food has generally become degraded, and the use of fertilisers binds minerals making them less available to the plants and to us when we eat them. The only way to mimic the Victorian kind of intake today would be to supplement your diet. You really can't get all the nutrients you need from a well-balanced diet. If anyone says you can, ask them for the evidence – we haven't seen it.

All this only gets you back to square one. It neither addresses reversing disease processes, as we have discussed in Part Two, nor a more progressive approach to extending your healthy life span.

THE VITAMIN MULTI-TASKERS

As we have already seen, one of the encouraging facts that has emerged from studying the usual conditions that accumulate with age is the remarkable crossover of certain nutrients. You take omega-3, for example, for your aching joints, and it reduces your risk of heart disease and improves your mood. Or, you take vitamin A for your eyes and it rejuvenates your skin and reduces cancer risk. With each nutrient you climb up the ladder towards reaching a healthy 100 years of age, as the Snakes and Ladders illustration on page 54 shows.

From studying the cellular ageing process as well as genetics and animal studies that have successfully extended life span, the very same set of nutrients emerge as anti-ageing heroes. Although there is no definitive proof yet – nor is there likely to be in your lifetime, because we'll have to wait decades to see how today's research volunteers age – there is certainly a good logical case, backed up by a growing amount of research for taking supplements where appropriate and becoming an anti-ageing front-liner with us. We'd also like to track your progress through the years via your 100% Health Programme, if you choose to take this option, to feed results back to us along the way.

Of course, there is an argument that one should 'wait and see' what happens in long-term studies but, in the area of ageing, if you 'wait and see' for too long, you won't be around to find out. The alternative is to act now. But are there any downsides?

One researcher who had this concern is Dr Gladys Block, formerly with the National Cancer Institute. She was concerned that thousands of people take large quantities of supplements on a daily basis, so she decided to study them, alongside people who took none or a daily low-dose RDA multivitamin.[33] What the study showed was that the 'many supplement takers' had 73 per cent less diabetes risk than non-supplement takers; 52 per cent less heart disease risk than non-supplement takers and were 74 per cent more likely to rate their own health as good or excellent. Regarding hard biological markers of ageing, the many-supplement takers came out better.

For example, 45 per cent of non-supplement takers, 37 per cent of RDA-multi takers, and only 11 per cent of many-supplement takers had elevated levels of homocysteine (above 9). The same pattern applied to cholesterol. On hard measures of vitamin levels, 94 per cent of many-supplement takers had optimal blood vitamin C levels. None were sub-optimal. Thirty-two per cent of non-supplement takers and 11 per cent of the RDA-multi takers were sub-optimal.

The following table shows the main stars that keep coming up both for reversing disease processes and promoting healthy ageing.

The anti-ageing nutrients

Nutrient	Anti-ageing	Memory or mood booster	Good for heart
Vitamin A	✓		
Vitamin C	✓		✓
Vitamin E	✓		✓
Vitamin D	✓	✓	✓
B vitamins (B_{12}, folic acid, B_6)	✓	✓	✓
Omega-3	✓	✓	✓
Chromium		✓	
Zinc	✓	✓	
Magnesium	✓	✓	✓
Antioxidants (CoQ_{10}, glutathione, NAC, lipoic acid, resveratrol	✓	✓	✓
Anti-inflammatories (quercetin, turmeric, etc)	✓	✓	✓
Digestive enzymes, probiotics, glutamine			

Weight and blood sugar	Immune-booster	Good for skin	Good for eyes	Good for sleep and stress	Good for digestion
	✓	✓	✓		
✓	✓	✓	✓	✓	
	✓	✓	✓		
	✓	✓			
				✓	
	✓	✓	✓		✓
✓			✓	✓	
✓	✓	✓	✓	✓	✓
✓				✓	
	✓		✓		
	✓	✓	✓		✓
	✓				✓

If you wanted a shotgun approach to supplementing, you'd be taking most of these nutrients, with a few add-ons depending on your particular health issues. This is most easily achieved by taking a high-strength multivitamin–mineral, as well as extra vitamin C, essential omegas (particularly omega-3), an antioxidant formula (including nutrients if your eyesight is deteriorating, and brain-friendly B vitamins and phospholipids). We'll be giving you a tailor-made list of supplements later in this chapter.

You will also be able to add optional nutrients to cover:

Blood pressure	Heart
Bones	Joints
Brain	Memory
Cancer	Mood
Digestion	Skin
Eyes	Weight and blood sugar

What kind of daily intake should we be shooting for? In the chart opposite you'll see the basic optimal supplemental levels for some of these more vital nutrients that are advisable for everyone to achieve from a good daily supplement programme (assuming you are eating a reasonably good diet). Then, there is the restoration level for correcting imbalances for the conditions listed above. Finally, there is the highest level for maximising anti-ageing. We'll be including these in your easy-to-use supplement programme on page 347.

Supplement levels

Nutrient	Optimum supplemental	Restoration	Maximum anti-ageing
Vitamin A	2,500mcg	5,000mcg	15,000mcg
Vitamin C	1,800mg	3,000mg	6,000mg
Vitamin E	300mg	600mg	800mg
Vitamin D	15mcg	25–50mcg	25–50mcg+
Vitamin B_{12}	10mcg	250–750mcg*	250–750mcg*
Folic acid	200mcg	400–800mcg*	400–800mcg*
Vitamin B_6	20mg	40mg	40mg
Magnesium	200mg	300mg	400mg
Zinc	15mg	25mg	35mg
Chromium	35mcg	200–600mcg	200–400mcg
Selenium	35mcg	100–200mcg	100–200mcg
CoQ_{10}	10mg	90–120mg	90–120mg
Glutathione or NAC	25mg	50–200mg	50–500mg
Lipoic acid	10mg	100–200mg	100–500mg
Omega-3 (DHA, EPA)	500mg	750–1,000mg	1,000mg

+ Your ideal intake of vitamin D is that which brings your blood level to above 100 and ideally around 125nmol/l. For most people 50mcg on a daily basis is too much, but can be good during the winter or for a few months to build up vitamin D stores. Otherwise don't exceed 25mcg on a daily basis.
* These high levels are only appropriate if you have raised homocysteine. We do not recommend supplemental folic acid above 200mcg if you have any risk of colorectal or other cancers. Your ideal intake is that which brings homocysteine below 7 mcmol/l.

GETTING THE LEVEL RIGHT

To give you an example of how these figures are derived, the basic RDA of vitamin A is a mere 800mcg. This is in sharp contrast to our ancestors' intake of an estimated 10,000mcg. We think a basic optimum intake is 3,500mcg. If you eat meat, fish and eggs, which provide retinol, you may achieve an intake of 750mcg. By eating beta-carotene-rich fruit and vegetables, you may achieve a further 750mcg. That adds up to 1,500mcg, which is 2,000mcg short of the basic optimum. That's why our basic optimum for supplementing is 2,500mcg, made up from both retinol and beta-carotene (the vegetable form). So, in a multivitamin, you want to add these two together to see what it provides. Now let's go to the other end of the scale. Skin expert Dr Des Fernandes supplements 15,000mcg vitamin A a day. That's the kind of level that is also most likely to help if you've got seriously deteriorating eyesight. Apart from being good for the skin and the eyes, vitamin A drives all cellular growth, all cell differentiation, improves apoptosis (that's the ability of cancer cells to commit suicide) and may increase telomere length. So, the chances are an increased intake will slow down the ageing process. A similar story can be told for each of these nutrients.

ARE THESE QUANTITIES DANGEROUS?

Of all the nutrients listed above, the one that has supposedly been given the most caution is vitamin A – but only for pregnant women; we assume that, if you are over 50, this is not a likelihood. Vitamin D, in very high levels, can be toxic. If you live in the northern hemisphere, this is unlikely to be an issue even at the highest supplemental doses; however, we advise a maximum of 50mcg (2,000iu) on a regular basis, with 50mcg a day for up to three months to restore normal levels (125 nmol/l). In the winter, in the northern hemisphere, even this amount is unlikely to be excessive. If you live in the northern hemisphere, and have dark skin, you are going to need these higher levels to maintain a healthy vitamin D status.

There is some concern, although not everyone agrees, with high-dose folic acid in people who have pre-cancerous cells, especially in the colon, indicated by polyps. The reason for this caution is that although folic acid prevents healthy cells from becoming cancerous, there is evidence that high doses of folic acid encourage the growth of pre-cancerous cells to cancer cells. Whether or not this occurs when supplementing a combination of homocysteine-lowering nutrients is not yet known. Given that high homocysteine levels also increase cancer risk, it is hard to say whether the benefit of supplementing such nutrients to lower a raised homocysteine level is of greater benefit than the possible risk of high-dose folic acid increasing cancer risk.

These are the only cautions we are aware of. Needless to say, even these cautions pale into insignificance against the risks of either doing nothing or taking the usual plethora of medical drugs.

BUILDING YOUR OWN ANTI-AGEING SUPPLEMENT PROGRAMME

How do you put all this together into your own personal daily supplement programme? There are two ways to do this. If you have completed the free 100% Health Check and then paid for your personal 100% Health Programme, your supplement will have been calculated for you. If not, you can more or less create your own in the following way:

RECOMMENDED FOR ALL:

- 2 × high-strength multivitamin–mineral tablets (taken one with breakfast and one at lunchtime). (Note most high-strength multis are taken in two doses – follow the pack instructions.)
- 2 × vitamin C 900mg, ideally with extra zinc (taken one with breakfast and one at lunchtime).
- 2 × essential omega-3 and omega-6: dosage 500mg of omega-3 (EPA+DPA+DHA); 50mg GLA (taken one with breakfast and one at lunchtime).
- 1 × 'antioxidant formula' (containing resveratrol, lipoic acid, glutathione, CoQ_{10}) (taken with breakfast).
- 1 × 'brain-friendly formula' with extra B vitamins and phospholipids (taken with breakfast).

(The above is what I (Patrick) take daily.)

OPTIONAL EXTRAS

Vitamin D If you live in the northern hemisphere, or have decreased bone mass or an increased cancer risk (that is, you have had cancer or a pre-cancer diagnosis), and depending on your blood level of vitamin D (which should ideally be around 125nmol/l) you would be wise to add 1 × 25mcg capsule or drop of vitamin D.

Vitamin A There is good reason for anyone to add 2–5 (small) capsules of vitamin A (retinol): 2,000–5,000mcg in total.

Lutein and zeathanthin If your eyesight is deteriorating, in addition to vitamin A, there is good reason to add lutein 20mg and zeathanthin 300mcg. Note: these often come with vitamin A as a supplement designed for supporting healthy eyes.

B vitamins and homocysteine-lowering supplements If you have memory concerns, cardiovascular risk or decreased bone-mass density, get your homocysteine level checked. If your homocysteine level is raised (above 7, or above 10, or above 15) take the levels of homocysteine-lowering nutrients shown on page 105. Then add the appropriate number of homocysteine-lowering nutrient complexes. You may also wish to double up on a brain-friendly formula containing phospholipids and an antioxidant formula if you want to maximise brain recovery.

L-carnitine and CoQ$_{10}$ If you have cardiovascular disease, poor heart function, or concerns about your ageing brain and eyesight, add 500–1,000mg of l-carnitine together with 60–90mg of CoQ$_{10}$.

Joint support If you have chronic pain or inflammation, for example arthritis, add a joint-support supplement providing natural anti-inflammatories such as turmeric, quercetin, olive and hop extracts, glucosamine and MSM. If you have joint pain or decreasing bone mass you may also wish to add a bone-support supplement providing extra calcium (250mg), magnesium (150mg), vitamin D (25mcg), vitamin K (250mcg), zinc (10mg) and boron (2mg). Also add omega-3 (500mg EPA).

Overweight or blood-sugar support If you are overweight, or have sugar cravings or diabetes, add chromium (400–600mcg), 5-HTP (100–200mg) and HCA (1,000–2,500mg) available in combination in some supplements. Also add a teaspoon (5g) of a super-soluble fibre such as glucomannan or PGX.

Sleep support If you are having difficulty sleeping, add 5-HTP 100mg (or melatonin 3mg), GABA 1,000mg and 200mg of magnesium an hour before bed. Some sleep formulas contain combinations of these, or the precursors of GABA – taurine and glutamine. Alternatively, try valerian – 150–300mg about 45 minutes before bedtime.

Skin support If your skin is ageing or sun damaged, add an antioxidant formula and vitamin A (5,000mg) plus transdermal vitamin A and C cream (see Resources).

Cancer support If you have cancer concerns, ensure your blood vitamin D level is at least 100nmol/l, and supplement accordingly to achieve this. Also, increase your daily intake of vitamin C from 2g to 4g and add an antioxidant formula. If your concerns relate to the prostate, supplement both saw palmetto (120–360mg per day) and pygeum (40–120mg per day). Also consider supplementing salvestrols.

Digestion support If you have digestion problems (indigestion, heartburn, bloating, flatulence) add digestive enzymes, probiotics and glutamine. Some formulas contain all three in one. After a course of antibiotics, always have probiotics and glutamine (5g, which is a heaped teaspoonful, last thing at night in water) for at least a week.

If you have many of the above conditions, it is best to pick two main areas of concern and focus on bringing these into balance, then work on the next issue until you are healthy.

Of course, the intention is not that you'll need all of these, or any of them, for that long, but only until you start to improve your health and reverse the disease processes. You can't cheat death, but you can cheat ill health. Once you have improved your health, just stick with the basics.

We hope you will complete our free 100% Health Check, because it's a valuable way of monitoring the health of people as they age. We will contact you every year to find out how you are doing. In this way we can work out what makes the most difference to thousands of people like us as we surf the Silver Tsunami.

Chapter 8

CORRECTING HORMONAL DEFICIENCIES

By the time you are 60 – and for many people before that – there is a good chance that you will be suffering from some hormonal deficiencies. After the menopause, a woman's body virtually stops producing progesterone, while oestrogen levels decline by about half, although oestrogen can also be made in fat cells. Testosterone levels also decline in both women and men.

There are all sorts of opinions about supplementing hormones, ranging from 'it's not natural' to 'we all need them'. It is hard to know what is natural. You could argue that we aren't designed to live into our eighties and nineties, and that once we are past procreating, biology doesn't care whether we have a good time or not. But do we have to put up with that?

In truth, the less virtuous you've been with your diet, drinking, exercise, stress and weight control over the years, the greater is the chance that you will suffer from the effects of hormone deficiencies. For some, simply improving your nutrition and lifestyle can perk you up enough (see below). But for many, a small dose of natural hormones designed to top you up to previous levels can make a remarkable difference. For both men and women, a trial period of three to six months of hormones can usually show you how effective they are likely to be for you. We have discussed the use of hormones and how to obtain them in Secret 10.

EAT FOR HORMONE HEALTH

Your hormonal balance will be greatly helped by eating a low-GL diet and following a healthy lifestyle.

CASE STUDY: LESLIE

'I started this way of eating [the low-GL diet] when I was a year off my fiftieth Birthday and my goal was not to be fat at 50. My goal was to lose two stone [12.7kg/28lb]. In just under a year, I actually lost about 3½ stone [22.2kg/49lb]. I never looked on it as a diet. It was easy. It was very straightforward, the recipes were fantastic, and I just kept going, and in the end I lost about 5 stone [31.7kg/70lb].

'But that's not all. I also have better nails, better skin, better hair, much more energy – and it's just a way of life for me now. I followed all the recipes and I took all the supplements, and I got rid of any menopausal symptoms that were lurking in the background – in fact, I can't even remember what they were, now!'

Here are some key diet pointers that help menopausal symptoms – and they help men as well as women.

- Eat good sources of phytoestrogens every day, including beans, chickpeas, or fermented soya products such as miso, tempeh, natto and tamari (not too much of the latter, as it is high in salt). You probably need the equivalent of 30–40g a day for an effect, which is about a cupful.

- Increase your intake of anti-ageing antioxidants by eating lots of brightly coloured fruits and vegetables.

- Balance your blood sugar by eating a low-GL diet and possibly supplementing chromium, 200mcg in the morning.

- Get fit with frequent weight-bearing exercise; also use 'belly breathing' such as Diakath Breathing (see page 335).

- Check your homocysteine level. If it's high, supplement additional folic acid, B_6 and B_{12} accordingly.

- Try these herbs: black cohosh (50mg a day) or dong quai (600mg a day) or vitex agnus-castus (4mg a day of a standardised extract).

TESTOSTERONE – BOTH MEN AND WOMEN NEED IT

Without testosterone sex drive dwindles in both men and women. You can get yourself tested, and symptoms are a good yardstick. If you want to pursue this option it is best to work with a well-informed doctor or health practitioner. In any event you'll need to get a prescription, the dose required being higher in men than women. Women are usually given between 1mg and 2.5mg a day. In the US some more adventurous hormone therapists give 5mg. Too much testosterone can make some people feel more aggressive. This is exceedingly rare at a lower dose, below 2.5mg, however. Adult males typically make 15mg a day. Testosterone cream can also be used locally to increase sensitivity and prevent dryness in women.

FOR MEN

As with all hormones it is important to find expert help. Because of the decreasing availability of testosterone treatment within the NHS, your best bet is to go privately to a Centre for Men's Health Clinic located in both London and Manchester. The centres use the latest on-line internet technology to enable patients to fill in their own histories and complete diagnostic questionnaires and blood tests prior to seeing specialist consultants for examination and treatment. This enables you to play a greater role in your own diagnosis and treatment. Details on these clinics and doctors, who are well informed about hormones, are given in Resources.

There are now internationally accepted guidelines for safe testosterone therapy, and these are given in many publications such as those of the International Society for the Study of Men's Health (ISSAM). It must be emphasised, however, that a simple questionnaire such as the AMS (ageing male symptoms), which has identified many cases by on-line screening, is better for detecting testosterone deficiency than blood tests because of the resistance to the hormone which is present in most cases.

THE WARNING SIGNS IN MEN

Besides a drop off in sex drive, the symptoms of a deficiency in men can include mild to moderate depression and irritability as well as the ones usually associated with heart problems, such as overweight, raised levels of glucose and fats in the blood. If one relies purely on the so-called lower level of blood testosterone, research shows that over 80 per cent of cases of the andropause (male menopause) would be missed, says leading testosterone expert Dr Malcolm Carruthers.

Testosterone pellets, which last for six months, are a bit like putting a tiger in your tank, but are expensive and have been largely replaced by injections called Nebido (Bayer-Schering), which last three months. Many men prefer oral preparations, Restandol (Testocaps) by Organon, or transdermal gels such as Testogel (Bayer-Schering) or Tostran (Pro-Strakan).

Afterword

A GOOD END

Although it is a subject we try to avoid thinking about, life is a one-way ticket with death at the end of the line. Although we may joke about it, the truth is that most fears can be traced back to our fear of death. Fear of losing your money, your job, your family or your health, or of being in pain – behind these concerns is often the fear of death or losing your sense of self. Going crazy, or developing Alzheimer's, are examples of such worries that lurk as possibilities at the end of our lives. But the more immediate problem is that fear steals happiness and makes it more likely that we'll fall ill.

Those whose lives and deaths I (Patrick) have most admired often become lighter towards the end, unburdened by the feeling that they are leaving business unfinished. Someone who has led a good life and made a difference, and who has avoided prolonged suffering, seems to find it easier to let go. There is more room for gratitude and less for grief and regrets.

As we saw in Part Three, Chapter 6, having a sense of meaning and purpose, with loving connections to others, seems to be both important for healthy ageing and for dealing well with the process of physical degeneration.

Like birth, death is a natural process, and it is easier to come to terms with the less you resist it. The big question is whether one's consciousness or essential self continues to exist afterwards. Personally, I think it does, based on experiences that I've had. Jerome is not convinced, however. But, whatever we believe, we have the possibility of a good healthy life and a swift and painless death.

In the Indian tradition, the process of dying well is about letting go of attachments – to people and ideas, and ultimately to the body with which we strongly identify. A wonderful example of this was the story of the local holy man, Zipruanna, who died in Nasirabad in India in the 1930s. One day, he knocked on the door of a family in the village and asked if he could have a bath and a meal. After completing his meal, he said, 'Zipru is leaving. You can cry now, but it won't make any difference,' and he closed his eyes. He was gone.

His last act was to wash his body and feed his body. It is through our body that we experience all the great sights, sounds, tastes and smells, and the sheer joy of physical movement. I consider 'optimum nutrition' to be a simple act of respect for this amazing vehicle that we one day must leave. It is disrespectful to feed your body junk, and it has terrible consequences, regardless of how much money you have. Modern medicine's marvels cannot stop you falling sick and suffering. You have a far better chance of staying well by caring for your body in the way that we suggest in this book.

Some might find the idea of an afterlife, or reincarnation, comforting and so they will be less fearful of death, but others may feel more like me (Jerome); I don't find the idea so terrible that I am simply a tiny bit-player, lasting the equivalent of a few nanoseconds in the life of this extraordinary universe that has been in existence for thirteen or so billion years. The philosophy that works for me is: look at the world with kind eyes, be as present as you can, and know that everything changes. Oh, and laugh a lot. The hope is to have a rewarding life, and still be delighted by new things to the end. And I hope this book brings you something similar.

DYING WELL

We have been impressed and inspired by the deaths of the first generation of scientists and doctors who founded the discipline of optimum nutrition (or orthomolecular medicine).

My (Patrick's) first teacher, Dr Carl Pfeiffer, suffered a massive heart attack in his fifties, which damaged his heart; he was given a maximum of ten years to live if he had a pacemaker fitted. He never did, and he died in his eighties. He was working six days a week and building a brick wall outside his house. He called me a few months before he died and said, 'Patrick, you know I am running on borrowed time?' He finally had another heart attack, but discharged himself from hospital to go back to work. He died of his third heart attack a few days later.

Dr Roger Williams, discovered pantothenic acid (vitamin B_5), co-discovered folic acid and first crystallised the idea of how our genes interact with our environment, creating our biochemical individuality. And hence he recognised the inadequacy of a recommended daily allowance (RDA) for everyone. He died in his nineties and we had been corresponding on points of science until his last few months, when his eyesight was failing.

Dr Linus Pauling, who put high-dose vitamin C on the map, died in his nineties, from prostate cancer, and was actively writing and researching until a few weeks before his death. I interviewed him months before his death and he was right on the cutting edge, generating new theories in relation to heart disease that are only now starting to be accepted.

Two years ago, Dr Abram Hoffer, who discovered the power of high-dose niacin (vitamin B_3), both for mental illness and for lowering cholesterol, died in his nineties. He was an active member of my Scientific Advisory Board, and he was as sharp as a razor until the end, still seeing patients weeks before his death. About four days before his passing he started to feel unwell. Two days before his death he was admitted to hospital and died, without pain, in peace – not of heart disease, cancer or Alzheimer's, but of old age, having led a full and active life, helping millions of people. Messages of gratitude, not so much of grief, poured in to his family from all over the world.

A story that touched me recently was the father of a woman at one of my workshops who, as he approached his death at close to a hundred years old, asked to be taken into the garden. His eyes lit up. He said one word, then he was gone. It was 'love'.

Whatever your views about whether there is life *after* death, our hope for you with this book is to give you the means to have a healthy life *before* death and to live a long one, with the maximum engagement at the end. In the words of the Vulcan Spock, who would no doubt appreciate the logic of our approach: live long and prosper.

Patrick Holford and Jerome Burne

REFERENCES

INTRODUCTION

1   From the UK Office for National Statistics. Available at http://www.ons.gov.uk. Go to publications and enter 'Focus on Older People 2010'
2   BBC News Channel, *'Older People on Drug Cocktail'*, Tuesday 28 July 2009
3   P. Rosch, 'Stress due to medical care and FDA failures', *2010 Health and Stress*, November;11:1–12
4   M. Pirmohamed, et al., 'Adverse drug reactions as cause of admission to hospital: Prospective analysis of 18,820 patients', *British Medical Journal*, 2004;329:15–19
5   Dr R. Lippman, *'Stay forty without diet or exercise'*, Outskirts Press in Boulder Colorado, 2008

PART ONE

1   J. Krska and T. Avery, 'Citizen medicine and why we must try it', *New Scientist*, 20 June 2011
2   K. Archibald, et al., 'Open letter to UK Prime Minister David Cameron and Health Secretary Andrew Lansley on safety of medicines', *Lancet,* 2011;377(9781):1915
3   L. Wolpert, *You're Looking Very Well: The Surprising Nature of Getting Old*, Faber and Faber, 2011
4   'Dramatic rise in pensioners as baby boomers enter golden years'. Press release from the Department of Work and Pensions, 21 Sept. 2010, www.dwp.gov.uk/newsroom/press-releases/2010/sep-2010/dwp121-10-210910.shtml
5   J. Kirkup, 'Baby-boomers own half of Britain's Wealth', *Daily Telegraph*, 27 Jan 2010
6   K. T. Khaw, et al., 'Combined Impact of Health Behaviours and Mortality in Men and Women: The EPIC-Norfolk Prospective Population Study', *PLoS Med,* 2008;5(1): e12
7   H. Dobnig, 'Independent association of low serum 25-hydroxyvitamin D and 1,25-dihydroxyvitamin D levels with all-cause and cardiovascular mortality', *Archives of Internal Medicine*, 2008;168(12):1340–9
8   C. Garland, et al., 'Vitamin D supplement doses and serum 25-hydroxyvitamin D in the range associated with cancer prevention', *Anticancer Research*, 2011;31(2):607–11
9   T. Byers, 'Anticancer vitamins du jour—The ABCED's so far', *American Journal of Epidemiology*, 2010;172(1):1–3
10 J. N. Hathcock, 'Risk assessment for vitamin D', *American Journal of Clinical Nutrition*, 2007;85(1):6–18
11 A. Dalgleish, 'Yes! A dose of sun CAN protect you against skin cancer', *Daily Mail Online*, 24 May 2011, available at: http://www.dailymail.co.uk/health/article-1390243/Sun-CAN-protect-skin-cancer.html?ito=feeds-newsxml
12 M. D. Peterson and P. M. Gordon, 'Resistance exercise for the aging adult: Clinical implications and prescription guidelines', *The American Journal of Medicine*, 2011;124(3):194–8

13   S. Al-Majid and H. Waters, 'The biological mechanisms of cancer-related skeletal muscle wasting: The role of progressive resistance exercise', *Biological Research for Nursing*, 2008;10(1):7–20

14   S. B. Solerte, et al., 'Improvement of blood glucose control and insulin sensitivity during a long-term (60 weeks) randomized study with amino acid dietary supplements in elderly subjects with type 2 diabetes mellitus', *American Journal of Cardiology*, 2008;101(11A): 82E–88E

15   B. N. Ames, 'Low micronutrient intake may accelerate the degenerative diseases of aging through allocation of scarce micronutrients by triage', *Proceedings of the National Academy of Sciences of the United States of America*, 2006;103(47)17589–94

16   M. C. Morris and C. C. Tangney, 'A potential design flaw of randomised trials of vitamin supplements', *JAMA*, 2011;305(13):1348–9

17   A. D. Smith, et al., 'Homocysteine-lowering by B vitamins slows the rate of accelerated brain atrophy in mild cognitive impairment', *PLoS One*, 2010;5(9):e12244

18   Ray Moynihan, 'Surrogates under scrutiny: fallible correlations, fatal consequences', *British Medical Journal*, 2011; 343:d5160

19   Antithrombotic Trialists' (ATT) Collaboration, C. Baigent, L. Blackwell, R. Collins, J. Emberson, et al., 'Aspirin in the primary and secondary prevention of vascular disease: Collaborative meta-analysis of individual participant data from randomised trials', *Lancet*, 30 May 2009;373(9678):1849–60

20   Helen Barnett, Peter Burrill, Ike Iheanacho, 'Don't use aspirin for primary prevention of cardiovascular disease', *British Medical Journal*, 2010; 340:c1805

21   Chun Shing Kwok and Yoon K. Loke, 'Critical overview on the benefits and harms of aspirin', *Pharmaceuticals*, 2010, 3;1491–1506;doi:10.3390/ph3051491

22   C. Fox, et al., 'Anticholinergic medication use and cognitive impairment in the older population: The Medical Research Council Cognitive Function and Ageing Study', *Journal of the American Geriatrics Society*, 2011;doi:10.1111/j.1532–5415.2011.03491.x. [Epub ahead of print]

23   I. Whitcroft, 'Some combinations of common drugs can cause early death', *Daily Mail*, 27 June 2011

24   Letitia Dobranici, 'Anticholinergic medication use in patients with Alzheimer's dementia: Results from a Romanian longitudinal study', *Timisoara Medical Journal*, 2010, Vol. 60, No. 2–3

25   S. Cohen, *Drug Muggers: Which Medications are Robbing Your Body of Essential Nutrients*, Rodale Books, 2011

26   J. Shoshana, M.D. Herzig, M.P.H. Byron, et al., 'Acid-suppressive medication use and the risk for nosocomial gastrointestinal tract bleeding', *Archives of Internal Medicine*, 2011;171(11):991–7

27   Bo Abrahamsen, Pia Eiken, Richard Eastell, et al., 'Proton pump inhibitor use and the antifracture efficacy of alendronate', *Archives of Internal Medicine*, 2011;171(11):998–1004

28   Teppo Jarvinen, et al., 'The true cost of pharmacological disease prevention', *British Medical Journal* 2011; 342:d2175

29   E.L. Fosbøl, F. Folke, S. Jacobsen, J.N. Rasmussen, et al., 'Cause-specific cardiovascular risk associated with nonsteroidal antiinflammatory drugs among healthy individuals', *Circulation: Cardiovascular Quality and Outcomes*, 2010 Jul;3(4):395–405

30 Paul Dieppe, Christopher Bartlett, Peter Davey, et al., 'Balancing benefits and harms: The example of non-steroidal anti-inflammatory drugs', *British Medical Journal*, 2004, 3 Jul.;329:31–4

31 D.J. Frey, et al., 'Influence of zolpidem and sleep inertia on balance and cognition during nighttime awakening: A randomized placebo-controlled trial', *Journal of the American Geriatrics Society*, 2011 Jan;59(1):73–81

32 C. Fox, K. Richardson, I.D. Maidment, G.M. Savva, 'Anticholinergic medication use and cognitive impairment in the older population: The Medical Research Council Cognitive Function and Ageing Study', *Journal of the American Geriatrics Society*, 2011 Jun 24;doi:10.1111/j.1532–5415.2011.03491.x.

33 F. Taylor, et al., 'Statins for the primary prevention of cardiovascular disease', *Cochrane Database of Systematic Reviews*, 2011;(1):CD004816

34 ibid

35 ibid

36 S. Banerjee, 'The use of antipsychotic medication for people with dementia: Time for action', *Department of Health*, 3 October 2009

37 T. R. Fried, et al., 'Effects of benefits and harms on older persons' willingness to take medication for primary cardiovascular prevention', *Archives of Internal Medicine*, 2011;171(10):923–8, Epub

38 T. L. Jarvinen, et al., 'The true cost of pharmacological disease prevention', *British Medical Journal*, 2011; 342:d2175

39 ibid

40 D. J. Llewellyn, et al., 'Vitamin D and risk of cognitive decline in elderly persons', *Archives of Internal Medicine*, 2010;170(13):1135–41

41 C. Vermeer, et al., 'Beyond deficiency: Potential benefits of increased intakes of vitamin K for bone and vascular health', *European Journal of Nutrition*, 2004;43(6):325–35

42 S. Cockayne, et al., 'Vitamin K and the prevention of fractures: Systematic review and meta-analysis of randomized controlled trials', *Archives of Internal Medicine*, 2006;166(12):1256–61

43 M. F. Holick, et al., 'Evaluation, Treatment, and Prevention of Vitamin D Deficiency: an Endocrine Society Clinical Practice Guideline', *Journal of Clinical Endocrinology and Metabolism*, 2011 [Epub ahead of print]

44 D. J. Llewellyn, et al., 'Vitamin D and risk of cognitive decline in elderly persons', *Archives of Internal Medicine*, 2010;170(13):1135–41

45 A. G. Pittas, et al., 'The role of vitamin D and calcium in type-2 diabetes: A systematic review and meta-analysis', *Journal of Clinical Endocrinology and Metabolism*, 2007; 92(6):2017–20; see also S. Kayaniyil, et al., 'Association of 25(OH)D and PTH with metabolic syndrome and its traditional and nontraditional components', *Journal of Clinical Endocrinology and Metabolism*, 2010 Oct 27 [Epub ahead of print]; see also 'Older people need more sun, expert urges', *Science Daily*, 12 May 2009 (Available at: http://www.sciencedaily.com/releases/2009/05/090511090940.htm)

46 G. Bjelakovic, et al., 'Vitamin D supplementation for prevention of mortality in adults', *Cochrane Database of Systematic Reviews*, 2011(7):CD007470

47 Y. L. Michael, et al., 'Primary care-relevant interventions to prevent falling in older adults: A systematic evidence review for the U.S. Preventive Services Task Force', *Annals of Internal Medicine*, 2010;153(12):815–25

48 S. N. Meydani, et al., 'Serum zinc and pneumonia in nursing home elderly', *American Journal of Clinical Nutrition*, 2007;86(4):1167–73

49 S. N. Meydani, et al., 'Vitamin E and respiratory tract infections in elderly nursing home residents: a randomized controlled trial', *JAMA*, 2004;18292(7):828–36

50 C. J. Bates, et al., 'Redox-modulatory vitamins and minerals that prospectively predict mortality in older British people: the National Diet and Nutrition Survey of people aged 65 years and over', *The British Journal of Nutrition*, 2011 Jan;105(1):123–32

51 B. N. Ames, 'Prevention of mutation, cancer, and other age-associated diseases by optimizing micronutrient intake', *Journal of Nucleic Acids*, 2010;2010:ppi:725071

52 A. D. Smith, et al., 'Homocysteine-Lowering by B Vitamins Slows the Rate of Accelerated Brain Atrophy in Mild Cognitive Impairment: A Randomized Controlled Trial', *PLoS One*, 2010;5(9):e12244

53 A. Vogiatzoglou, et al., 'Vitamin B12 status and rate of brain volume loss in community-dwelling elderly', *Neurology*, 2008;71:826–32

54 J. Lewis, et al., 'The potential of probiotic fermented milk products in reducing the risk of antibiotic associated diarrhoea and *Clostridium difficile* disease', *International Journal of Dairy Technology*, 2009;62(4):461–71

55 M. M. Soong, et al., 'Observational study of the effects of probiotics in the treatment of constipation in the elderly', poster presented at the 19th World Congress of Gerontology and Geriatrics, Paris 2009

56 H.S. Gill, K.J. Rutherfurd, M.L. Cross, 'Dietary probiotic supplementation enhances natural killer cell activity in the elderly: An investigation of age-related immunological changes', *Journal of Clinical Immunology*, 2001; 21:264–71

57 'Thousands eat so badly they're dangerously undernourished (… and hospital makes it WORSE)', *Daily Mail*, 27 Oct. 2009. http://www.dailymail.co.uk/health/article-1223173/Malnutrition-epidemic-Thousands-eat-badly-theyre-dangerously-undernourished---hospital-makes-WORSE.html

58 M. H. Rabadi, et al., 'Intensive nutritional supplements can improve outcomes in stroke rehabilitation', *Neurology*, 2008;71(23):1856–61

59 Y. Okamoto, et al., 'Attenuation of the systemic inflammatory response and infectious complications after gastrectomy with preoperative oral arginine and omega-3 fatty acids supplemented immunonutrition', *World Journal of Surgery*, 2009;33(9):1815–21

60 K. Sriram and V. A. Lonchyna, 'Micronutrient supplementation in adult nutrition therapy: Practical considerations', *Journal of Parenteral and Enteral Nutrition*, 2009;33(5);548–62

61 L. Wolpert, *You're looking very well: the surprising nature of getting old*, Faber and Faber, 2011

62 E. L. Robb, et al., 'Mitochondria, cellular stress resistance, somatic cell depletion and lifespan', *Current Aging Science*, 2009;2(1):12–27

63 W. Chowanadisai, et al., 'Pyrroloquinoline quinone stimulates mitochondrial biogenesis through cAMP response element-binding protein phosphorylation and increased PGC-1alpha expression', *Journal of Biological Chemistry*, 2010;285(1):142–52; R. Rucker, et al., 'Potential physiological importance of pyrroloquinoline quinone', *Alternative Medicine Review*, 2009;14(3):268–77

64 F. J. Larsen, et al., 'Dietary inorganic nitrate improves mitochondrial efficiency in humans', *Cell Metabolism*, 2011;13(2):149–59

65   R. Farzaneh-Far, et al., 'Prognostic value of leukocyte telomere length in patients with stable coronary artery disease', *Arteriosclerosis, Thrombosis, and Vascular Biology*, 2008;28(7):1379–84

66   J. B. Richards, et al., 'Higher serum vitamin D concentrations are associated with longer leukocyte telomere length in women', *American Journal of Clinical Nutrition*, 2007;86(5):1420–5

67   S. W. Brouilette, et al., 'West of Scotland Coronary Prevention Study Group. Telomere length, risk of coronary heart disease, and statin treatment in the West of Scotland Primary Prevention Study: a nested case-control study', *Lancet*, 2007;369(9556):107–14

68   M. Jaskelioff, et al., 'Telomerase reactivation reverses tissue degeneration in aged telomerase-deficient mice', *Nature*, 2011;469(7328):102–6

69   M. Fossel, et al., *The Immortality Edge: Realise the Secrets of Your Telomeres for a Longer Healthier Life*, Wiley, 2010

70   W. de Ruijter, R.G.J. Westendorp, W.J.J. Assendelft, 'Use of Framingham risk score and new biomarkers to predict cardiovascular mortality in older people: Population based observational cohort study', *British Medical Journal* 2009, 8 Jan; 338:a3083 doi: 10.1136/bmj.a3083

71   A. D. Smith, et al., 'Homocysteine-lowering by B vitamins slows the rate of accelerated brain atrophy in mild cognitive impairment: A randomized controlled trial', *PLoS One*, 2010;5(9):e12244

72   C. A. De Jager, et al., 'Cognitive and clinical outcomes of homocysteine-lowering B vitamin treatment in mild cognitive impairment: A randomized controlled trial', *International Journal of Geriatric Psychiatry*, 2011, 21 July; doi:10.1002/gps.2758. [Epub ahead of print]

73   B. N. Ames, 'Prevention of Mutation, Cancer, and Other Age-Associated Diseases by Optimizing Micronutrient Intake', *Journal of Nucleic Acids*, 2010;2010: 725071

74   J. C. McCann and B. N. Ames, 'Adaptive dysfunction of selenoproteins from the perspective of the triage theory: why modest selenium deficiency may increase risk of diseases of aging', *The FASEB Journal*, 2011;25(6):1793–814

75   B. N. Ames, 'Prevention of Mutation, Cancer, and Other Age-Associated Diseases by Optimizing Micronutrient Intake', *Journal of Nucleic Acids*, 2010; 2010:725071

76   C. J. McMackin, et al., 'Effect of combined treatment with alpha-Lipoic acid and acetyl-L-carnitine on vascular function and blood pressure in patients with coronary artery disease', *Journal of Clinical Hypertension*, 2007;(4):249–55.

77   C.T. Loy and S.M. Twigg, 'Growth factors, AGEing, and the diabetes link in Alzheimer's disease', *Journal of Alzheimer's Disease*, 2009;16(4):823–31

78   B. Y. Li, et al., 'Induction of lactadherin mediates the apoptosis of endothelial cells in response to advanced glycation end products and protective effects of grape seed procyanidin B2 and resveratrol', *Apoptosis*, 2011;16(7):732–45

79   P. Balakumar, et al., 'The multifaceted therapeutic potential of benfotiamine', *Pharmacological Research*, 2010;61(6):482–8

80   S. Bengmark, et al., 'A plant-derived health: The effects of turmeric and curcuminoids', *Nutricion Hospitalaria*, 2009;24(3):273–81

81   Rachel Ellis, 'Could the Atkins diet help you keep diabetes at bay?' *Daily Mail*, 9 August 2011

82   K. Lin, et al., 'Regulation of the *Caenorhabditis elegans* longevity protein DAF-16 by insulin/IGF-1 and germline signaling', *Nature Genetics*, 2001;28(2):139–45

83 J. Guevara-Aguirre, et al., 'Growth hormone receptor deficiency is associated with a major reduction in pro-aging signaling, cancer, and diabetes in humans', *Science Translational Medicine*, 2011;3(70):70ra13

84 H. A. Hirsch, et al., 'A Transcriptional Signature and Common Gene Networks Link Cancer with Lipid Metabolism and Diverse Human Diseases', *Cancer Cell*, 2010;17(4):348–61

85 R. M. Anson, et al., 'Intermittent fasting dissociates beneficial effects of dietary restriction on glucose metabolism and neuronal resistance to injury from calorie intake', *Proceedings of the National Academy of Sciences of the U.S.A*, 2003;100(10):6216–20

86 J. B. Johnson, et al., 'Alternate day calorie restriction improves clinical findings and reduces markers of oxidative stress and inflammation in overweight adults with moderate asthma', *Free Radical Biology & Medicine*, 2007;42(5):665–74

87 K. A. Varady, et al., 'Improvements in body fat distribution and circulating adiponectin by alternate-day fasting versus calorie restriction', *Journal of Nutritional Biochemistry*, 2010;21(3):188–95. Epub

88 Michael Rose, 'Life begins at 90', *New Scientist*, 6 Aug. 2011

89 S. J. Olshansky, et al., 'Position statement of human aging', *Journals of Gerontology, Series A: Biological Sciences and Medical Sciences* 57, 2002 Aug (8): B292–B297

90 R. N. Butler, et al., 'New model of health promotion and disease prevention for the 21st century', *British Medical Journal*, 2008;337:a399

91 R. K. Minor, et al., 'Dietary interventions to extend life span and health span based on calorie restriction', *Journals of Gerontology, Series A: Biological Sciences and Medical Sciences*, 2010;65(7):695–703

92 S. V. Ramagopalan, et al., 'A ChIP-seq defined genome-wide map of vitamin D receptor binding: Associations with disease and evolution', *Genome Research*, 2010;20(10):1352–60

93 S. Bocklandt, et al., 'Epigenetic predictor of age', *PLoS One*, 2011;6(6):e14821

94 M. Ristowa and K. Zarsedo, 'How increased oxidative stress promotes longevity and metabolic health: The concept of mitochondrial hormesis (mitohormesis)', *Experimental Gerontology*, 2010;45(6):410–18

95 J. Holt-Lunstad, et al., 'Social relationships and mortality risk: A meta-analytic review', *PLoS Medicine*, 2010;7(7):e1000316

96 G. Miller, 'Epigenetics: The seductive allure of behavioral epigenetics', *Science (New York)*, 2010;329(5987): 24–7

97 S. S. Gehani, et al., 'Polycomb group protein displacement and gene activation through MSK-dependent H3K27me3S28 phosphorylation', *Molecular Cell*, 2010 Sep 24;39(6):886–900

98 G. Miller, 'Epigenetics: The seductive allure of behavioral epigenetics', *Science (New York)*, 2010;329(5987): 24–7

PART TWO

1 Editorial, 'Why are drug trials in Alzheimer's disease failing?', *Lancet*, 2010 Aug 28;376(9742):658 doi:10.1016/S0140–6736(10)61316–5

2 A. D. Smith, letter in *Lancet*, 2010 30 Oct;376:1466

3 K. Yaffe, 'Glycosylated hemoglobin level and the development of cognitive impairment or dementia in older women', *Journal of Nutrition, Health and Ageing*, 2006;10(4):293–5

4 S. A. Lipton, et al., 'Neurotoxicity associated with dual actions of homo-cysteine at the

N-methyl-D-aspartate receptor', *Proceedings of the National Academy of Sciences of the USA*, 1997;94:5923–8; see also M. F. Beal, et al., 'Neurochemical characterization of excitotoxin lesions in the cerebral cortex', *Journal of Neuroscience*, 1991;11:147–58

5   D. A. Snowdon, et al., 'Serum folate and the severity of atrophy of the neo-cortex in Alzheimer disease: Findings from the Nun Study', *The American Journal of Clinical Nutrition*, 2000;71(4):993–8

6   D. E. Zylberstein, et al., 'Midlife homocysteine and late-life dementia in women: A prospective population study', *Neurobiology of Aging*, March 2009;32(3):380–6

7   A. D. Smith, 'The worldwide challenge of the dementias: a role for B vitamins and homocysteine?', *Food Nutrition Bulletin*, June 2008;29(2 Suppl):S143–72

8   S. J. Duthie, et al., 'Homocysteine, B vitamin status, and cognitive function in the elderly', *American Journal of Clinical Nutrition*, May 2002;75(5):908–13; see also D. Kado, et al., 'Homocysteine levels and decline in physical function', *American Journal of Medicine*, November 2002;113(7):537–42; see also A. McCaddon, et al., 'Total serum homocysteine in senile dementia of Alzheimer's type', *International Journal of Geriatric Psychiatry*, 1998;13:235–9

9   A. McCaddon, et al., 'Analogues, ageing and aberrant assimilation of vitamin B_{12} in Alzheimer's disease, dementia and geriatric cognitive disorders', *Dementia and Geriatric Cognitive Disorders*, 2001;12(2):133–7; see also (2); see also A. Oulhaj, et al., 'Homocysteine as a predictor of cognitive decline in Alzheimer's disease', *International Journal of Geriatric Psychiatry*, 2010;25(1):82–90

10 E. Nurk, et al., 'Plasma total homocysteine and memory in the elderly: The Hordaland Homocysteine Study', *Annals of Neurology*, December 2005;58(6):847–57

11 S. Seshadri, et al., 'Plasma homocysteine as a risk factor for dementia and Alzheimer's disease', *New England Journal of Medicine*, 2002;346(7):466–8

12 J. H. Williams, et al., 'Minimal hippocampal width relates to plasma homo-cysteine in community-dwelling older people', *Age and Ageing*, 2002;31:440–4; see also (2); see also (1) and (6) – A. Oulhaj, et al.; see also P. S. Sachdev, et al., 'Relationship between plasma homocysteine levels and brain atrophy in healthy elderly individuals', *Neurology*, 2002;58:1539–41; see also H. X. Wang, et al., 'Vitamin B(12) and folate in relation to the development of Alzheimer's disease', *Neurology*, 2001;56(9):1188–94; see also T. Matsui, et al., 'Elevated plasma homocysteine levels and risk of silent brain infarction in elderly people', *Stroke*, 2001;32:1116.

13 See (17) below.

14 A. McCaddon, et al., 'Homocysteine and cognitive decline in healthy elderly', *Dementia and Geriatric Cognitive Disorders*, 2001;12(5):309–13; see also (2) and A. Vogiatzoglou, et al., 'Vitamin B_{12} status and rate of brain volume loss in community-dwelling elderly', *Neurology*, 2008;71(11):826–32; see also H. Refsum, 'Low vitamin B-12 status in confirmed Alzheimer's disease as revealed by serum holotranscobalamin', *Journal of Neurology Neurosurgery and Psychiatry*, 2003;74:959–61; see also (1); see also J.A. Luchsinger, et al., 'Relation of higher folate intake to lower risk of Alzheimer disease in the elderly', *Archives of Neurology*, 2007;64(1):86–92

15 P. Aisen, et al., 'High-dose B vitamin supplementation and cognitive decline in Alzheimer disease', *Journal of the American Medical Association*, 2008;300(15):1774–83

16 A. D. Smith, et al., 'Homocysteine-lowering by B vitamins slows the rate of accelerated brain atrophy in mild cognitive impairment: A randomized controlled trial', *Public Library of Science ONE*, 2010;5(9)e12244

17   C. A. Jager, et al., 'B vitamin treatment in mild cognitive impairment', *Public Library of Science MEDICINE*, 2011;Pending Publication

18   J. Durga, et al., 'The effect of 3-year folic acid supplementation on cognitive function in older adults in the FACIT trial: A randomized, double blind, controlled trial', *Lancet*, 2007; 369:208–16.

19   A. Vogiatzoglou, et al.,'Vitamin B_{12} status and rate of brain volume loss in community-dwelling elderly', *Neurology*, 2008 Sep 9;71(11):826–32

20   S. J. Eussen, et al., 'Oral cyanocobalamin supplementation in older people with vitamin B_{12} deficiency a dose-finding trial', *Archives of Internal Medicine*, 2005;165:1167–72

21   K. Koyama, et al., 'Efficacy of methylcobalamin on lowering total homo-cysteine plasma concentrations in haemodialysis patients receiving high dose folate supplementation', *Nephrology Dialysis Transplantation*, 2002;17:916–22

22   D. O. McGregor, et al., 'Betaine supplementation decreases post-methionine hyperhomo-cysteinemia in chronic renal failure', *Kidney International*, 2002;61(3):1040–6

23   S. Seshadri, et al., 'Plasma homocysteine as a risk factor for dementia and Alzheimer's disease', *New England Journal of Medicine*, 2002;346(7):466–8

24   M. C. Morris, et al., 'Consumption of fish and n-3 fatty acids and risk of incident Alzheimer disease', *Archives of Neurology*, 2003;60(7):940–6

25   K. Yurko-Mauro, et al., 'Beneficial effects of docosahexaenoic acid on cognition in age-related cognitive decline', *Alzheimer's and Dementia: The Journal of the Alzheimer's Association*, 2010;6:456–64

26   J. F. Quinn, et al., 'Docosahexaenoic acid supplementation and cognitive decline in Alzheimer disease: a randomized trial', *Journal of the American Medical Association*, November 2010;304(17):1903–11

27   J. Alvarez-Sabín and G. C. Román, 'Citicoline in vascular cognitive impairment and vascular dementia after stroke', *Stroke*, 2011 Jan;42(1 Suppl):S40–3

28   S. K. Tayebati, et al., 'Effect of choline-containing phospholipids on brain cholinergic transporters in the rat', *Journal of the Neurological Sciences*, 2011;302(1–2):49–57. See also R. Schliebs and T. Arendt, 'The cholinergic system in aging and neuronal degeneration', *Behavioural Brain Research*, 2010;221(2):555–63. See also S. Ladd, et al., 'Effect of phosphatidylcholine on explicit memory', *Clinical Neuropharmacology*, December 1993;16(6):540–9. See also F. Amenta, et al., 'The cholinergic approach for the treatment of vascular dementia: evidence from pre-clinical and clinical studies', *Clinical and Experimental Hypertension*, 2002;24(7–8):697–713

29   P. M. Kidd, 'Dietary phospholipids as anti-aging nutraceuticals', in R.A. Klatz and R. Goldman, eds, *Anti-Aging Medical Therapeutics*, Health Quest Publications; 2000:283–301

30   G. Murilado, et al., 'Circadian secretion of melatonin and thyrotropin in hospitalized aged patients', *Aging (Milano)*, February 1993;5(1);39–46

31   S. Schreiber, et al., 'An open trial of plant-source derived phosphatidylserine for treatment of age-related cognitive decline', *Israel Journal of Psychiatry Related Sciences*, 2000;37(4)302–7

32   B. L. Jorisse, et al., 'The influence of soy-derived phosphatidylserine on cognition in age-associated memory impairment', *Nutritional Neuroscience*, 2001;4(2):121–34

33   O. Blin, et al., 'Effects of dimethylaminoethanol pyroglutamate (DMAE p-Glu) against memory deficits induced by scopolamine: evidence from preclinical and clinical studies', *Psychopharmacology (Berl)*, 2009 Dec;207(2):201–12.

34   P. P. Zandi, et al., 'Reduced risk of Alzheimer disease in users of antioxidant vitamin supplements: the Cache County Study', *Archives of Neurology*, 2004;61:82–98

35   R. Petersen, et al., 'Vitamin E and donepezil for the treatment of mild cognitive impairment', *New England Journal of Medicine*, 2005;352:2379–88

36   A. Maczurek, et al., 'Lipoic acid as an anti-inflammatory and neuroprotective treatment for Alzheimer's disease', *Advance Drug Delivery Review*, 2008;60(13–14):1463–70

37   A. McCaddon and P. R. Hudson, 'L-methylfolate, methylcobalamin, and N-acetylcysteine in the treatment of Alzheimer's disease-related cognitive decline', *CNS Spectrum*, 2010;15(1 Suppl 1):2–5;discussion 6

38   P. Scheltens, et al., 'Efficacy of a medical food in mild Alzheimer's disease: A randomized, controlled trial', *Alzheimer's and Dementia*, 2010;6(1):1–10.e1

39   A Vogiatzoglou, et al., 'Dietary sources of vitamin B-12 and their association with plasma vitamin B-12 concentrations in the general population: The Hordaland Homocysteine Study', *American Journal of Clinical Nutrition*, 2009;89(4):1078–87

40   S. S. Karuppagounder, et al., 'Dietary supplementation with resveratrol reduces plaque pathology in a transgenic model of Alzheimer's disease', *Neurochemistry International*, 2009 Feb;54(2):111–18

41   C. Christine, et al., 'Adherence to a Mediterranean-type dietary pattern and cognitive decline in a community population', *American Journal of Clinical Nutrition*, 2011;93:1–7

42   P. Verhoef, et al., 'Contribution of caffeine to the homocysteine-raising effect of coffee: A randomized controlled trial in humans', *American Journal of Clinical Nutrition*, 2002;76(6):1244–8

43   M. J. Grubben, et al., 'Unfiltered coffee increases plasma homocysteine concentrations in healthy volunteers: a randomized trial', *American Journal of Clinical Nutrition* 2000;71(2):480–4

44   A. Ulvik, et al., 'Coffee consumption and circulating B-vitamins in healthy middle-aged men and women', *Clinical Chemistry*, 2008;54(9):1489–96

45   D. Panagiotakos, et al., 'The association between coffee consumption and plasma total homocysteine levels: The "ATTICA" study', *Heart Vessels*, 2004;19(6):280–6; see also R. Gelber, et al., 'Coffee intake in midlife and risk of dementia and its neuropathologic correlates', *Journal of Alzheimer's Disease*, 2011;23(4):607–15

46   J. A. Luchsinger, et al., 'Hyperinsulinemia and risk of Alzheimer diesase', *Neurology*, 2004;63(7):1187–92

47   A. M. Abbatecola, et al., 'Insulin resistance and executive dysfunction in older persons', *Journal of the American Geriatrics Society*, 2004;52(10):1713–18

48   W. L. Xu, et al., 'Diabetes mellitus and risk of dementia in the Kungsholmen project: A 6-year follow-up study', *Neurology*, 2004;63(7):1181–6. See also K. Yaffe, et al., 'Diabetes, impaired fasting glucose, and development of cognitive impairment in older women', *Neurology*, 2004;63(4):658–63

49   W. L. Xu, et al., 'Diabetes mellitus and risk of dementia in the Kungsholem project: a 6-year follow-up study', *Neurology*, 2004;63(7):1181–6; L. B. Hassing, et al., 'Type 2 diabetes mellitus contributes to cognitive decline in old age: A longitudinal population-based study', *Journal of the International Neuropsychology Society*, 2004;10(4):599–607; see also K. Yaffe, 'Glycosylated hemoglobin level and the development of cognitive impairment or dementia in older women', *Journal of Nutrition, Health and Ageing*, 2006;10(4):293–5; see also Z. Arvanitakis, et al., 'Diabetes mellitus and risk of Alzheimer disease and decline in cognitive function', *Archives of Neurology*, 2004;61(5):661–6; see also R. O. Roberts, et al., 'Metabolic syndrome, inflammation, and nonamnestic mild cognitive impairment in older persons: A population-based study', *Alzheimer Disease and Associated Disorder*, 2010;24(1):11–18; see

also J.M. Garcia-Lara, et al., 'The metabolic syndrome, diabetes, and Alzheimer's disease', *Revista de Investigacion Clinica*, 2010;62(4):343–9

50 K. Yaffe, et al., 'The Metabolic Syndrome and Development of Cognitive Impairment among Older Women', *Archives of Neurology,* 2009;66(3):324–8

51 J. W. Bijlsma, F. Berenbaum, F. P. Lafeber, 'Osteoarthritis: An update with relevance for clinical practice', *Lancet*, 2011 Jun 18;377(9783):2115–26

52 L. Teppo, N. Järvinen, et al., 'The true cost of pharmacological disease prevention', *British Medical Journal*, 2011; 342:d2175 doi:10.1136/bmj.d2175

53 B. Abrahamsen, et al., 'Proton pump inhibitor use and the antifracture efficacy of alendronate', *Archives of Internal Medicine*, 2011;171(11):998–1004

54 Research presented by Professor Richard Bockman chief of endocrinology at Weill Cornell Medical College in New York at the Endocrine Society's 93rd annual meeting in Boston June 2011

55 D. Cohen, 'Out of joint: The story of the ASR', *British Medical Journal*, 2011 14 May; 342:d2905 doi: 10.1136/bmj.d2905

56 M. Spangler, et al., 'Calcium supplementation in postmenopausal women to reduce the risk of osteoporotic fractures', *American Journal of Health-System Pharmacy*, 2011;68(4):309–18

57 M. Nestle, 'Eating made simple: How do you cope with a mountain of conflicting diet advice?', *Scientific American*, 2007 Aug 8; http://www.scientificamerican.com/article.cfm?id=eating-made-simple

58 M. J. Bolland, et al., 'Calcium supplements with or without vitamin D and risk of cardiovascular events: Reanalysis of the Women's Health Initiative limited access dataset and meta-analysis', *British Medical Journal*, 2011 Apr 19;342:d2040. doi: 10.1136/bmj.d2040

59 Reference taken from *Women's Health Weekly* and distributed via NewsRex.com.

60 C. G. Gjesdal, et al., 'Plasma total homocysteine level and bone mineral density', *Archives of Internal Medicine*, 2006;166:88–94; see also R. R. Maclean, et al., 'Homocysteine as a predictive factor for hip fracture in older persons', *New England Journal of Medicine*, 2004;350:2042–9; see also J. B. Van Meurs, et al., 'Homocysteine levels and the risk of osteoporotic fracture', *New England Journal of Medicine*, 2004;350:2033–41; see also M. Hermmann, et al., 'The role of hyperhomocysteinemia as well as folate, vitamin B_6 and B_{12} deficiencies in osteoporosis: A systematic review', *Clinical Chemistry Laboratory Medicine*, 2007;45(12):1621–32; see also Z. Krivosíková, et al., 'The association between high plasma homocysteine levels and lower bone mineral density in Slovak women: The impact of vegetarian diet', *European Journal of Nutrition,* 2010;49(3):147–53

61 Y. Sato, et al., 'Effect of folate and mecobalamin on hip fractures in patients with stroke', *Journal of the American Medical Association*, 2005;293:1082–8; see also Z. Ouzzif, et al., 'Relation of plasma total homocysteine, folate and vitamin B_{12} levels to bone mineral density in Moroccan healthy postmenopausal women', *Rheumatology International*, 2010 Jul 31. [Epub ahead of print]; Ouzzif, et al., [20676649]

62 R. Thaler, et al., 'Homocysteine suppresses the expression of the collagen cross-linker lysyl oxidase involving IL-6, Fli1, and epigenetic DNA methylation', *Journal of Biological Chemistry*, 2011;286(7)5578–88

63 T. Ito, R. T. Jensen, 'Association of long-term proton pump inhibitor therapy with bone fractures and effects on absorption of calcium, vitamin B_{12}, iron, and magnesium', *Current Gastroenterology Reports*, 2010 Dec;12(6):448–57

64 Y. X. Yang, et al., 'Long-term proton pump inhibitor therapy and risk of hip fracture', *Journal of the American Medical Association*, 2006 Dec 27;296(24):2947–53

65   J. Prior, 'Progesterone as bone-trophic hormone', *Endocrine Reviews*, 1990;11(2):386–98

66   J. Prior, et al., 'Spinal bone loss and ovulatory disturbances', *New England Journal of Medicine*, 1990;323(18):1221–7

67   J. Rossouw, et al., 'Risks and benefits of estrogen plus progestin in healthy postmenopausal women: Principal results from the Women's Health Initiative randomized controlled trial', *Journal of the American Medical Association*, 2002 Jul 17;288(3):321–33

68   Medicines and Healthcare products Regulatory Agency (MHRA), 'Further advice on safety of hormone replacement therapy (HRT)', press release, 3 December 2003, see: http://www.mhra.gov.uk/NewsCentre/Pressreleases/CON002044

69   D. Felson, et al., 'The effect of postmenopausal estrogen therapy on bone density in elderly women', *New England Journal of Medicine*, 1993 Oct. 14;329(16):1141–6; J. Rossouw, et al., 'Risks and benefits of estrogen plus progestin in healthy postmenopausal women: Principal results from the Women's Health Initiative randomized controlled trial', *Journal of the American Medical Association*, 2002 Jul 17;288(3):321–33

70   A. Katsnelso, 'The bones of contention', *Nature*, 2010;466(19):914–15

71   K. H. Wenger, et al., 'Effect of whole-body vibration on bone properties in aging mice', *Bone*, 2010 Oct;47(4):746–55

72   A. A. Bavry, A. Khaliq, Y. Gong, E. M. Handberg, 'Harmful Effects of NSAIDs among Patients with Hypertension and Coronary Artery Disease', *Am. J. Med.*, 2011 Jul;124(7):614–20

73   J. M. Bjordal, et al., 'Non-steroidal anti-inflammatory drugs, including cyclo-oxygenase-2 inhibitors, in osteoarthritic knee pain: Meta-analysis of randomised placebo controlled trials', *British Medical Journal*, 2004;329(7478):1317

74   P.R. Ush and M.U. Naidu, 'Randomised, double-blind, parallel, placebo-controlled study of oral glucosamine, methylsulfonylmethane and their combination in osteoarthritis', *Clinical Drug Investigation*, 2004;24(6):353–63

75   J. Reginster, et al., 'Long-term effects of glucosamine sulphate on osteoarthritis progression: A randomised, placebo-controlled clinical trial', *Lancet*, 2001;357(9252):251–6

76   Results presented at the American College of Rheumatology Annual Scientific Meeting (2005). Available at http://arthritis.about.com/od/glucosamine/a/glucosaminesulf.htm

77   P. Wilkens, et al., 'Effect of glucosamine on pain-related disability in patients with chronic low back pain and degenerative lumbar osteoarthritis: A randomized controlled trial', *Journal of the American Medical Association*, 2010;304(1):45–52

78   S. Wandel, et al., 'Effects of glucosamine, chondroitin, or placebo in patients with osteoarthritis of hip or knee: Network meta-analysis', *British Medical Journal*, 2010;341:c4675

79   J. Gruenwald, et al., 'Effect of glucosamine sulphate with or without omega-3 fatty acids in patients with osteoarthritis', *Advances in Therapy*, 2009;26(9):858–71

80   P. R. Usha and M. U. Naidu, 'Randomised, double-blind, parallel, placebo-controlled study of oral glucosamine, methylsulfonylmethane and their combination in osteoarthritis', *Clinical Drug Investigation*, 2004;24(6)353–63

81   No authors listed, 'Methylsulfonylmethane (MSM) monograph', *Alternative Medicine Review*, 2003;8(4):1514–22

82   S. W. Jacob and J. Appleton, *MSM: The Definitive Guide. A comprehensive review of the science and therapeutics of methylsulfonylmethane*, Freedom Press, 2003:107–21

83   M. G. Signorello, et al., 'Effect of homocysteine on arachidonic acid release in human platelets', *European Journal of Clinical Investigation*, 2002;32(4):279–84

84   R. Roubenoff, et al., 'Abnormal homocysteine metabolism in rheumatoid arthritis', *Arthritis and Rheumatism*, 1997;40(4):718–22

85   X. M. Gao, et al., 'Homocysteine, ankylosing spondylitis and reactive arthritis: Homocysteine modification of HLA antigens and its immunological consequences', *European Journal of Immunology*, 1996;26(7):1443–50

86   A. Hernanz, et al., 'Increased plasma levels of homocysteine and other thiol compounds in rheumatoid arthritis women', *Clinical Biochemistry*, 1999;32(1):65–70

87   P. E. Lazzerini, et al., 'Homocysteine enhances cytokine production in cultured synoviocytes from rheumatoid arthritis patients', *Clinical and Experimental Rheumatology*, 2006;24(4):387–93

88   M. A. Flynn, et al., 'The effect of folate and cobalamin on osteoarthritic hands', *Journal of the American College of Nutrition*, 1994;13(4):351–6

89   For further information read, J. M. Ellis's book, *Free of Pain: A Proven Inexpensive Treatment for Specific Types of Rheumatism*, Southwest Publishing, 1983

90   R. Goldberg and J. Katz, 'A meta-analysis of the analgesic effects of omega-3 polyunsaturated fatty acid supplementation for inflammatory joint pain', *Pain*, 2007;129(1–2):210–23

91   C. M. Bitler, et al., 'Hydrolyzed olive vegetation water in mice has anti-inflammatory activity', *Journal of Nutrition*, 2005;135(6):1475–9

92   E. M. Matheson, 'The association between onion consumption and bone density in perimenopausal and postmenopausal non-Hispanic white women 50 years and older', *Menopause*, 2009;16(4):756–9

93   R. Wilken, et al., 'Curcumin: A review of anti-cancer properties and therapeutic activity in head and neck squamous cell carcinoma', *Molecular Cancer*, 2011;10:12

94   B. White and D. Z. Judkins, 'Clinical Inquiry. Does turmeric relieve inflammatory conditions?', *Journal of Family Practice*, 2011;60(3):155–6

95   Y. B. Shaik, et al., 'Role of quercetin (a natural herbal compound) in allergy and inflammation', *Journal of Biological Regulators and Homeostatic Agents*, 2006;20(3–4):47–52

96   J. A. Welsh, et al., 'Caloric sweetener consumption and dyslipidemia among US adults', *Journal of the American Medical Association*, 2010;303(15):1490–7

97   I. Shai, et al., 'Weight loss with a low-carbohydrate, Mediterranean, or low-fat diet', *New England Journal of Medicine*, 2008;359(3):229–41

98   L. Hooper, et al., 'Reduced or modified dietary fat for preventing cardiovascular disease (Review)', *The Cochrane Collaboration and published in The Cochrane Library*, 2011;7

99   A. Astrup, et al., 'The role of reducing intakes of saturated fat in the prevention of cardiovascular disease: Where does the evidence stand in 2010?', *American Journal of Clinical Nutrition*, 2011;93(4):684–8

100   E. Balk, et al., 'Effect of chromium supplementation on glucose metabolism and lipids: A systematic review of randomized controlled trials', *Diabetes Care*, 2007 Aug;30(8):2154–63

101   L. Flicker, et al., 'Body mass index and survival in men and women aged 70 to 75', *Journal of the American Geriatrics Society*, 2010;58(2):234–41

102   C. Hublin, MD, et al., 'Sleep and mortality: A population-based 22-year follow-up study', *Sleep*, 2007;30(10):1245–53

103   J. E. Gangwisch, et al., 'Inadequate sleep as a risk factor for obesity: Analyses of the NHANES I', *Sleep*, 2005;28(10):1289–96

104   I. N. Karatsoreos, et al., 'Disruption of circadian clocks has ramifications for metabolism, brain, and behavior', *Proceedings of the National Academy of Sciences of the United States of America*, 2011;108(4):1657

105   J. Glass, et al., 'Sedative hypnotics in older people with insomnia: Meta-analysis of risks and benefits', *British Medical Journal*, 2005;331:1169 doi: 10.1136/bmj.38623.768588.47

106 A. N. Siriwardena, et al., 'GPs' attitudes to benzodiazepine and "Z-drug" prescribing: A barrier to implementation of evidence and guidance on hypnotics', *British Journal of General Practice*, 2006;56(533):964–7

107 C. Baglioni, et al., 'Sleep and emotions: A focus on insomnia', *Sleep Medicine Reviews*, 2010;14(4):227–38

108 L. Shilo, et al., 'The effects of coffee consumption on sleep and melatonin secretion', *Sleep Medicine*, 2002;3(3):271–3

109 E. Mills, et al., 'Melatonin in the treatment of cancer: A systematic review of randomized controlled trials and meta-analysis', *Journal of Pineal Research*, 2005 Nov.;39(4):360–6

110 A. Brzezinski, et al., 'Effects of exogenous melatonin on sleep: A meta-analysis', *Sleep Medicine Reviews*, 2005;9(1):41–50

111 S. A. Rahman, et al., 'Antidepressant action of melatonin in the treatment of Delayed Sleep Phase Syndrome', *Sleep Medicine*, February 2010;11(2):131–6

112 T. C. Birdsall, '5-Hydroxytryptophan: A clinically-effective serotonin precursor', *Alternative Medicine Review*, 1998;3(4):271–80

113 W. Shell, et al., 'A randomized, placebo-controlled trial of an amino acid preparation on timing and quality of sleep', *American Journal of Therapeutics*, 2010;17(2):133–9

114 M. Hornyak, 'Magnesium therapy for periodic leg movements-related insomnia and restless legs syndrome: An open pilot study', *Sleep*, 1998;21(5):501–5

115 M. Rondanelli, 'The effect of melatonin, magnesium, and zinc on primary insomnia in long-term care facility residents in Italy: A double-blind, placebo-controlled clinical trial', *Journal of the American Geriatrics Society*, 2011 Jan;59(1):82–90. doi: 10.1111/j.1532–5415.2010.03232

116 M. Spinella, *The Psychopharmacology of Herbal Medicine*, MIT Press, 2001

117 M. Dorn, 'Valerian versus oxazepam: Efficacy and tolerability in nonorganic and nonpsychiatric insomniacs – A randomized, double-blind clinical comparative study', *Forschende Komplementarmedizin und Klassische naturheilkunde*, 2000;7:79–81

118 E. Vorbach, et al., 'Treatment of insomnia: Effectiveness and tolerance of a valerian extract', *Psychopharmakotheraphie*, 1996;3:109–15

119 S. Bent, et al., 'Valerian for sleep: A systematic review and meta-analysis', *American Journal of Medicine* 2006;119(12):1005–12

120 C. Aboa-Eboule, et al., 'Job strain and risk of acute recurrent coronary heart disease events', *Journal of the American Medical Association*, 2007;298(14):1652–60

121 N. Vogelzangs, et al., 'Urinary cortisol and six-year risk of all-cause and cardiovascular mortality', *Journal of Clinical Endocrinology and Metabolism*, 2010;95(11):4959–64

122 A.K. Eriksson, et al., 'Psychological distress and risk of pre-diabetes and type 2 diabetes in a prospective study of Swedish middle-aged men and women', *Diabetic Medicine*, 2008;25:834–42

123 L. Johansson, et al., 'Midlife psychological stress and risk of dementia: A 35-year longitudinal population study', *Brain*, 2010;133:2217–24

124 M. Kivmaki, et al., 'Common mental disorder and obesity: Insight from four repeat measures over 19 years: Prospective Whitehall II cohort study', *British Medical Journal*, 2009;339:b3765

125 H. Kuper, et al., 'Job strain and risk of breast cancer', *Epidemiology*, 2007;18(6):764–8

126 100% Health Survey, Holford & Associates, 2010 – see www.patrickholford.com/index.php/shop/bookdetail/614/

127 D. Childre and D. Rozman, *Transforming Stress: The HeartMath Solution for Relieving Worry, Fatigue and Tension*, New Harbinger Publications, 2005

128 ibid

129 *HeartMath Intervention for Counselors, Therapists, Social Workers and Health Care Professionals: Establishing a New Baseline for Sustained Behavioral Change*, published by HeartMath LLC, 2008

130 R. McCraty and D. Tomasino, 'Emotional stress, positive emotions and psychophysiological coherence' in *Stress in Health and Disease*, Wiley 2006: 342–65

131 R. McCraty, et al., 'The impact of a new emotional self-management program on stress, emotions, heart-rate variability, dhea and cortisol, integrative', *Physiological and Behavioural Science*, 1998;33(2):151–70

132 R. McCraty, et al., 'Emotional self-regulation program enhances psychological health and quality of life in patients with diabetes', HeartMath Research Centre, Institute of HeartMath, Boulder Creek, CA, available at: http://www.renetobe.nl/1e%20nivo%20mediteren/8e%20 meditatie/bestanden/diabetes-patient-study.pdf

133 R. McCraty, et al., 'Impact of workplace stress reduction program on blood pressure and emotional health in hypertensive employees', *Journal of Alternative and Complementary Medicine*, 2003;9(3):355–69

134 Study carried out at the Pacemaker Clinic for Kaiser Hospitals in Orange County, California and featured in the Heartmath Interventions manual, HeartMath LLC, 2008:46

135 L. Yai, '"Brain music" in the treatment of patients with insomnia', *Neuroscience and Behavioural Physiology*, 1998;28:330–5

136 I. Olszewska and M. Zarow, 'Does Music During Dental Treatment Make a Difference?' Available at: www.silenceofmusic.com/pdf/dentists.pdf

137 R. Kafi, et al., 'Improvement of naturally aged skin with vitamin A (retinol)', *Archives of Dermatology*, 2007;143:606–12

138 M. Richelle, et al., 'Skin bioavailability of dietary vitamin E, carotenoids, polyphenols, vitamin C, zinc and selenium', *British Journal of Nutrition*, 2006;96: 227–38

139 D. Fernandes, 'Understanding and treating photoageing', cited in: I. J. Peled and E. K. Manders (eds), *Esthetic Surgery of the Face*, Informa Healthcare, 2004

140 M. C. Aust, et al., 'Percutaneous collagen induction – Regeneration in place of cicatrisation', *Journal of Reconstructive and Aesthetic Surgery*, 2011;64(1):97–107

141 ibid

142 B. C. Melnik and G. Schmitz, 'Role of insulin, insulin-like growth factor-1, hyperglycaemic food and milk consumption in the pathogenesis of acne vulgaris', *Experimental Dermatology*, 2009;18(10):833–41

143 S. Wright, 'Essential fatty acids in clinical dermatology', *Journal of Nutrition Medicine*, 1990;1:301–13

144 R. Osborne, et al., 'Understanding metabolic pathways for skin anti-aging', *Journal of Drugs in Dermatology*, 2009;8(7 Suppl):s4–7.

145 K. A. Tadini and P. M. Campos, 'In vivo skin effects of a dimethylaminoethanol (DMAE) based formulation', *Die Pharmazie*, December 2009;64(12):818–22

146 R. Grossman, 'The role of dimethylaminoethanol in cosmetic dermatology', *American Journal of Clinical Dermatology*, 2005;6(1):39–47

147 G. Morissette, et al., 'The anti-wrinkle effect of topical concentrated 2-dimethylaminoethanol involves a vacuolar cytopathology', *British Journal of Dermatology*, 2007;156(3):433–9

148 F. Bray, et al., 'The changing global patterns of female breast cancer incidence and mortality', *Breast Cancer Research*, 2004;6:229–39

149 P. Lichtenstein, et al., 'Environmental and heritable factors in the causation of cancer-analyses of cohorts of twins from Sweden, Denmark, and Finland', *New England Journal of Medicine*, 2000;343(2):78–85

150 C. A. Gonzalez and E. Riboli, 'Diet and cancer prevention: Contributions from the European Prospective Investigation into Cancer and Nutrition (EPIC) study', *European Journal of Cancer*, 2010;46(14)2555–62

151 G. Morgan, et al., 'The contribution of cytotoxic chemotherapy to 5-year survival in adult malignancies', *Clinical Oncology*, 2004;16(8):549–60

152 D.H. Howard, et al., 'The value of new chemotherapeutic agents for metastatic colorectal cancer', *Archives of Internal Medicine*, 2010;170(6):537–42

153 S. Epstein, 'Winning the war against cancer? ... Are they even fighting it?', *Ecologist*, 1998;28(2):69–80

154 C. F. Garland, et al., 'Vitamin D supplement doses and serum 25-hydroxyvitamin D in the range associated with cancer prevention', *Anticancer Research*, 2011;31(2):607–11

155 J. E. Manson, et al., 'Vitamin D and prevention of cancer: Ready for prime time?', *New England Journal of Medicine*, 2011;364(15):1385–7

156 R. P. Ojha, et al., 'Vitamin D for cancer prevention: Valid assertion or premature anointment?', *American Journal of Clinical Nutrition,* 2007;86(6):1804–5

157 S. Epstein, 'Winning the war against cancer? ... Are they even fighting it?' *Ecologist*, 1998;28(2):69–80

158 A. Baron, 'Typescript of interview with Simon Wolff', 13 May 1993, cited in: M. Walker, 'Sir Richard Doll: A questionable pillar of the cancer establishment', *Ecologist*, 1998;28(2):82–92

159 J. G. Hogervorst, et al., 'Dietary acrylamide intake and the risk of renal cell, bladder, and prostate cancer', *American Journal of Clinical Nutrition*, 2008;87(5):1428–38

160 R. B. Shekelle, et al., 'Dietary vitamin A and risk of cancer in the Western Electric study', *Lancet*, November 1982(8257):1185–90

161 World Cancer Research Fund, *Food Nutrition and the Prevention of Cancer*, 1997, p.138

162 B. Buijsse, et al., 'Plasma carotene and alpha-tocopherol in relation to 10-y all-cause and cause-specific mortality in European elderly: The Survey in Europe on Nutrition and the Elderly, a Concerted Action (SENECA)', *American Journal of Clinical Nutrition*, 2005;82(4):879–86

163 G. Omenn, et al., 'The Beta-Carotene and Retinol Efficacy Trial (CARET)', *New England Journal of Medicine*, 1996;334:1150–5

164 SuViMax study at news.bbc.co.uk/go/em/fr/-/1/hi/health/3122033.stm

165 J. Baron, et al., Neoplastic and antineoplastic effects of beta-carotene on volorectal adenoma, *Journal of the National Cancer Institute*, 2003;95(10):717–22

166 S. Mannisto, et al., 'Dietary carotenoids and risk of lung cancer in a pooled analysis of seven cohort studies', *Cancer Epidemiology Biomarkers and Prevention*, 2004;13(1):40–8

167 B. Frei, 'Efficacy of dietary antioxidants to prevent oxidative damage and inhibit chronic disease', *Journal of Nutrition*, 2004;134:3196S–3198S

168 L. Mingetti, et al., 'Peripheral reductive capacity is associated with cognitive performance and survival in Alzheimer's disease', *Journal of Neuroinflammation*, 2006;3:4

169 G. Block, 'Vitamin C and cancer prevention: The epidemiologic evidence', *American Journal of Clinical Nutrition*, 1991;53(1 Suppl):270S–82S

170 G. Block, 'Epidemiologic evidence regarding vitamin C and cancer', *American Journal of Clinical Nutrition*, 1991;54(6 Suppl):1310S–4S

171 K. A. Head, 'Ascorbic acid in the prevention and treatment of cancer', *Alternative Medicine Review*, 1998;3(3):174–86

172 M. Eichholzer, et al., 'Prediction of male cancer mortality by plasma levels of interacting vitamins: 17-year follow-up of the prospective Basel study', *International Journal of Cancer*, 1996;66(2):145–50; see also C. M. Loria, et al., 'Vitamin C status and mortality in US adults', *American Journal of Clinical Nutrition*, 2000;72(1):139–45; see also K. T. Khaw, et al., 'Relation between plasma ascorbic acid and mortality in men and women in EPIC-Norfolk prospective study: A prospective population study, European Prospective Investigation into Cancer and Nutrition', *Lancet*, 2001;357(9257):657–63

173 E. Cameron and L. Pauling, 'Supplemental ascorbate in the supportive treatment of cancer: Prolongation of survival times in terminal human cancer', *Proceedings of the National Academy of Sciences of the United States of America*, October 1976;73(10):3685–9

174 Q. Chen, et al., 'Pharmacologic doses of ascorbate act as a prooxidant and decrease growth of aggressive tumor xenografts in mice', *Proceedings of the National Academy of Sciences of the United States of America*, 2008;105(32):11105–9

175 M. G. Espey, et al., 'Pharmacologic ascorbate synergizes with gemcitabine in preclinical models of pancreatic cancer', *Free Radical Biology Medicine*, 2011;50(11):1610–19

176 A. Tavani, et al., 'Consumption of sweet foods and breast cancer risk in Italy', *Annals of Oncology*, 2006 Feb;17(2):341–5

177 A. Tavani, et al., 'Consumption of sweet foods and breast cancer risk in Italy', *Annals of Oncology*, 2006 Feb;17(2):341–5; and C. A. Krone and J. T. Ely, 'Controlling hyperglycemia as an adjunct to cancer therapy', *Integrative Cancer Therapies*, 2005 Mar.;4(1):25–31; and S. C. Larsson, et al., 'Glycemic load, glycemic index and breast cancer risk in a prospective cohort of Swedish women', *International Journal of Cancer*, 2009 Jul. 1;125(1):153–7; and W. Wen, et al., 'Dietary carbohydrates, fiber, and breast cancer risk in Chinese women', *American Journal of Clinical Nutrition*, 2009 Jan.;89(1):283–9; and S. Sieri, et al., 'Dietary glycemic index, glycemic load, and the risk of breast cancer in an Italian prospective cohort study', *American Journal of Clinical Nutrition*, 2007 Oct.;86(4):1160–6; and M. Lajous et al., 'Carbohydrate intake, glycemic index, glycemic load, and risk of postmenopausal breast cancer in a prospective study of French women', *American Journal of Clinical Nutrition*, 2008 May;87(5):1384–91; and S. E. McCann, et al., 'Dietary patterns related to glycemic index and load and risk of premenopausal and postmenopausal breast cancer in the Western New York Exposure and Breast Cancer Study', *American Journal of Clinical Nutrition*, 2007 Aug.;86(2):465–71

178 M. L. Slattery, et al., 'Dietary sugar and colon cancer', *Cancer Epidemiology, Biomarkers and Prevention*, 1997 Sept.;6(9):677–85

179 D. S. Michaud, et al., 'Dietary sugar, glycemic load, and pancreatic cancer risk in a prospective study', *Journal of the National Cancer Institute*, 2002 Sept. 4;94(17):1293–300

180 S. A. Silvera, et al., 'Glycaemic index, glycaemic load and ovarian cancer risk: A prospective cohort study', *Public Health Nutrition*, 2007 Oct.;10(10):1076–81

181 G. Randi, et al., 'Glycemic index, glycemic load and thyroid cancer risk', *Annals of Oncology*, 2008 Feb.;19(2):380–3

182 S. A. Silvera, et al., 'Glycaemic index, glycaemic load and risk of endometrial cancer: A prospective cohort study', *Public Health Nutrition*, 2005 Oct.;8(7):912–19; S. C. Larsson

et al., 'Carbohydrate intake, glycemic index and glycemic load in relation to risk of endometrial cancer: A prospective study of Swedish women', *International Journal of Cancer*, 2007 Mar. 1;120(5):1103–7

183 P. Bertuccio, et al., 'Dietary glycemic load and gastric cancer risk in Italy', *British Journal of Cancer*, 2009 Feb. 10;100(3):558–61

184 A. W. Barclay, et al., 'Glycemic index, glycemic load, and chronic disease risk: A meta-analysis of observational studies', *American Journal of Clinical Nutrition*, 2008 Mar.;87(3):627–37

185 G. C. Kabat et al., 'Repeated measures of serum glucose and insulin in relation to postmenopausal breast cancer', *International Journal of Cancer*, 2009 June 2 [Epub ahead of print]; see also M. J. Gunter, et al., 'Insulin, insulin-like growth factor-I, and risk of breast cancer in postmenopausal women', *Journal of the National Cancer Institute*, 2009 Jan. 7;101(1):48–60

186 V. W. Ho, et al., 'A low carbohydrate, high protein diet slows tumor growth and prevents cancer initiation', *Cancer Research*, 2011;71(13):4484–93

187 M. J. Gunter, et al., 'Insulin, insulin-like growth factor-I, and risk of breast cancer in postmenopausal women', *Journal of the National Cancer Institute*, 2009;101(1):48–60

188 T. M. Brasky, et al., 'Specialty supplements and breast cancer risk in the VITamins And Lifestyle (VITAL) Cohort', *Cancer Epidemiology Biomarkers & Prevention*, 2010;19(7):1696–708

189 N. J. West, et al., 'Eicosapentaenoic acid reduces rectal polyp number and size in familial adenomatous polyposis', *Gut*, 2010;59(7):918–25

190 V. Fradet, et al., 'Dietary omega-3 fatty acids, cyclooxygenase-2 genetic variation, and aggressive prostate cancer risk', *Clinical Cancer Research*, 2009;15(7):2559–66

191 M. Johansson, et al., 'Serum B vitamin levels and risk of lung cancer', *Journal of the American Medical Association*, 2010;303(23):2377–85

192 E. Ruden, et al., 'Exercise behavior, functional capacity, and survival in adults with malignant recurrent glioma', *Journal of Clinical Oncology*, 2011; 29(21):2918–23

193 G. A. Potter, et al., 'The cancer preventative agent resveratrol is converted to the anticancer agent piceatannol by the cytochrome P450 enzyme CYP1B1', *British Journal of Cancer*, March 2002;86(5):774–8

194 See www.patrickholford.com/salvestrolcasestudies

195 Coronary heart disease statistics in England, February 2011, British Heart Foundation. Available at: www.bhf.org.uk

196 H. Tunstall-Pedoe, et al., 'Contribution of trends in survival and coronary-event rates to changes in coronary heart disease mortality: 10-year results from 37 WHO MONICA project populations. Monitoring trends and determinants in cardiovascular disease', *Lancet*, 1999;353(9164):1547–5

197 W. Willetts, 'The great fat debate: Total fat and health', *Journal of the American Medical Association*, 2011;111(5)660–2

198 L. Hooper, et al., 'Reduced or modified dietary fat for preventing cardiovascular disease', *Cochrane Database Systematic Reviews*, 2011;(7):CD002137

199 M. Kendrick, *The Great Cholesterol Con: The Truth about What Really Causes Heart Disease and How to Avoid it*, John Blake, 2008

200 A. I. Qureshi, et al., 'Regular egg consumption does not increase the risk of stroke and cardiovascular diseases', *Medical Science Monitor*, 2006;13(1):CR1–8; also L. Djoussé and J. M. Gaziano, 'Egg consumption and cardiovascular disease and mortality, The Physicians'

Health Study', *American Journal of Clinical Nutrition*, 2008 Apr.;87(4):964–9; also D. K. Houston, et al., 'Dietary fat and cholesterol and risk of cardiovascular disease in older adults: The Health ABC Study', *Nutrition, Metabolism and Cardiovascular Disease*, 2011 Jun.;21(6):430–7; also C. Scrafford, et al., 'Egg consumption and CHD and stroke mortality: A prospective study of US adults', *Public Health*, 2011 Feb.;14(2):261–70

201 N. L. Harman, et al., 'Increased dietary cholesterol does not increase plasma low density lipoprotein when accompanied by an energy-restricted diet and weight loss', *European Journal of Nutrition*, 2008;47(6):287–93

202 14 March 2006, *Metro* newspaper, front page

203 F. Taylor, et al., 'Statins for the primary prevention of cardiovascular disease', *Cochrane Database Systematic Review* 2011;1:CD004816

204 J. Abramson and J. Wright, 'Are lipid-lowering guidelines evidence-based?', *Lancet* 2007;369:168–9

205 K. Kausik, et al., 'Statins and All-Cause Mortality in High-Risk Primary Prevention. A Meta-analysis of 11 Randomized Controlled Trials Involving 65 229 Participants', *Archives of Internal Medicine*, 2010;170(12):1024–31

206 L. Teppo, et al., 'The true cost of pharmacological disease prevention', *British Medical Journal*, 2011;342:doi:10.1136/bmj.d2175

207 U. Ravnskov, et al., 'Analysis and comment controversy: Should we lower cholesterol as much as possible?', *British Medical Journal*, 2006;332:1330–2

208 B. Golomb, et al., 'Physician response to patient reports of adverse drug effects: Implications for patient-targeted adverse effect surveillance', *Drug Safety*, 2007;30(8)669–75

209 A. A. Alsheikh-Ali, et al., 'Effect of the magnitude of lipid lowering on risk of elevated liver enzymes, rhabdomyolysis, and cancer: Insights from large randomized statin trials', *Journal of the American College of Cardiology*, 2007;50409–18

210 D. Mangin, et al., 'Preventive health care in elderly people needs rethinking', *British Medical Journal*, 2007;335:285–7

211 P. H. Langsjoen, et al., 'Treatment of statin adverse effects with supplemental Coenzyme Q10 and statin drug discontinuation', *Biofactors*, 2005;25(1–4):147–52

212 K. Jones, et al., 'Coenzyme Q-10 and cardiovascular health', *Alternative Therapies in Health & Medicine*, 2004;10(1):22–30; see also M. Dhanasekaran and J. Ren, 'The emerging role of coenzyme Q-10 in aging, neurodegeneration, cardiovascular disease, cancer and diabetes mellitus', *Current Neurovascular Research*, 2005;2(5):447–59

213 P. Langsjoen and A. Langsjoen, 'Overview of the use of CoQ10 in cardiovascular disease', *Biofactors*, 1999;9(21–4):273–84

214 I. Gissi-HF, et al., 'Effect of n-3 polyunsaturated fatty acids in patients with chronic heart failure (the GISSI-HF trial): A randomised, double-blind, placebo-controlled trial', *Lancet*, 2008;372(9645):1223–30

215 R. De Caterina, 'n-3 Fatty Acids in Cardiovascular Disease', *New England Journal of Medicine*, 2011;364(25):2439–50

216 P. M. Kris-Etherton, et al., 'Omega-3 fatty acids and cardiovascular disease: New recommendations from the American Heart Association', *Arteriosclerosis, Thrombosis and Vascular Biology*, 2003;23(2):151–2

217 D. Thomas, et al., 'Low glycaemic index or low glycaemic load diets for overweight and obese', *Cochrane Database Systematic Reviews*, 2007;(3):CD005105

218 I. Gigleux, et al., 'Comparison of a dietary portfolio diet of cholesterol-lowering foods and a statin on LDL particle size phenotype in hypercholesterolaemic participants', *British Journal of Nutrition*, 2007 Dec;98(6):1229–36

219 S. Cohen, *Drug Muggers: Which Medications Are Robbing Your Body Of Essential Nutrients*, Rodale, 2011

220 W. J. Mroczek, et al., 'Effect of magnesium sulfate on cardiovascular hemodynamics', *Angiology*, 1977;28:720–4

221 B. T. Altura and B. M. Altura, 'Magnesium in cardiovascular biology an important link between cardiovascular risk factors and atherogenesis', *Cellular & Molecular Biology Research,* 1995;41(5)28–36

222 M. D. Ashen and R. S. Blumentahl, 'Clinical Practice. Low HDL cholesterol levels', *New England Journal of Medicine,* 2005;353(12):1252–60

223 M. J. Chapman, et al., 'Niacin and fibrates in atherogenic dyslipidemia: Pharmacotherapy to reduce cardiovascular risk', *Pharmacology & Therapeutics,* 2010;126(3):314–45

224 S. Hughes, 'What future for niacin after AIM-HIGH?', 4 July 2011. Available at: http://www.theheart.org/article/1248191.do

225 W. De Ruijter, et al., 'Use of Framingham risk score and new biomarkers to predict cardiovascular mortality in older people: Population based observational cohort study', *British Medical Journal*, 2009;338:a3083

226 ibid

227 X. Wang, et al., 'Efficacy of folic acid supplementation in stroke prevention: A meta-analysis', *Lancet*, 2007;369(9576):1876–81

228 D. S. Wald, et al., 'Reconciling the evidence on serum homocysteine and ischaemic heart disease: A meta-analysis', *PLoS ONE,* 2011;6(2):e16473

229 M. Rath and L. Pauling, 'Unified theory of human cardiovascular disease leading the way to the abolition of this disease as a cause for human mortality', *Journal of Orthopaedic Medicine*, 1992;7:5–15

230 B. G. Nordestgaard, et al., 'Lipoprotein(a) as a cardiovascular risk factor: Current status', *European Heart Journal*, 2010;31(23):2844–53

231 K. A. Lysend-Williamson, 'Niacin Extended Release (ER)/Simcastatin (Simcor) (Simcor®): A guide to its use in lipid regulation', *Drugs in R&D*, 2010;10(4):253–60

232 D. Holmes, 'An answer to angina', *Holistic Health*, 1995;49:20–3

233 Y. Kubota, et al., 'Dietary intakes of antioxidant vitamins and mortality from cardiovascular disease: The Japan Collaborative Cohort (JACC) study', *Stroke*, 2011;42(6):1665–72

234 J. Breilmann, et al., 'Effect of antioxidant vitamins on the plasma homocysteine level in a free-living elderly population', *Annals of Nutrition and Metabolism*, 2010;57(3–4):177–82

235 E. Mah, et al., 'Vitamin C status is related to proinflammatory responses and impaired vascular endothelial function in healthy, college-aged lean and obese men', *Journal of American Diet Association*, 2011;111(5):737–43

236 D. Grimes, *Vitamin D and Cholesterol: The Importance of the Sun*, Tennison Publishing, 2009

237 J. H. Lee, et al., 'Vitamin D deficiency: An important, common, and easily treatable cardiovascular risk factor?', *Journal of the American College of Cardiology*, 2008;52(24):1949–56

238 J. H. Lee, et al., 'Prevalence of vitamin D deficiency in patients with acute myocardial infarction', *American Journal of Cardiology*, 2011;107(11):1636–8

239 S. Maiya, et al., 'Hypocalcaemia and vitamin D deficiency: An important, but preventable, cause of life-threatening infant heart failure', *Heart*, 2008; 94(5):581–4

240 I. Al Mheid, et al., 'Vitamin D status is associated with arterial stiffness and vascular dysfunction in healthy humans', *Journal of the American College of Cardiology*, 2011;58(2):186–92

241 W. B. Grant, 'An estimate of the global reduction in mortality rates through doubling vitamin D levels', *European Journal of Clinical Nutrition*, 2011 Jul 6. doi:10.1038/ejcn.2011.68

242 N. Vogelzangs, et al., 'Urinary cortisol and six-year risk of all-cause and cardiovascular mortality', *Journal of Clinical Endocrinology & Metabolism*, 2010;95(11):4959–64

243 R. McCraty, et al., 'Impact of workplace stress reduction program on blood pressure and emotional health in hypertensive employees', *Journal of Alternative and Complementary Medicine*, 2003;9(3):355–69

244 'Study carried out at the Pacemaker Clinic for Kaiser Hospitals in Orange County, California and featured in the HeartMath Interventions manual', HeartMath LLc, 2008:46

245 R. H. Schneider, et al., 'Long-term effects of stress reduction on mortality in persons > or = 55 years of age with systemic hypertension', *American Journal of Cardiology*, 2005 May 1;95(9):1060–4

246 W. Atkinson, et al., 'Food elimination based on IgG antibodies in irritable bowel syndrome: A randomised controlled trial', *Gut*, 2004;53:1459–64

247 M. Wilders-Truschnig, et al., 'IgG antibodies against food antigens are correlated with inflammation and intima media thickness in obese juveniles', *Experimental and Clinical Endocrinology and Diabetes*, 2008;116(4):241–5

248 S. Buhner, et al., 'Activation of human enteric neurons by supernatants of colonic biopsy specimens from patients with irritable bowel syndrome', *Gastroenterology*, 2009;137(4):1425–34

249 F. Guarner, et al., 'Consensus statements from the workshop "Probiotics and Health: Scientific Evidence"', *Nutricion Hospitalaria*, 2010;25(5):700–4

250 D. B. Silk, et al., 'Clinical trial: The effects of a trans-galactooligosaccharide prebiotic on faecal microbiota and symptoms in irritable bowel syndrome', *Aliment Pharmacology and Therapeutics*, 2009;29(5):508–18

251 P. Moayyedi, et al., 'The efficacy of probiotics in the treatment of irritable bowel syndrome: A systematic review', *Gut*, 2010;59(3):325–32

252 'Influenza vaccines: Poor evidence for effectiveness in elderly', *Science Daily*, Retrieved Jul. 7, 2011,Wiley-Blackwell, Feb. 17 2010

253 F. Guarner, et al., 'Consensus statements from the workshop "Probiotics and Health: Scientific Evidence"', *Nutricion Hospitalaria*, 2010;25(5):700–4

254 M. Lyte, 'Probiotics function mechanistically as delivery vehicles for neuroactive compounds: Microbial endocrinology in the design and use of probiotics', *BioEssays*, Wiley-Blackwell, July 2011, doi: 10.1002/bies.201100024

255 Y. X. Yang, et al., 'Long-term proton pump inhibitor therapy and risk of hip fracture', *Journal of the American Medical Association*, 2006;296:2947–295

256 E. Andrès, et al., 'Vitamin B_{12} (cobalamin) deficiency in elderly patients', *CMAJ*, August 2004;171(3):251–9

257 Y. Cheng, et al., 'Alpha-lipoic acid alters post-translational modifications and protects the chaperone activity of lens alpha-crystallin in naphthalene-induced cataract', *Current Eye Research*, 2010;35(7):620–30

258 J. Qu, et al., 'Coenzyme Q10 in the human retina', *Investigative Ophthalmology and Visual Sciences*, 2009;50(4):1814–18

259 Chung-Jung Chiu, et al., 'Dietary carbohydrate and the progression of age-related macular degeneration: A prospective study from the Age-Related Eye Disease Study', *American Journal of Clinical Nutrition*, 2007;86:180–8

260 W.G. Christen, et al., 'Dietary carotenoids, vitamins C and E, and risk of cataract in women: A prospective study', *Archive Ophthalmology*, 2008;126(1):102–9

261 L. Ma, et al., 'Lutein and zeaxanthin intake and the risk of age-related macular degeneration: a systematic review and meta-analysis', *British Journal of Nutrition*, 2011 Sep 8 doi:10.1017/S0007114511004260, published online

262 J. Hippisley-Cox, 'Unintended effects of statins in men and women in England and Wales: Population based cohort study using the QResearch database', *British Medical Journal*, 2010;340:c2197 doi:10.1136/bmj.c2197

263 No authors listed, 'Drug-induced cataracts', *Prescrire International*, 2011;20(113):41–3

264 R. M. Santaella and F. W. Fraunfelder, 'Ocular adverse effects associated with systemic medications: Recognition and management', *Drugs*, 2007;67(1):75–93

265 M. Larkin, 'Vitamins reduce risk of vision loss from macular degeneration', *Lancet*, 2001;358(9290):1347; 'National Eye Institute of America, Age-Related Eye Disease Study (AREDS)', *Archives of Ophthalmology*, 2001;119:1417–36

266 N. Krishnadev, et al., 'Nutritional supplements for age-related macular degeneration', *Current Opinion in Ophthalmology*, 2010;21(3):184–9

267 V. Agte and K. Tarwadi, 'The importance of nutrition in the prevention of ocular disease with special reference to cataract', *Ophthalmic Research*, 2010;44(3):166–72

268 W. G. Christen, et al., 'Folic acid, pyridoxine, and cyanocobalamin combination treatment and age-related macular degeneration in women: the Women's Antioxidant and Folic Acid Cardiovascular Study', *Archives of Internal Medicine*, 2009;169(4):335–41

269 J. M. Seddon, et al., 'Dietary fat and risk for advanced age-related macular degeneration', *Archives of Opthalmology*, 2001;119:1191–9

270 W. G. Christen, et al., 'Dietary ω-3 fatty acid and fish intake and incident age-related macular degeneration in women', *Archives of Opthalmology*, 2011 Jul;129(7):921–9

271 J. Feher, et al., 'Improvement of visual functions and fundus alterations in early age-related macular degeneration treated with a combination of acetyl-L-carnitine, n-3 fatty acids, and coenzyme Q10', *Ophthalmologica*, 2005;219(3):154–66

272 A. E. Millen, et al., 'Vitamin D status and early age-related macular degeneration in postmenopausal women', *Archives of Ophthalmology*, 2011;129(4):481–9

273 B. Hammond, et al., 'Eat fruits and vegetables for better vision', Institute of Food Technologists, *Science Daily*, 19 Dec. 2009

274 C. Tamer, et al., 'Serum dehydroepiandrosterone sulphate level in age-related macular degeneration', *American Journal of Ophthalmology*, 2007;143(2):212–16

275 P. Guarneri, et al., 'Neurosteroids in the retina: neurodegenerative and neuroprotective agents in retinal degeneration', *Annals of the New York Academy of Sciences*, 2003;1007:117–28

276 E. L. Paul, 'The treatment of retinal diseases with Micro Current Stimulation and nutritional supplementation', Presented to The International Society for Low-vision research and rehabilitation, Goteborg University, 1997

277 J. Hippisley-Cox, et al., 'Unintended effects of statins in men and women in England and

Wales: Population based cohort study using the QResearch database', *British Medical Journal*, 2010;340:c2197

278 J. A. Mares, et al., 'Healthy diets and the subsequent prevalence of nuclear cataract in women', *Archives of Ophthalmology*, 2010;128[6]:738–49

279 S. M. Bouton, 'Vitamin C and the ageing eye', *Archives of Internal Medicine*, 1939;63:930–45; see also J. Blondin, et al., 'Prevention of eye lens protein damage by dietary vitamin C', *Federal Proceedings*, 1986,45:478

280 R. D. Ravindran, et al., 'Inverse association of vitamin C with cataract in older people in India', *Ophthalmology*, 2011 Oct; 118(10):1958–1965.e2. Epub 2011 Jun 25

281 M. Kernt, et al., 'Coenzyme Q10 prevents human lens epithelial cells from light-induced apoptotic cell death by reducing oxidative stress and stabilizing BAX / Bcl-2 ratio', *Acta Ophthalmologica*, 2010;88(3):e78–86

282 J. Zhang and S. Wang, 'Topical use of coenzyme Q10-loaded liposomes coated with trimethyl chitosan: Tolerance, precorneal retention and anti-cataract effect', *International Journal of Pharmacology*, 2009;372(1–2):66–75

283 K. M. Cornish, et al., 'Quercetin metabolism in the lens: role in inhibition of hydrogen peroxide', *Free Radical Biology and Medicine*, 2002;33(1):63–70

284 A. Jacadzadeh, et al., 'Preventive effect of onion juice on selenite-induced experimental cataract', *Indian Journal of Ophthalmology*, 2009;57(3):185–9

285 R. D. Steigerwalt, et al., 'Mirtogenol potentiates latanoprost in lowering intraocular pressure and improves ocular blood flow in asymptomatic subjects', *Clinical Ophthalmology*, 2010;4:471–6

286 I. Cecilia, et al., 'Allosteric Modulation of Retinal GABA Receptors: Ascorbic acid', *Journal of Neuroscience*, 2011;31(26): 9672–82; doi: 10.1523/?JNEUROSCI.5157–10.2011

287 H. Ohguro, et al., 'High levels of MSG can damage the retina', *New Scientist and Experimental Eye Research*, 2002;75(3):307–15

288 L. Quaranta, et al., 'Effect of ginkgo biloba extract on preexisting visual field damage in normal tension glaucoma', *Ophthalmology*, 2003;110(2):359–62

289 M. S. Passo, et al., 'Exercise training reduces intraocular pressure among subjects suspected of having glaucoma', *Archives of Ophthalmology*, 1991;109:1096–109

290 J. Hoberman, *Testosterone Dreams: Rejuvenation, Aphrodisia, Doping*, University of California Press, 2005

291 J. E. Rossouw, et al., 'Risks and benefits of estrogen plus progestin in healthy postmenopausal women: Principal results from the Women's Health Initiative randomized controlled trial', *Journal of the American Medical Association*, 2002;288:321–33

292 S. Tehillah, et al., 'Rates of Atypical Ductal Hyperplasia Have Declined with Less Use of Postmenopausal Hormone Treatment: Findings from the Breast Cancer Surveillance Consortium', *Cancer Epidemiol Biomarkers Prev*, 2009:2822–8; doi:10.1158/1055–9965. EPI-09-0745

293 J. V. Wright, 'Bio-identical steroid hormone replacement: Selected observations from 23 years of clinical and laboratory practice', *Ann N Y Acad Sci*, 2005;1057:506–24

294 K. Holtorf, 'The bioidentical hormone debate: Are bioidentical hormones (estradiol, estriol, and progesterone) safer or more efficacious than commonly used synthetic versions in hormone replacement therapy?', *Postgraduate Medical Journal*, 2009 Jan;121(1):73–85

295 R. T. Chlebowski, et al., 'Estrogen plus progestin and breast cancer incidence and mortality in postmenopausal women', *Journal of the American Medical Association*, 2010;304[15]:1684–92

296 T. Rowan, et al., 'Oestrogen plus progestin and lung cancer in postmenopausal women (Women's Health Initiative trial): A post-hoc analysis of a randomised controlled trial', *Lancet*, 2009;374(9697)1243–51

297 E. T. Schwartz and K. Holtorf, 'Hormones in wellness and disease prevention: common practices, current state of the evidence, and questions for the future', *Prim Care*, 2008;35(4):669–705

298 J. Prior, et al., 'Spinal bone loss and ovulatory disturbances', *New England Journal of Medicine*, 1990;323(18)1221–7

299 J. Lee, 'Osteoporosis reversal: The role of progesterone', *International Clinical Nutritional Review*, 1990;10:384–91; see also J. Lee, 'Osteoporosis reversal with transdermal progesterone', *Lancet*, 1990;336(8726):1327

300 A. Cooper, et al., 'Systemic absorption of progesterone from Progest cream in postmenopausal women', *Lancet*, 1998;351(9111):1255–6

301 A. Fournier, et al., 'Unequal risks for breast cancer associated with different hormone replacement therapies: results from the E3N cohort study', *Breast Cancer Res Treat*, 2008;107(1):103–11

302 R. McCraty, et al., 'The impact of a new emotional self-management program on stress, emotions, heart rate variability, DHEA and cortisol', *Integrative and Physiological and Behavioral Science*, 1998;33(2):151–70

303 J. W. Lin, et al., 'Metabolic syndrome, testosterone, and cardiovascular mortality in men', *Journal of Sexual Medicine*, 2011 doi: 10.1111/j.1743–6109.2011.02343

304 N. Bassil, et al., 'The benefits and risks of testosterone replacement therapy: A review', *Journal of Therapeutics and Clinical Risk Management*, 2009;5(3):427–48

305 A. Morgentaler, et al., 'Testosterone therapy in men with untreated prostate cancer', *J Urol*, 2011;185(4):1256–60

PART THREE

1   K. T. Khaw, et al., 'Combined impact of health behaviours and mortality in men and women: The EPIC–Norfolk prospective population study', *PLoS Medicine*, 2008;5(1)e12

2   L. L. Moisey, et al., 'Caffeinated coffee consumption impairs blood glucose homeostasisin response to high and low glycemic index meals in healthy men', *Journal of Clinical Nutrition*, 2008; 87(5)1254–61

3   E. Cheraskin, 'The Breakfast/Lunch/Dinner Ritual', *Journal of Orthomolecular Medicine*, 1993;8:1st Quarter

4   R. Lappalainen, et al., 'Drinking water with a meal: A simple method of coping with feelings of hunger, satiety and desire to eat', *European Journal of Clinical Nutrition*, 1993;47(11):815–19

5   B. J. Rolls, et al., 'Volume of food consumed affects satiety in men', *American Journal of Clinical Nutrition*, 1998;67(6):1170–7

6   M. Boschmann, et al., 'Water-induced thermogenesis', *Journal of Clinical Endocrinology and Metabolism*, 2003;88(12):6015–19; see also M. Boschmann, et al., 'Water drinking induces thermogenesis through osmosensitive mechanisms', *Journal of Clinical Endocrinology and Metabolism*, 2007;92(8):3334–7

7   M. A. Shafiee, et al., 'Defining conditions that lead to the retention of water: The importance of the arterial sodium concentration', *Kidney International*, 2005;67(2):613–21

8   J. R. Claybaugh, et al., 'Effects of time of day, gender, and menstrual cycle phase on the human response to a water load', *American Journal of Physiology: Regulatory, Integrative and Comparative Physiology*, 2000;279(3):R966–73

9   D. O. Baliunas, et al., 'Alcohol as a risk factor for type 2 diabetes: A systematic review and meta-analysis', *Diabetes Care*, 2009;32(11):2123–32

10   D. Mozaffarian, et al., 'Changes in diet and lifestyle and long-term weight gain in women and men', *New England Journal of Medicine*, 2011;364(25):2392–404

11   R. Weiler, et al., 'Should health policy focus on physical activity rather than obesity? Yes', *British Medical Journal*, 2010;340:c2603

12   G. Reynolds, ' Phys Ed: How exercising keeps your cells young', *New York Times*, 27 Jan. 2010. Available at: http://well.blogs.nytimes.com/2010/01/27/phys-ed-how-exercising-keeps-your-cells-young/

13   W. McArdle, Chapter in *Medical Aspects of Clinical Nutrition*, Keats Publishing, 1983

14   J. D. Edinger, et al., 'Aerobic fitness, acute exercise and sleep in older men', *Sleep*, 1993;16(4):351–9. See also K. A. Kubitz, et al., 'The effects of acute and chronic exercise on sleep. A meta-analytic review', *Sports Medicine*, 1996;21(4):277–91; see also E. Naylor et al., 'Daily social and physical activity increases slow-wave sleep and daytime neuropsychological performance in the elderly', *Sleep*, 2000 Feb 1;23(1):87–95; C. M. Shapiro et al., 'Slow-wave sleep: a recovery period after exercise', *Science*, 1981 Dec 11; 214(4526):1253–4

15   C. Hollenbeck, et al., 'Effect of habitual exercise on regulation of insulin stimulated glucose disposal in older males', *Journal of the American Geriatrics Society*, 1986;33:273–7

16   P. Ebelin, et al., 'Mechanism of enhanced insulin sensitivity in athletes', *American Society for Clinical Investigations*, 1993; 92:1623–31

17   R. Kurzweil and T. Grossman, *Transcend: Nine Steps to Living Well Forever*, Rodale 2010

18   J. Cannell, B. Hollis, M. Sorenson, et al., 'Athletic Performance and vitamin D', *Medicine and Science in Sports and Exercise*, 2009 May;41(5):1102–10

19   M. Ohayon, 'Epidemiology study on insomnia in the general population', *Sleep*, 1996;19(3 Suppl):S7–S15

20   G. Hajak, et al., 'Epidemiology of severe insomnia and its consequences in Germany', *European Archives of Psychiatry and Clinical Neuroscience*, 2001;251(2):49–56

21   R. G. Rosenfield and S. E. Gargosky, 'Assays for insulin-like growth factors and their binding proteins: Practicalities and pitfalls', *Journal of Pediatrics*, 1996;128(5 Pt2):S532–7

22   J. D. Edinger, et al., 'Aerobic fitness, acute exercise and sleep in older men', *Sleep*, 1993;16(4):351-9; see also K. A. Kubitz, et al., 'The effects of acute and chronic exercise on sleep: A meta-analytic review', *Sports Medicine*, 1996;21(4):277-91; E. Naylor et al, 'Daily social and physical activity increases slow-wave sleep and daytime neuropsychological performance in the elderly', *Sleep*, 2000;23(1):87–95; see also C. M. Shapiro, et al., 'Slow-wave sleep: A recovery period after exercise', *Science*, 1981;214(4526):1253–4

23   E. Langer, *Mindfulness*, Addison Wesley, 1989

24   M. D. Rablen, A. J. Oswald, 'Mortality and immortality: The Nobel Prize as an experiment into the effects of status upon longevity', *Journal of Health Economics*, 2008;27(6):1462–71

25   E. J. Giltay, et al., 'Dispositional optimism and all-cause and cardiovascular mortality in a prospective cohort of elderly Dutch men and women', *Archives of General Psychiatry*, 2004;61:1126–35

26   G. V. Ostir, et al., 'Emotional well-being predicts subsequent functional independence and survival', *Journal of American Geriatric Society*, 2000;48(5):473–8

27   C. Tregear et al., 'Positive emotions and attitudes: precious keys to longevity', *Journal of European Anti-Ageing Medicine*, Issue 4, Oct 2006;31–2

28   N. Ranjit, et al., 'Psychosocial factors and inflammation in the multi-ethnic study of atherosclerosis', *Archives of Internal Medicine*, 2007;167:174–81

29   M. E. Register, et al., 'Development and Psychometric Testing of the Register – Connectedness Scale for Older Adults', *Research in Nursing & Health*, 2011;34(1)60–72

30   M. E. Register, and J. Herman, 'A middle range theory for generative quality of life for the elderly', *Advances in Nursing Science*, 2006;29(4):340–50

31   J. W. Rowe, et al., 'Successful aging', *Gerontologist*, 1997;37:433–40. See also J. W. Rowe and R. L. Kahn, 'Human aging: Usual and successful', *Science*, 1987; 237:143–9

32   P. Clayton and J. Rowbotham, 'An unsuitable and degraded diet? Part one: Public health lessons from the mid-Victorian working class diet', *Journal of the Royal Society of Medicine*, 2008:101:282–9

33   G. Blocks, et al., 'Usage patterns, health, and nutritional status of long-term multiple dietary supplement users: A cross-sectional study', *Nutrition Journals*, 2007;6:30

RECOMMENDED READING

GENERAL

Marc E. Agronin, *How We Age: A Doctor's Journey into the Heart of Growing Old*, Da Cappo (2012)

Suzy Cohen, *The Drug Muggers: Which Medications are Robbing Your Body of Essential Nutrients and Natural Ways to Restore Them*, Rodale (2011)

Michael Fossel, Greta Blackburn, Dave Woynarowski, *Immortality Edge: Realize the Secrets of Your Telomeres for a Longer Healthier Life*, Wiley (2010)

Richard C. Francis, *Epigenetics: The Ultimate Mystery of Inheritance*, Norton (2011)

Patrick Holford, *The Optimum Nutrition Bible*, Piatkus (2004)

Patrick Holford, *The 10 Secrets of 100% Healthy People*, Piatkus (2009)

Patrick Holford and Fiona McDonald Joyce, *The 10 Secrets of 100% Health Cookbook*, Piatkus (2012)

Ray Kurzweil and Terry Grossman, *Transcend: Nine Steps to Living Well For Ever*, Rodale (2009)

David Stipp, *The Youth Pill: Scientists At The Brink of an Anti-Aging Revolution*, Current (2010)

Jonathan Weiner, *Long for this World: The Strange Science of Immortality*, Ecco (2010)

Lewis Wolpert, *You're Looking Very Well: The Surprising Nature of Getting Old*, Faber and Faber (2012)

PART 2

Secret 1

Patrick Holford, *The Alzheimer's Prevention Plan*, Piatkus (2011)

Secret 2

Patrick Holford, *Say No to Arthritis*, Piatkus (2010)

Secret 3

Patrick Holford, *The Low-GL Diet Bible*, Piatkus (2005)

Patrick Holford and Fiona McDonald Joyce, *The Low-GL Diet Cookbook*, Piatkus (2005)

Patrick Holford, *Say No to Diabetes*, Piatkus (2011)

Secret 4

Doc Childre and Deborah Rozman, *Transforming Stress: The HeartMath Solution for Relieving Worry, Fatigue, and Tension*, New Harbinger Publications (2005)

Patrick Holford, *The Feel Good Factor*, Piatkus (2010)

Patrick Holford, *How to Quit Without Feeling S**t*, Piatkus (2008)

Secret 6

Patrick Holford and Liz Efiong, *Say No to Cancer*, Piatkus (2010)

Patrick Holford and Jennifer Meek, *Boost Your Immune System*, Piatkus (2010)

Secret 7

Patrick Holford, *Say No to Heart Disease*, Piatkus (2010)

Secret 8

Patrick Holford, *Improve Your Digestion*, Piatkus (2009)

Secret 9

Jonathan Barnes, *Improve Your Eyesight: A Guide to the Bates Method for Better Eyesight without Glasses*, Souvenir Press (2000)

Secret 10

Dr Malcolm Carruthers, *The Testosterone Revolution*, Thorsons (2001)

Dr Marion Gluck and Viki Edgson, *It Must Be My Hormones: Getting Your Life Back with Bio-Identical Hormone Therapy*, Michael Joseph (2012)

Patrick Holford, *Balance Your Hormones*, Piatkus (2011)

PART 3

Phil Campbell, *Ready Set Go! Synergy Fitness for Time-crunched Adults*, Pristine Publishers Inc. (2002)

RESOURCES

GENERAL INFORMATION

bioage check Are you ageing faster or slower than your real age? Find out by completing our online questionnaire and tests at www.patrickholford.com/bioage.

The Brain Bio Centre is an outpatient clinic of the charitable Food for the Brain Foundation in London, that specialises in the nutritional treatment of mental health issues, ranging from depression and insomnia to Alzheimer's and Parkinson's disease, under the direction of Patrick Holford. The Centre's team of expert nutritional therapists, backed up by a psychiatrist and neurologist, works with you to identify any nutritional or biochemical imbalances that may be contributing to your symptoms and the consultation provides you with a tailored programme to correct these issues and restore your health. Through a process of nutritional and psychiatric assessment, appropriate clinical tests, dietary advice and/or supplements will then be recommended. Visit www.brainbiocentre.com or tel.: +44 (0) 20 8332 9600.

The Food for the Brain Foundation is a non-profit educational charity directed by Patrick Holford, which aims to promote awareness of the link between learning, behaviour, mental health and nutrition; and to educate and provide educational material to children, parents, teachers, schools, the public, the catering industry, health professionals and the government. The website has a free online Cognitive Function Test. It takes 15 minutes to complete and is validated for anyone over the age of 50. Depending on your score, it tells you what to do to improve your memory. For more information visit www.foodforthebrain.org.

Nutritional therapy and consultations To find a recommended nutritional therapist near you, visit the 'advice' section on www.patrickholford.com. This service gives details on whom to see in the

UK as well as internationally. If there is no one available nearby, you can always take an online assessment – see below.

Online 100% Health Programme Are you 100% healthy? Find out with our FREE Health Check and comprehensive personalised 100% Health Programme giving you a personalised action plan, including diet and supplements. The 100% Health Programme costs £24.95 but, as a reader of this book, at the time of going to press you can save £5 by putting in the following discount code: 10SECUK187. Visit www.patrickholford.com.

Zest4Life is a health and nutrition club, based on low-GL principles, which provides advice, coaching and support for losing weight and gaining health through a series of weekly meetings offered throughout the UK, Ireland and in selected countries abroad. For more information, visit www.zest4life.eu.

Psychocalisthenics is an excellent exercise system that takes less than 20 minutes a day, and develops strength, suppleness, stamina as well as generating vital energy. The best way to learn it is to do the Psychocalisthenics Training. See www.patrickholford.com (events) for details. Also available is the Psychocalisthenics CD and DVD, available from www.patrickholford.com (shop). For further information please see www.pcals.com.

Silence of Peace CD Based on centuries-old use of specific musical scales and arrangements, the music of John Levine helps you enter a more peaceful state of mind – excellent as an aid for a good night's sleep. To find out more and purchase visit www.patrickholford.com (shop).

STRESS-BUSTING AND EXERCISE

HeartMath You can attend a 'Transforming Stress' half-day workshop. We run these twice a year. See the events section of www.patrickholford.com. The EmWave Personal Stress Reliever is also available from this website. For further details on HeartMath visit www.heartmath.com.

Yoga To find a hatha yoga class (which usually includes meditation) near to you, visit www.bwy.org.uk for The British Wheel of Yoga, to find an accredited teacher. Or for an Iyengar yoga class (which uses props to help with the postures), visit www.iyengaryoga.org.uk for The Iyengar Yoga Association.

EYE HEALTH

MCS for protection against age-related macular degeneration. Electrical stimulation, which encourages cellular regeneration, is applied using a micro-current stimulator (MCS) to acupressure points around the eyes. Visit www.dovehealth.com.

Pinhole glasses can help with most focusing problems, even if you already use spectacles or lenses. Visit www.trayner.co.uk.

HORMONAL HEALTH

FOR WOMEN

Hormonal assessment: to find a doctor experienced in using bio-identical hormones visit www.bio-hormone-health.com. This is a site dedicated to offering women information, news and expert opinion and access to doctors and experienced professionals working in the field of women's health and natural bio-identical hormones.

The Natural Progesterone Information Society also has a list of practitioners in the UK; visit www.npis.info.

Dr Marion Gluck, who is quoted in Secret 10, has a website that provides information on bio-identical hormones as well as contact details for other practitioners; www.mariongluck.bradlangdon. co.uk/. She has also set up an independent pharmacy in London that specialises in supplying individually prescribed bio-identical hormone prescriptions and vitamin supplements for health and beauty; www. specialist-pharmacy.com.

FOR MEN

The Centre for Men's Health focuses on the treatment of testosterone deficiency syndrome, a condition that can lead to premature ageing as well as the loss of vitality and virility. Testosterone replacement therapy (TRT) has been shown to dramatically reverse these symptoms and restore the patient's health, drive and libido. Patients complete an online diagnostic questionnaire and health history, and organise blood tests prior to seeing specialist consultants for examination and treatment. The Centre has clinics in London, Manchester and Glasgow. Visit www.centreformenshealth.co.uk or tel.: +44 (0)20 7636 8283.

LABORATORY TESTS

Food Allergy (IgG ELISA), Homocysteine, GLCheck (measures your level of glycosylated haemoglobin, also called HbA1C) are available through YorkTest Laboratories, using a home-test kit where you can take your own pinprick blood sample and return it to the lab for analysis. Visit www.yorktest.com, or call freephone (UK) 0800 074 6185. These test kits are also available from www.totallynourish.com.

At the time of going to press, if you enter the discount code HCY GL PH (and live in the UK or Eire) you can save £48 by having both your homocysteine and GLCheck tested at once from www.yorktest.com.

In South Africa, IgG food allergy testing is available from www.msdafrica.net.
Homocysteine testing is available from a number of laboratories such as Lancet Labs and Ampath.

In Canada, IgG food allergy testing is available from www.yorktest.ca. **Homocysteine testing** is available from www.lifelabs.com and www.gamma-dynacare.ca.

Vitamin D can be tested for £20 from www.vitamindtest.org.uk and is available through your doctor.

Telomere-length testing is currently only available in the US from www.spectracell.com/telomere-testing/.

HEALTH PRODUCTS

Sugar alternative – XyloBrit (xylitol) is a low-GL natural sugar alternative – available from health-food stores and www.totallynourish. com.

Chia seeds, the highest vegetarian source of omega-3, are available online and from www.totallynourish.com.

Cherry Active is sold in a highly concentrated juice format. Mix a 30ml serving with 250ml water to make a deliciously healthy, low-GL cherry juice. Each 946ml bottle contains the juice from over 3,000 cherries – that's half a tree's worth – and contains a month's supply. Cherry Active is also available as a dried cherry snack and in capsules. Available online or for more information and to order, visit www.totallynourish. com (see below).

Salvestrols To find a practitioner near you who is knowledgeable in the use of salvestrols or to obtain both maintenance and higher therapeutic dosage levels of salvestrols, contact www.1880life.com or tel.: 0845 0896470.

SUPPLEMENTS AND SUPPLIERS

Finding your own perfect supplement programme can be confusing, but the website www.patrickholford.com offers useful guidance in the 'supplements' section.

In this section are examples of supplements that provide the herbs and nutrients at the levels discussed in this book. The addresses of the companies whose products we've referred to are given at the end.

MULTIVITAMINS AND MINERAL SUPPLEMENTS

Supplementing the right multivitamin is the most important supplement decision you make. Most multis are based on RDA levels of nutrients, which are not the same as optimum nutrition levels. A good multivitamin–mineral based on optimum nutrition levels is Patrick Holford's Optimum Nutrition Formula. Another is Solgar's VM2000. Both of these recommend taking two tablets a day. Optimum Nutrition Formula has higher mineral levels, especially for calcium and magnesium, as well as more vitamin D. Ideally, take a multivitamin–mineral with an extra 2 × 900mg of vitamin C. Patrick Holford's Optimum Nutrition Pack provides the multivitamin, extra vitamin C and essential omega-3 and 6 oils all in a daily strip. Their 100% Health Pack also provides AGE Antioxidants and Brain Food.

In South Africa, Patrick Holford's Optimum Nutrition Formula, ImmuneC and Essential Omegas are available from www.holforddirect. co.za.

BONE AND JOINT SUPPORT

Patrick Holford's Bone support provides extra calcium (250mg), magnesium (150mg), vitamin D (25mcg), vitamin K (250mcg), zinc (10mg) and boron (2mg).

In South Africa, this formula is available as OsteoFood.

Joint support nutrients such as turmeric, quercetin, olive and hop extracts, glucosamine and MSM are available in Patrick Holford's Joint Support, also available in South Africa.

DIGESTIVE ENZYMES AND SUPPORT

A good digestive enzyme combination should contain protease, amylase and lipase, which digest protein, carbohydrate and fat respectively. Some also contain amyloglucosidase (which helps to digest glucosides found in certain beans and vegetables) and lactase (which helps to digest milk sugars). If you get bloated after lentils or beans, such as soya products, choose an enzyme that contains alpha-galactosidase. Try Solgar's Vegan Digestive Enzymes. You can also buy digestive enzymes with probiotics – Patrick Holford's DigestPro contains all these enzymes and probiotics.

ESSENTIAL FATS AND FISH OIL SUPPLEMENTS

The most important omega-3 fats are DHA, DPA and EPA, found both in oily fish and in cod liver oil. The most important omega-6 fat is GLA, the richest source being borage (also known as starflower) oil. Try Patrick Holford's Essential Omegas, which provides a highly concentrated mix of EPA, DHA, DPA and GLA. They also produce Mega-EPA, a high-potency omega-3 fish oil supplement. Seven Seas produce Extra High Strength Cod Liver Oil.

In South Africa Essential Omegas are available from www. holforddirect.co.za.

EYE SUPPORT

Nutrients that support eye health include almost all antioxidants, available in combination formulas such as Patrick Holford's AGE Antioxidant and CoQ_{10}+Carnitine also available in **South Africa** from www.holforddirect.co.za. Solgar provide lutein supplements. High-dose vitamin A (see below) is also helpful.

HOMOCYSTEINE-FRIENDLY B VITAMINS

A good methyl nutrient complex should contain at least B_6, B_{12} and folic acid in high doses. Some formulas also contain vitamin B_2, tri-methyl-glycine (TMG), zinc, and N-acetyl-cysteine. Three products that fulfil these criteria are Patrick Holford's Connect which contains them all; or Solgar's Gold Specifics Homocysteine Modulators, which contains TMG, vitamin B_6, vitamin B_{12} and folic acid; or Higher Nature's H Factors which contains vitamins B_2, B_6, B_{12}, folic acid and zinc, plus TMG (see www.highernature.co.uk).

In South Africa, Patrick Holford's H Factor is available from www. holforddirect.co.za.

FOR THE BRAIN

Brain Food Formula, providing phospholipids and B vitamins, is available from www.totallynourish.com and www.holforddirect.co.za in **South Africa**.

PROBIOTICS/DIGESTIVE ENZYMES/GUT REPAIR

Probiotics are supplements of beneficial bacteria, the two main strains being *Lactobacillus acidophilus* and *Bifidobacterium bifidus*. There are various types of strains within these two – some more important in children, others in adults. There is quite some variability in amounts of bacteria (some labels say, for example, 'a billion viable organisms per capsule') and quality. A very good product is Patrick Holford's Bio-Acidophilus and also Digestpro, which also contains digestive enzymes and glutamine.

In South Africa, Patrick Holford's Digestpro is available from www.holforddirect.co.za.

D-Mannose: to alleviate urinary tract infections like cystitis. See www.sweet-cures.com.

SLEEP SUPPORT

Nutrients that support good sleep include 5-HTP, the amino acid GABA, magnesium and the herbs valerian, passiflora and hops. GABA is not available in the UK. Try Patrick Holford's Chill Food Formula.

In South Africa, Patrick Holford's Chill Food Formula is available from www.holforddirect.co.za.

SUGAR BALANCE AND WEIGHT CONTROL

Patrick Holford's Cinnachrome provides 200mcg of chromium with cinnamon high in MCHP (Cinnulin PF® is the name of a concentrated extract of cinnamon that is especially high in MCHP).

In South Africa, Cinnachrome is available from www.holforddirect.co.za.

Patrick Holford's GL Support provides Chromium, 5HTP, and HCA.

In South Africa, a similar formula, called Appestop, is also available from www.holforddirect.co.za.

Carboslow – 1 teaspoon (5g) of a super-soluble fibre such as glucomannan is also available in South Africa from www.holforddirect.co.za and from www.totallynourish.com in the UK.

VITAMIN A

Vitamin A is available in tablets and drops. Solgar provide 1,500mcg (5,000iu) vitamin A per tablet; BioCare's BiomulsionA provides 1,500mcg (5,000iu) per drop.

VITAMIN D

Vitamin D can be purchased easily from good health stores from suppliers including Higher Nature, Viridian and Solgar. For quick absorption, you might want to consider sublingual (under the tongue) BiomulsionD drops from BioCare. Each drop provides 25mcg (1,000iu).

SKINCARE PRODUCTS

Environ products were developed by the cosmetic surgeon Dr Des Fernandes, to prevent skin cancer and address the damaging effects of the environment on our skin. Formulated with scientifically proven active ingredients, including vitamin A and the antioxidant vitamins C, E and beta-carotene, which are used in progressively higher concentrations, Environ will help maintain a normal healthy skin, especially where there are signs of ageing, pigmentation, problem skin and scarring. If you look at Environ's website, www.environ.co.za and go to the 'results' section, you will see some extraordinary skin transformations achieved with transdermal vitamins. Dr Fernandes also pioneered the concept of micro-needling to help more of the vitamins to penetrate the skin and promote collagen for plumper, smoother skin. He created Roll-CIT (CIT stands for collagen induction therapy) rollers for use at home. Environ products are available from www.totallynourish.com or direct from an Environ skincare therapist. See www.iiaa.eu or call 020 8450 2020 to find one near you in the UK and Ireland. In South Africa, call 0800 220 402. For international enquiries, call +27 11 2685711 or email tollfree@environ.co.za or visit www.environ.co.za.

SUPPLEMENT SUPPLIERS

The following companies produce good-quality supplements that are widely available in the UK.

BioCare offers an extensive range of nutritional and herbal supplements. Visit www.biocare.co.uk; tel 0121 433 3727.

Patrick Holford's range, including daily 'packs', which are good for travelling or when you are away from home, are stocked by Holland and Barrett and most good health-food stores. They are also available by mail order from Totally Nourish (www.totallynourish.com) – see below.

Higher Nature Available in most independent health-food stores or visit www.highernature.co.uk; tel.: 0800 458 4747 (freephone in the UK).

Solgar Available in most independent health-food stores or visit www.solgar-vitamins.co.uk; tel.: +44 (0) 1442 890355.

Viridian For stockists visit www.viridian-nutrition.com; tel.: +44 (0) 1327 878050.

Totally Nourish is an 'e'-health shop that stocks many high-quality health products, including home-test kits and supplements. Visit www.totallynourish.com; tel.: 0800 085 7749 (freephone within the UK).

AND IN OTHER REGIONS

South Africa

The original Patrick Holford vitamin and supplement brand from the UK is now available in South Africa through leading health-food stores, Dis-Chem and Clicks retail pharmacies. They are also available online direct from www.holforddirect.co.za; tel.: 011 2654 554 and are delivered by post or by courier direct to your door.

Australia

Solgar supplements are available in Australia. Visit www.solgar.com.au; tel.: 1800 029 871 (free call) for your nearest supplier. Another good brand is Blackmores.

New Zealand

BioCare (see above) and Patrick Holford products are available in New Zealand through Pacific Health, PO Box 56248, Dominion Road, Auckland 1446. Visit www.pachealth.co.nz; tel.: 0064 9815 0707.

Singapore

BioCare (see above), Patrick Holford and Solgar products are available in Singapore through Essential Living. Visit www.essliv.com; tel.: 6276 1380.

UAE

BioCare (see above) and Patrick Holford supplements are available in Dubai and the UAE from Organic Foods & Café, PO Box 117629, Dubai, United Arab Emirates; visit www.organicfoodsandcafe.com; tel.: +971 44340577.

Kenya

Patrick Holford supplements are available in all Healthy U stores. Visit www.healthy-U2000.com.

INFORMATIVE WEBSITES

Institute for Ageing and Health Located at Newcastle University, the Institute for Ageing and Health is very much focused on the research side of ageing, rather than the immediately practical. Its stated aim is to bring together basic, clinical, social and computer scientists, engineers, and researchers to address how and why we age and the treatment of associated disease and disability. Recent research includes computer modelling the brain's defences against damaging free radicals (oxidants) and protein build-up in Alzheimer's – research which suggests that lifestyle changes to prevent damage from free radicals may help to fight dementia and other brain disorders. The Institute does not, however, make any recommendations. Visit www.ncl.ac.uk/iah.

Institute of Healthy Ageing Located at University College London, this institute is devoted to research: 'An interdisciplinary centre for research on the biology of ageing and ageing-related disease that aims to develop a new translational biogerontology to protect against the diseases of old age.' The research projects include using *C. elegans* worms to find out how turning down the genes involved in insulin/IGF-1 signalling, as well as calorie restriction, is able to increase life span. Visit www.ucl. ac.uk/iha.

Annual Anti-ageing Conference London, brings together mainly American and European academics and clinicians with lectures on such topics as the use of growth hormone, mineral and vitamin deficiencies, and cutting heart risk by reducing insulin levels. See list of previous speakers and topics on the website. Visit www.antiageingconference. com.

The British Longevity Society was founded nearly 20 years ago with the aim of educating the public about ways to counteract the effects of ageing. The website is a modest affair with a few links to practitioners. Visit www.thebls.org/index.htm.

For a newsletter that contains detailed reports on some of the more exotic supplements, visit www.thebls.org/newsletter.htm.

American Academy of Anti-Aging Medicine (A4M) is a good example of the differences between US and UK approaches to anti-ageing. This is huge and relentlessly commercial. Last August there was a big ad on the home page for a conference on bio-identical hormones with links to sign up for courses in 'Anti-Aging, Functional and Regenerative Medicine and Integrative Cancer'. In the following four months there were 'A4M' conferences in five American cities as well as Melbourne, Bangkok and Bali. Visit www.worldhealth.net.

Anti Aging Systems Describes itself as 'the world's largest supplier of specialist medicines, bio-identical hormones and nutrition, concentrating on anti-aging medicine, nutrition and information'. Here you will find all the most exotic supplements taken by ultra-anti-agers, complete with fairly detailed accounts of why they might be useful. Visit www.antiaging-systems.com/ or www.antiaging-nutrition.com/.

Professor Michael Rose has a website setting out his evolutionary theory that explains how eating a Stone Age-type diet could dramatically increase your life span. Attractively set out, readable and well informed. Visit www.55theses.org.

The Bulletproof Executive A remarkably heavyweight self-improvement site. Reports from a 15-year single-minded crusade to upgrade the human being using every available technology. It claims that the author has done it and so can you; upgrade your IQ by 20 points; get healthier by sleeping less than four hours a night; and so on. Visit www.bulletproofexecutive.com.

For serious discussions and posts on latest anti-ageing developments, visit groups.google.com/forum/#!forum/sci.life-extension.

Nutra Ingredients USA An American site with a specialist take on supplements. Visit www.nutraingredients-usa.com.

The Anti Aging Source An American site devoted to an extensive range of supplements. Contains interviews with anti-ageing celebs, such as Greta Blackburn – telomere expert. Visit www.anti-aging-source.com.

Mind and Muscle A site devoted to body builders, but anti-agers in the know are increasingly interested in the connection between maintaining muscle mass and ageing well. Visit www.mindandmuscle.net/articles.

BLTC Research A site on the wildest shores of anti-ageing devoted to 'paradise-engineering'. This involves: 'abolishing the biological substrates of suffering in both humans and all sentient life', which will be achieved by rewriting the vertebrate genome, redesigning the global ecosystem and delivering genetically pre-programmed well-being. For the fantasy end of high-tech anti-ageing, visit www.bltc.com.

Dr Sahelian writes about dietary supplements and natural medicine and treats his patients with them. The site claims 10,000 hits a day. There's a wealth of intelligent reviews on a wide range of supplements that acknowledges when research/evidence is weak. Visit www. RaySahelian.com.

Anti-aging Guide Detailed coverage of most of the main anti-ageing approaches – calorie reduction, supplements, exercise, and so on, although it seems rather out of date. The list of cited papers are rarely more recent than 2005. Visit www.anti-aging-guide.com.

Fight Aging One of the most comprehensive and up-to-date sites. The opening page has well informed descriptions of the latest research. There is also lots of background material and links to over 40 blogs and no commercial links at all. Visit www.fightaging.org.

SENS Foundation Home to the foundation mentioned in Part One, Chapter 6 that is dedicated to a high-tech solution to making major increases in life span. Visit www.sens.org.

Ray & Terry's Set up by two high-profile American anti-agers, Ray Kurzweil (described as a 'restless genius' by the *Wall Street Journal*), and Dr Terry Grossman, who runs a longevity clinic in Denver, Colorado. The site essentially offers a wide range of products. Visit www.rayandterry.com.

Aging Sciences – Anti-Aging Firewalls. A blog that's firmly based in recent research and regularly updated. It's centred on the idea that there are at least 14 (and rising) processes that start to run down or become less efficient as we age, and the different biochemical and lifestyle approaches that can help to erect a 'firewall' against each of them. Visit anti-agingfirewalls.com.

Life Extension Foundation One of the very first organisations set up to develop anti-ageing methods. It offers a lot of supplements but also a magazine and a daily newsletter. Visit www.lef.org.

Maximum Life Foundation Another site related to the Life Extension Foundation where 'Biotech, Infotech and Nanotech Meet to Reverse Aging'. There's a wide range of ageing topics covered, ads for conferences and a free downloadable pdf file setting out an anti-ageing programme. Visit www.maxlife.org.

Senescence.info A personal site set up by a researcher involved in the biology and genetics of ageing with a passion for explaining it to the general public. It's idiosyncratic but with a lot of very accessible background material. Visit www.senescence.info.

CR Society International Everything you need to know about the science and practice of a calorie-restricted diet from those who are already doing it. Visit www.crsociety.org.

INDEX

Ever wish you were better informed?

Join my 100% Health Club today and you'll receive:

✔ My newsletter, plus Special Reports on vital health topics

✔ Immediate access to hundreds of health articles and special reports.

✔ Have your questions answered in our Members Only blogs.

✔ Save money on supplements, books and other health products.

✔ Save up to £50 on Patrick Holford's **100% Health Workshop**.

✔ Become part of a community of like-minded people and help others.

JOIN TODAY at **www.patrickholford.com**

❝ Being a member has transformed my life, and that of many of my family and friends. Patrick's information is always spot on and really practical. My member benefits and discounts save me much more than the subscription. Being a member is a must if you ❞ want to be and stay healthy.

Joyce Taylor

100%Health®
Weekend Intensive

The workshop that works.

D	C	B	A
NOT GOOD	AVERAGE	REASONABLY HEALTHY	SUPER HEALTHY

Karen before: **36%**

Karen after: **86%**

Learn how to go from 'average' to superhealthy in a weekend.

Do YOU want to:

✔ Take control of your own health?

✔ Master your weight?

✔ Turn back the clock?

✔ Prevent and reverse disease?

✔ Transform your diet, your health and your life?

Discover the **8 secrets of optimum living** - and put them into action with your own individualised personal health and fitness programme with **Patrick Holford**.

"I thought I was healthy. I feel absolutely fantastic. It's changed my life." Karen S.

" Learnt more in a day than a lifetime. Definitely recommended.**"** Sarah F.

" It worked miraculously. I lost 5 stones in 5 months. Life has become very good.**"** Fiona F.

" I have so much more energy. I wake up raring to go. It's changed my life.**"** Matthew F.

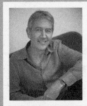

"You can wake up full of energy, with a clear mind and balanced mood, never gain weight and stay disease free. Having worked with over 60,000 people I know what changes are going to most rapidly transform how you feel."
Patrick Holford

"Visionary." Independent

"Health guru Patrick Holford addresses the true causes of illness." Guardian

"One of the world's leading authorities on new approaches to health" Daily Mail

Thousands of people have transformed their health.
Why not become one of them?
For more information see **www.patrickholford.com**

100%Health® is the registered trademark of Holford & Associates